Infant and Early Childhood Mental Health

Core Concepts and Clinical Practice

Infant and Early Childhood Mental Health

Core Concepts and Clinical Practice

Edited by

Kristie Brandt, C.N.M., M.S.N., D.N.P.
Bruce D. Perry, M.D., Ph.D.
Stephen Seligman, D.M.H.
Ed Tronick, Ph.D.

Foreword by

T. Berry Brazelton, M.D.

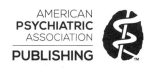

AMERICAN
PSYCHIATRIC
ASSOCIATION
PUBLISHING

Copyright © 2014 American Psychiatric Association
ALL RIGHTS RESERVED

Manufactured in the United States of America on acid-free paper
21   5   4
First Edition

Typeset in Adobe's Antique Olive and Bembo Std.

American Psychiatric Association Publishing
800 Maine Ave. SW, Suite 900
Washington, DC 20024-2812
www.appi.org

Library of Congress Cataloging-in-Publication Data
Infant and early childhood mental health : core concepts and clinical practice / Kristie Brandt, Bruce D. Perry, Stephen Seligman, Ed Tronick ; foreword by T. Berry Brazelton. — First edition.
    p. ; cm.
Includes bibliographical references and index.
ISBN 978-1-58562-455-3 (pbk. : alk. paper)
    I. Brandt, Kristie, editor of compilation. II. Perry, Bruce Duncan, editor of compilation. III. Seligman, Stephen, editor of compilation. IV. Tronick, Edward, editor of compilation. V. American Psychiatric Association, issuing body.
    [DNLM: 1. Child Psychology. 2. Child Development. 3. Child, Preschool. 4. Infant. 5. Mental Disorders—diagnosis. 6. Mental Disorders—therapy. WS 105]
    RJ502.5
618.92′89—dc23   2013023288
British Library Cataloguing in Publication Data
A CIP record is available from the British Library.

Contents

Contributors

Marie E. Anzalone, Sc.D., O.T.R./L., F.A.O.T.A.
Occupational Therapist in Private Practice, Richmond, Virginia

Kristie Brandt, C.N.M., M.S.N., D.N.P.
Assistant Clinical Professor of Pediatrics, UC Davis School of Medicine, Sacramento, California; Director, Parent-Infant and Child Institute, Napa, California; Co-Developer and Director, University of Massachusetts Boston Infant-Parent Mental Health Fellowship/ Postgraduate Certificate Program

T. Berry Brazelton, M.D.
Clinical Professor of Pediatrics Emeritus, Harvard Medical School; Founder and Faculty, Brazelton Touchpoints Center, Division of Developmental Medicine, Boston Children's Hospital, Boston, Massachusetts

Cailey Bromer, B.S.
Graduate Student, Brown Center for the Study of Children at Risk, Warren Alpert Medical School of Brown University, Women and Infants Hospital of Rhode Island, Department of Neuroscience, Brown University, Providence, Rhode Island

James Diel, M.Ed., M.F.T.
Director of Mental Health, Aldea Children and Family Services, Napa, California

George Downing, Ph.D.
Clinical Faculty, Salpêtrière Hospital and Paris University VIII, Paris, France

Joshua Feder, M.D.
Director of Research, Interdisciplinary Council on Developmental and Learning Disorders, Kentfield, California

Tiffany Field, Ph.D.
Director, Touch Research Institute, University of Miami Medical School, Miami, Florida

Carol George, Ph.D.
Professor of Psychology, Mills College, Oakland, California

Linda Gilkerson, Ph.D.
Professor, Erikson Institute, Chicago, Illinois

Larry Gray, M.D.
Assistant Professor, Department of Pediatrics, University of Chicago, Chicago, Illinois

Alexandra Murray Harrison, M.D.
Assistant Clinical Professor, Harvard Medical School; Training and Supervising Analyst, Cambridge Health Alliance, Boston Psychoanalytic Society and Institute, Cambridge, Massachusetts

Stephen P. Hinshaw, Ph.D.
Professor, Department of Psychology, University of California, Berkeley, California

John Hornstein, Ed.D.
Research Associate, The Children's Hospital Boston, Division of Developmental Medicine, Harvard Medical School, Boston, Massachusetts; Affiliate Professor, Department of Education, University of New Hampshire, Durham, New Hampshire

Wolfgang Jordan, M.B.A., M.I.M.
Professor, Otto-von-Guericke University, Magdeburg; Chief Psychiatrist, Clinic for Psychiatry and Psychotherapy, Magdeburg Hospital, Germany

Cassandra L. Joubert, Sc.D.
Professor, Department of Public Health, California State University, Fresno, California

Barry M. Lester, Ph.D.
Professor of Psychiatry and Human Behavior and Pediatrics; Director, Center for the Study of Children at Risk, Warren Alpert Medical School of Brown University, Women and Infants Hospital of Rhode Island, Providence, Rhode Island

Connie Lillas, Ph.D., M.F.T., R.N.
Director, Interdisciplinary Training Institute, Pasadena, California; Training and Supervising Analyst at the Institute of Contemporary Psychoanalysis, Los Angeles, California, and the Newport Psychoanalytic Institute, Tustin, California; Chief Faculty for the Early Intervention Training Institute at Los Angeles Child Guidance Clinic, Los Angeles, California

Mark Ludwig M.S.W., L.C.S.W.
Core Faculty, Somatic Psychology Program, California Institute of Integral Studies, San Francisco, California

Carmen J. Marsit, Ph.D.
Associate Professor, Departments of Pharmacology and Toxicology and Community and Family Medicine, Geisel School of Medicine at Dartmouth, Hanover, New Hampshire

Barbara McCarroll, Ph.D.
Facilitator Mentor, California Infant-Family Early Childhood Mental Health Specialist and Reflective Practice, Napa County Therapeutic Child Care Center, Napa, California

Michael M. Morgan, Ph.D., L.M.F.T.
Associate Professor, University of Wyoming, Laramie, Wyoming

Benjamin W. Nelson, B.A.
Ph.D. Candidate, University of Oregon, Eugene; Research Assistant/Coordinator, UCLA Semel Institute for Neuroscience and Human Behavior, Los Angeles, California

Cherise Northcutt, Ph.D.
Director of Mental Health Programs, A Better Way, Inc., Berkeley, California; Faculty, University of Massachusetts Boston Infant-Parent Mental Health Fellowship/Postgraduate Certificate Program in Napa, California, and Boston, Massachusetts

Suzanne C. Parker, B.A.
Department of Psychology, University of Miami, Florida

Bruce D. Perry, M.D., Ph.D.
Senior Fellow, ChildTrauma Academy, Houston, Texas; Adjunct Professor, Department of Psychiatry and Behavioral Sciences, Feinberg School of Medicine, Northwestern University, Chicago, Illinois

Corinna Reck, Ph.D.
Head Psychologist, Clinic for Psychiatry and Psychotherapy, University of Heidelberg Medical School, Heidelberg, Germany

Margaret Ritchey, M.A., R.P.T., D.P.T.
Case Manager, Pediatric Physical Therapist, Neonatal Follow-Up Program, Children's Hospital and Research Center Oakland, Oakland, California

Ruby Moye' Salazar, L.C.S.W., B.C.D.
Founder and Director, Pennsylvania Lifespan Services, Clark's Summit, Pennsylvania

Stephen Seligman, D.M.H.
Clinical Professor of Psychiatry, Infant-Parent Program, University of California, San Francisco; Joint Editor-in-Chief, *Psychoanalytic Dialogues: International Journal of Relational Perspectives;* Training and Supervising Analyst, San Francisco Center for Psychoanalysis and Psychoanalytic Institute of Northern California, San Francisco, California

Daniel J. Siegel, M.D.
Founding Co-Director, Mindful Awareness Research Center, UCLA Mindsight Institute, Los Angeles, California

Mary Beth Steinfeld, M.D.
Associate Clinical Professor, Developmental-Behavioral Pediatrics, UC Davis Department of Pediatrics, UC Davis MIND Institute, Sacramento, California

Barbara Stroud, Ph.D.
Private Consultant, Barbara Stroud Training and Consultation, Palo Alto, California

Ed Tronick, Ph.D.
University Distinguished Professor, Department of Psychology, University of Massachusetts, Boston; Lecturer, Department of Newborn Medicine, Brigham and Women's Hospital, Harvard Medical School, Boston, Massachusetts

Regina von Einsiedel, M.D.
Chief Psychiatrist, Park Psychiatric Clinic, Westfalen, Bad Lippspringe, Germany

Susanne Wortmann-Fleischer, M.D.
Supervisor and Psychiatrist, Neuropsychiatric Center, Mannheim and Ludwigshafen, Germany

Disclosure of Competing Interests

The following contributors to this book indicated that they have no competing interests or affiliations to declare.

Marie E. Anzalone, Sc.D., O.T.R./L., F.A.O.T.A.
Kristie Brandt, C.N.M., M.S.N., D.N.P.
T. Berry Brazelton, M.D.
James Diel, M.Ed., M.F.T.
George Downing, Ph.D.
Joshua Feder, M.D.
Tiffany Field, Ph.D.
Carol George, Ph.D.
Linda Gilkerson, Ph.D.
Larry Gray, M.D.
Alexandra Murray Harrison, M.D.
Stephen P. Hinshaw, Ph.D.
John Hornstein, Ed.D.
Wolfgang Jordan, M.B.A., M.I.M.
Cassandra L. Joubert, Sc.D.
Barry M. Lester, Ph.D.
Connie Lillas, Ph.D., M.F.T., R.N.
Mark Ludwig M.S.W., L.C.S.W.
Carmen J. Marsit, Ph.D.
Barbara McCarroll, Ph.D.
Michael M. Morgan, Ph.D., L.M.F.T.

Benjamin W. Nelson, B.A.
Cherise Northcutt, Ph.D.
Suzanne C. Parker, B.A.
Bruce D. Perry, M.D., Ph.D.
Margaret Ritchey, M.A., R.P.T., D.P.T.
Ruby Moye' Salazar, L.C.S.W., B.C.D.
Stephen Seligman, D.M.H.
Daniel J. Siegel, M.D.
Mary Beth Steinfeld, M.D.
Barbara Stroud, Ph.D.
Ed Tronick, Ph.D.
Regina von Einsiedel, M.D.
Susanne Wortmann-Fleischer, M.D.

Foreword

For years, it has been my belief that the quality of the infant-parent and child-parent relationship is the best predictor of outcome for any child. Yet in the busy worlds of pediatrics, home visiting, nursing, early education, early intervention, occupational therapy, and other disciplines, this relationship is typically not attended to in the course of working with the family. Often, severe behavioral and relationship problems go unseen and unaddressed until a child starts kindergarten. At that point, therapeutic work is much harder than if such work had begun earlier in the life of the child and the development of the relationship. No professional group *regularly and typically in contact with families and young children* holds the specific responsibility for monitoring and supporting the parent-child relationship. How have we let such an important component of health and well-being go unaddressed for so long? In my view, this mission must be shared by all of us who are in regular contact with families from pregnancy through age 5.

Back in 1969, when I wrote my first book, *Infants and Mothers: Differences in Development* (New York, Delacorte Press), I began with the statement "Normal babies are not all alike" (p. xxi). This came as a surprise to parents and professionals at the time, but since then research in such areas as sensory processing, temperament, motor abilities, regulatory capacities, and engagement, including my own work in these areas, has shed significant light on these variations and on what makes for these individual differences in infant and child characteristics, capacities, and vulnerabilities. Most strikingly, though, I have found my early contention to be true across multiple domains: infants influence their environments as much as they are influenced by their environment. Infants shape and are shaped by relationships with their parents and other important adults in their lives, and they are partners in cocreating ways of being together.

Not only is every child different, but parents also bring to the relationship their own history of being parented, hopes and dreams, vulnerabilities, temperament, history of relationships, and general mental health. This unique relationship between every parent and child is what makes infant and early childhood mental health work both challenging and exciting.

Parents are hungry to see their children thrive, and I think we can offer them something very important. We can help them see the power they have in their child's optimal development through the processes of falling in love with their baby, delighting in their child, developing an understanding from birth of their child's behavior, wondering about the meaning of the behavior for both themselves and their child, and watching how the child's behavior is shaping parental behavior, thoughts, and meaning. The latter component is particularly important as the parent develops a deeper understanding of his or her own experience of being parented and of being a child, and then builds the ability to reflect on his or her own child's experience of being parented. So powerful is this experience that I have seen some parents who are challenged by addiction be motivated to stay clean and sober as they realize how important it is to provide their child with a good parent. This, I think, is the key to a healthy, functional parent–child relationship and a functional family system, and it is the core of infant-family and early childhood mental health.

Early in my work I saw how powerful the infant was at activating the parent and the family system. As a result, I realized that when I shared a newborn's behaviors with parents very early, they were able to learn that the infant could help them to be the child's unique parents. Infants impact their environment from the womb, but at birth the power of infants to shape their environment, and those in the system around them, becomes clear to any provider willing to observe. Infants let parents know what works and what does not work. This trial-and-error process is a dynamic feedback loop that calls on the parent and the child to be fully engaged in fulfilling their roles in this interactive system. Around the world I have seen that infants not only shape their direct caregiving environment, but ultimately play a role in shaping the larger culture around them, while at the same time the infants are adapting to and shaped by the caregiving they receive and the larger culture that they were born into.

My pediatric residency did not provide me with the foundation I felt a pediatrician needed for understanding a child's development, including the mental health concerns and implications of infancy and early childhood. My child psychiatry training at the James Jackson Putnam Children's Center opened my eyes to the effects on the child of relationally impoverished environments and to the desires of all parents to do well by their children, even while some struggle with their own mental health issues and/or histories of maltreatment in the process, or their children struggle with behavioral, regulatory, or other serious issues. In my 70 years of medical practice, I have seen the rich potential of skilled and caring providers to support optimal parent and child development even in the face of high risk and seemingly insurmountable obstacles. My hope is that you are one of those providers and that this book will further enhance your skills and commitment to that endeavor.

Sadly, children sometimes do experience mental illness in the early years from birth to age 5, and professionals must be adequately trained to detect such conditions and either treat them directly (as appropriate) or make a suitable referral for proper treatment. But such conditions, fortunately, are rare and most of the focus for providers during these early years is to work diligently in scaffolding the healthy trajectory of the parent and child as their relationship develops and as each is shaped as an individual and, together, as a dyad in the process. This early and primary relationship will shape the future for both of them in profound ways that we now know will impact health and well-being throughout their lives.

I believe this work should begin during pregnancy with getting to know what the parents' dreams, hopes, and worries are; what concerns them; and how they already envision the relationship they will have with their new baby. Forming this kind of collaborative connection and building a strong working alliance with families are critical as we learn to trust one another and are able to share together any challenges they are facing and work jointly to find the best possible course of action. This, to me, is the cornerstone of infant-parent and early childhood mental health work. However, our current health and social services systems often work against us in this endeavor. Our systems have become increasingly separate, driven by funding policies and the treatment of human beings according to their problem or diagnosis rather than the treatment of each person as a whole human being and of families as systems, not disconnected people. Even our health care payment systems, both Medicaid and private insurance, work against us at times: when providers cannot refer or consult with other providers outside their systems, when families lose health insurance while unemployed or for other reasons and must leave a provider's care, or when families are forced to change providers because their health care coverage changes or their provider withdraws from a payment system. Meanwhile, thousands of children and families are without any health care coverage and cannot pay out of pocket for health care. If we get too discouraged by such issues, it is to the detriment of the very important work of safeguarding and supporting children and families to grow and thrive. We are obliged to connect with families wherever and whenever we can, and to not miss any opportunity to inquire about and observe how the parent, the child, and the relationship are doing, and then to support and intervene as needed. In this pursuit, we must be advocates for providing all families with coverage for the services they need, or even provide services without payment in some cases.

Our best preparation is to ensure that every provider serving a family from pregnancy until the child starts kindergarten understands the basic concepts of infant-parent and early childhood mental health and has core competencies in this area for clinically working with families. One example of a basic competency for all providers is my Touchpoints approach, which focuses on cycles of disorganization, functional regression, and family stress that can precede each developmental step for the child, and the effect of this developmental process on the caregiver, the child, and the larger system around them (see www.brazeltontouch-points.org/about/what-is-touchpoints). The Touchpoints approach also involves predicting for parents when these cycles will likely occur, discussing what they can expect, and planning together with them what they can do when these cycles occur. Another example of a basic competency is the Newborn Behavioral Observations system, which is a relationship-building tool for use with parents at birth and any time in the first 12 weeks (adjusted age) after their baby is born (see www.brazelton-institute.com/clnbas.html). It is vital that we find ways to move training in such core competencies into professional education, as well as provide clinical support and reflective mentoring for providers working to advance and maintain related clinical skills after completing their formal professional education.

The Napa Infant-Parent Mental Health Fellowship/Postgraduate Certificate Program provides just such interdisciplinary training, and this book captures the essence of the program. I am proud to have participated in the development of the program, and since its inception I have been a faculty member working with and being inspired by each class of fellows. This program is a gold standard for training providers to address infant-parent and early childhood mental health needs in whatever setting and from whatever disciplinary perspective the child and family are being served. I have worked with Dr. Kristie Brandt since

1994 and have great admiration for her work in advancing the interdisciplinary field of infant-parent mental health. She has assembled here an excellent group of coeditors and chapter authors, all luminaries in this important field. This book will help guide our field for many years to come.

In this book, the editors and chapter authors describe from their perspective key concepts fundamental to infant-parent and early childhood mental health work. All of these facets and lenses are needed to construct and expand this comprehensive and interdisciplinary field. The core concepts are laid out in a coherent and clear way, with clinical applications provided to enhance the incorporation of these concepts into clinical practice. My dream is that every professional, regardless of discipline, will attend to and nurture the child's social and emotional development and the quality of the parent-child relationship in every contact with the family. I urge all providers working from the prenatal period through a child's first decade to read this book. I believe it will enhance that cause and advance the field of infant and early childhood mental health.

T. Berry Brazelton, M.D.
Professor of Pediatrics, Emeritus, Harvard Medical School;
Boston Children's Hospital; Founder, Brazelton Touchpoints Center

Preface

When discussions first began about writing this book, American Psychiatric Publishing expressed the desire to disseminate more broadly among professionals core concepts related to the infant and early childhood mental health field. The hope was to include content similar to what was included in the 15-month Napa Infant-Parent Mental Health Fellowship that began in 2002, became the Napa Infant-Parent Mental Health Fellowship/Postgraduate Certificate Program in 2008, and affiliated in 2009 with the University of Massachusetts Boston, where a sister program started that year. The curriculum for the Napa program was specifically created to 1) address the needs of professionals working in the field and wanting to expand their specialization skills and knowledge, 2) offer core competency training for professionals entering the field, and 3) create a groundswell movement within the field for world-class transdisciplinary training accessible, both by scheduling and cost, to working clinicians. The hope was to craft for the field a forum for discussion and study, a model of professional adult learning, and an extensive network of transdisciplinary professionals for consultation, referral, discussion, and expansion of the field. Through over 10 years of operation, that quest has been steadily pursued.

An additional essential element in the program's development was to assemble a multidisciplinary faculty willing and able to embrace a truly transdisciplinary approach that, according to Bruder (1994), "requires the team members to share roles and systematically cross discipline boundaries...so that more efficient and comprehensive assessment and intervention services may be provided" (p. 61). In this model, "professionals from different disciplines teach, learn, and work together to accomplish a common set of intervention goals for a child and her family" (Bruder 1994, p. 61). With this in mind, we editors sought contributions from a disciplinarily diverse group of authors, most of whom are faculty and/or graduates of the Napa program and all of whom have vastly different training, expertise, and clinical experience. In addition, throughout the book, words such as *clinician, therapist, provider, professional,* and *teacher* are intentionally used interchangeably to describe and unify all of us working in this important field.

This book is intended to be an overview of the infant and early childhood mental health field from both theoretical and clinical perspectives. Clinical practice must be solidly derived from and grounded in linkages to theory, research, scientific discoveries, other reported findings, and the thoughtful amalgamating work of the clinician in meeting the unique circumstances of each clinical situation. Thus, instead of trying to cover the entire field of infant-parent, family, and early childhood mental health, we determined that the greatest value to practicing clinicians would be to focus on key concepts related to serving children and families from pregnancy through age 5, to open conceptual windows, and to provide clinical basics across as broad a swath as practical given the page constraints. Some specific conditions, including, for example, maternal or paternal depression, special needs, preterm birth, grief and loss, child trauma, and regulatory challenges, were not given specific chapters. Rather, we decided to weave related core concepts throughout multiple chapters to create in the writing *and* the reading of this book a literary parallel for the multifaceted, multilayered, and interwoven complexity that resembles the real lives of real families, and the real work of real clinicians.

In Chapter 1, I provide a general introduction to the field of infant and early childhood mental health, dyadic functioning, and the developmental process. Key concepts are explored, including who is being served in infant and early childhood mental health (the child, the parent, the family, the relationship), the nature of therapy, and why transdisciplinary work is essential in this field. A transdisciplinary therapeutic approach model is provided in this chapter to support clinicians in exploring the gateways and pathways for therapeutic work.

Chapter 2 focuses on Perry's Neurosequential Model of Therapeutics and working with maltreated and/or traumatized children through the lens of neurodevelopment; an awareness of the impacts of maltreatment at various stages of development; and the therapeutic approaches inferred from the timing of deleterious experiences. Where working with maltreated children can often seem futile or too immense to undertake, this chapter brings hope.

Chapter 3 introduces Tronick's core concepts of mutual regulation, dyadic states of consciousness, mismatch and repair, and meaning making as they are evidenced in the seemingly simple dyadically interactive game of peek-a-boo. The dynamic nature of human connection and the "messiness" of interactional patterns in relationships are offered to readers as the typical, nonlinear way in which humans grow, change, interact, and connect.

Chapter 4 highlights Brazelton's neurodevelopmental and relational Touchpoints, with a focus on the developmental progression of young children and their caregivers through cycles of behavioral and interactional disorganization, bursts in development, and reorganizations, in a complex and contextual—yet predictable—pattern. Using a child's behavior to find entrance into a family system and form a therapeutic alliance for working with families is central to this chapter.

Chapter 5 introduces the Neurorelational Framework (NRF), which offers a novel transdisciplinary approach for optimizing early childhood services by providing a common language for team collaboration and a "parts to whole" perspective. The NRF is illustrated briefly in the chapter by examining toxic stress patterns through the lens of the four brain systems in order to map neurodevelopmental triggers and sources of resilience.

Chapter 6 gives readers an overview of attachment theory and the implications for clinical work. The chapter also examines the complex intergenerational nature of attachment as parents bring their own history of childhood relationships and their experience of being parented themselves into the process of parenting their own children.

Chapter 7 centers on understanding the history and contemporary thinking around psychoanalytic and psychodynamic theory, and presents Harrison's Parent Consultation Model, which embraces these concepts in a short, five-step format that can be used by most clinicians to support families with concerns about their child's behavior or the parent-child relationship.

Chapter 8 introduces Siegel's concept of mindsight and the triangle of wellness: the mind, the brain, and relationships. A definition of "mind" is provided, with an introduction to the field of interpersonal neurobiology, and attuned, mindfulness-informed therapeutic work is discussed from the perspectives of both the client and the clinician.

Chapter 9 provides a basic foundation of counseling skills for all disciplines working with families. In addition, the authors offer a description of psychotherapy, guidelines for knowing when a psychotherapy referral is indicated, and steps for determining whether a specific provider is the right match when making a referral for a child, parent, or family.

Chapter 10 lays out the basic concepts of epigenetics, introduces the concept of behavioral epigenetics, and presents a developmental origins model of child and adult mental health disorders. The influences of evolution and development on behavior are discussed in tandem with risk and protective factors that are relevant to working clinicians.

Chapter 11 focuses on diagnostic schemata for children ages 0–5 and highlights the *Diagnostic Classification of Mental Health and Developmental Disorders of Infancy and Early Childhood,* Revised Edition (DC:0-3R). For over 17 years, crosswalks have been in existence to facilitate billing DC:0-3 and DC:0-3R codes within DSM-IV, and this chapter provides a prototype for crosswalking DC:0-3R codes to DSM-5.

Chapter 12 concentrates on the phenomenon of problematic crying in infants in the first year. Data suggest troubling relationships between fussy babies and triggers for shaken baby syndrome, possible links with dyadic relational challenges, and later regulatory issues for the child. This chapter provides clinicians with core skills for early intervention and more advanced information for intervention, referral, and program development for helping families.

Chapter 13 emphasizes the impact of sensory processing, physical functioning, and sensory-based regulation on a child's development and dyadic functioning. Written by an occupational therapist and a physical therapist, this chapter offers every clinician in the field new insights into helping children and dyads when sensory or functional challenges exist or are suspected, and pinpoints specific mental health opportunities embedded in the work of occupational and physical therapists.

Chapter 14 presents core concepts about autism spectrum disorder (ASD) that are necessary for all clinicians in the field, but then advances the discussion into the unique dyadic challenges presented when an ASD is diagnosed, suspected, or feared by the parent. The quality of the dyadic relationship, which is central to optimal outcomes for the child but often lost or overlooked in the process of providing intervention services for ASD, is the focus of this chapter.

Chapter 15 brings the reader into the somatosensory world of the infant, where touch is a primary sensory modality for dyadic communication. Humans seek, exchange, process, and use touch to establish relationships, for regulation, and for social and personal communication. This chapter explores not only the experience of the infant, but also that of the parent, including physiological benefits to the parent and infant from massage and other forms of touch.

Chapter 16 focuses on developmental psychopathology, a field influenced by child and adolescent psychology and psychiatry and developmental science. Developmental psychopathology has contributed to understanding the etiology and underlying mechanisms of behavioral and emotional disorders, risk, resilience, and the impacts of environment and parenting. This chapter also discusses the impact of stigma on families seeking mental health services for their children.

Chapter 17 is an introduction to Downing's Video Intervention Therapy (VIT), a highly effective therapeutic approach in work with parents of children ages 0–5 that can be used across disciplines in a coaching, counseling, or psychotherapeutic mode. VIT facilitates rapid change in human relationships and typically involves viewing video segments of a dyad interacting, and working with the parent on what is seen and heard. This chapter can yield immediate VIT practice skills for clinicians.

Chapter 18 opens a dialogue on evidence-based treatments and evidence-based practices in the field, and distinguishes these two concepts that are often mistakenly used interchangeably. Among many topics is the issue of randomized controlled trials, a research standard that is often not feasible in infant mental health work or that is ethically prohibited despite being a standard applied to the field. The highly skilled professional standard of evidence-based practice is a primary focus.

Chapter 19 is a call to action for practitioners in the field to sustain or begin active reflective work to enhance and transform practice and improve outcomes for those served. The chapter discusses solo, one-to-one, and group reflective work; facilitation; opportunities to reflect; and neurobiological aspects of reflective processes.

Chapter 20 closes the book by exploring the experience of the child, the parent, and the therapist. Intersubjectivity, mentalization, attachment theory, intergenerational transmission of trauma and maltreatment, and a view of transactional thinking are richly interwoven to inform readers and expand their thinking and clinical work.

The field of infant-parent, family, and early childhood mental health is too vital to the health and well-being of individuals, families, and whole communities for us as practitioners to fall behind in the acquisition and application of new knowledge for practice, to lose the passion that drives our work, or to no longer feel inspired or gratified when we are witness to or a part of relieving some human suffering or improving any aspect of someone's life. If this book is helpful to you in your work, if it spurs you on with greater passion and commitment, or if it inspires you to transform your practice in small or large ways, then its purpose has been fulfilled.

Kristie Brandt, C.N.M., M.S.N., D.N.P

Reference

Bruder MB: Working with members of other disciplines: collaboration for success, in Including Children With Special Needs in Early Childhood Programs. Edited by Wolery M, Wilbers JS. Washington, DC, National Association for the Education of Young Children, 1994, pp 45–70

Acknowledgments

We want to express our gratitude to the many people who made this book possible. In particular, special thanks to John McDuffie, editorial director, and Robert Hales, M.D., editor-in-chief, from American Psychiatric Publishing, whose invitation in May 2011 led to the writing and publication of this book. Their faith in successful completion of the work never wavered. We also thank John Brandt for his tireless work and efforts toward the completion of the book. The editors also wish to acknowledge and thank the following:

- Clinicians and families everywhere, who generously open their lives and their work to generate new understandings of helping and healing
- The hundreds of current and past graduate fellows in the Napa and Boston Infant-Parent Mental Health Fellowship/Postgraduate Certificate Programs, now sponsored by the University of Massachusetts Boston, for their inspiration and for teaching us so much, and the extraordinary faculty for their support and commitment to all aspects of the programs
- The chapter authors, for the hours spent researching, writing, and revising chapters
- The late Louis Sander, M.D., a dear friend of the Napa program who provided consultation and mentoring to many, and attended gatherings of the fellowship from 2003 through 2012
- T. Berry Brazelton, M.D., for his passion, ceaseless effort, and scholarly pursuits while endeavoring for over 70 years to make things better for children and families everywhere

CHAPTER 1

Core Concepts in Infant-Family and Early Childhood Mental Health

Kristie Brandt, C.N.M., M.S.N., D.N.P.

Our earliest recallable memories from our lives as 3- to 5-year-olds may be diffuse and not fully formed. Some of us may recollect a few high-affect, punctate memories prior to age 3, but most of our experiences from the prenatal period through age 36–48 months cannot be recalled as adults (Fivush and Haden 2003). Nevertheless, we carry within us, as somatosensory or implicit memories and representations, the memory of having been a baby and a small child: the way we were handled and talked to, the quality of important relationships we had, and whether or not we felt safe, protected, and loved during that time. Although largely out of our adult awareness, these early childhood memories and experiences significantly influence the rest of our lives through our neural anatomy, neurobiology, and inner lives as human beings. Thus, infant and early childhood mental health touches and influences all of human experience.

Infant mental health (IMH) focuses on the early experience of the child from the prenatal period through age 5, as well as children over age 5 who are developmentally or functionally younger. The definitions, focus, core concepts, and therapeutic implications of IMH are discussed in this chapter. Although it is nearly impossible in this limited space to provide an IMH foundation that is wide enough and deep enough to do justice to the field, vital core concepts will be touched upon, inviting the reader into a deeper appreciation of the importance of the early years in supporting the development of healthy children and adults, recognizing early evidence of problems, and therapeutically intervening to protect and restore wellness.

Definitions and Basics of Infant Mental Health

Mental health has been defined as the capacity to experience "the full range of life's emotions at each developmental phase of life, in a broad, comprehensive, stable, and deep manner" (Greenspan 2009, p. 5). This field of working to support the mental health of children from birth to age 5 years and their families is known by a variety of names: infant mental health, infant-parent mental health, infant and early childhood mental health, infant-family and early childhood mental health, and social-emotional wellness, among others. The first use of the term *infant mental health* is attributed to Fraiberg in the late 1970s, when she developed a program for children ages 0–3 to treat problems in the infant-parent relationship (Fraiberg 1980). For the balance of this chapter, the acronym IMH will be used to describe this field of working with children, from conception through age 5, and with their parents, families, and other important caregivers.

Currently, the World Association for Infant Mental Health (2012) defines IMH as the ability of children "to develop physically, cognitively, and socially in a manner which allows them to master the primary emotional tasks of early childhood without serious disruption caused by harmful life events. Because infants grow in a context of nurturing environments, infant mental health involves the psychological balance of the infant-family system." Zero to Three National Center for Infants, Toddlers, and Families (2012) defines IMH as "the healthy social and emotional development of a child from birth to 3 years; and a growing field of research and practice devoted to the: promotion of healthy social and emotional development; prevention of mental health problems; and treatment of the mental health problems of very young children in the context of their families." This latter definition is particularly useful because it specifically addresses the four primary areas of service: promotion, prevention, early intervention, and treatment.

Every child must be provided with five essential ingredients for optimal development in all domains, but especially mental health: 1) a safe, healthy, and low-stress pregnancy; 2) the opportunity and ability to "fall in love" and "be in love" with a safe and nurturing adult; 3) support in learning to self-regulate; 4) support in learning to mutually regulate; and 5) nurturing, contingent, and developmentally appropriate care. Without these foundational experiences, children are at high risk for developmental, relational, and behavioral difficulties and are at increased risk for mental illness (Edwards et al. 2005; Radtke et al. 2011). Conversely, if this decisive period "gets off to a good enough start, the child's and family's futures will be on track to develop their full potential" (Barnard 2010, p. 54).

The Dyad, the Moment, and Dyadic Functioning

In IMH work, emphasis is focused on the dyad (parent and child) and dyadic functioning as the primal stratum of the child's development. Dyadic reciprocal exchanges form the foundation for the development of much of what makes people human (Birss 2007; Tronick 2003). The smallest of dyadic interactions continually shape the nature of the dyadic relationship, while at the same time these small interactions are representational of the entirety of the relationship to that point. Micro patterns of interaction assemble to construct the "whole" or macro relationship. Infants and young children typically negotiate a series of dyadic relationships, creating unique and intimate patterns of interaction with important people in their lives (e.g., parents, grandparents, siblings, other relatives, teachers), and such connections contribute to the child's overall development and repertoire for relationships (Brazelton 1992).

It follows, then, that the "moment" becomes the basic element of concern in IMH such that each moment enfolds all other moments, and the content of any moment implies the whole of the dyad's experience of being together (Bohm 1980; Sander 2008). Dyadic relationships are constructed moment by moment, and they can be therapeutically addressed moment by moment. For clinicians, observing *any moment* of a dyadic interchange provides clinical information about the whole of the dyad's relationship and therapeutic opportunities to be jointly explored, in such a way that there are implications for the larger relationship and all other dyadic moments.

In a reflective facilitation session with a clinician working to incorporate Video Intervention Therapy in her work (see Chapter 17, "Video Intervention Therapy for Parents With Psychiatric Disturbance"), the clinician described her case before starting a video of a dyad. She cautioned that the recorded mother-child interaction was not "typical" for this dyad, saying that the mother (Eva) was usually responsive and attentive, but in the video clip about to be seen, Eva was exasperated and upset with her older child after having been up all night with a second child, age 3 weeks. Such justifications or exceptions are often invoked by clinicians when negative affect or problematic interchanges are observed, as if these exchanges should be discounted as unimportant or are the negative exception to otherwise positive interactional patterns. However, each interaction is part of the entirety of the experience of the dyad and holds equal valence as part of their larger "whole" of being together. With the exception of harmful patterns, such as abuse or neglect, or patterns in which negative interactions predominate, the experience of navigating together a range of affects strengthens the dyad as well as both partners as individuals. From a typical positive, neutral, or negative interaction, each partner in the dyad experiences something and learns something both about himself or herself and about the other person relative to self-regulation, mutual regulation, asynchrony, and dissonance in relationships; through this process, the partners reachieve regulatory stability and move forward with a relationship that has been changed by the experience, yet can continue to achieve harmonious and reciprocally coordinated states and dyadic exchanges at a new level (Sander 1969). The ability of both partners in a dyadic exchange (child and caregiver) to coordinate their interactions, repair the frequent interactive errors that occur, and move from negative to positive affect is a key element in positive development (Tronick 1989).

Figure 1–1 shows four photos from a 7-second interaction between a 3-year-old girl and her great-grandmother. In photo 1, the child throws her arm back while laughing after

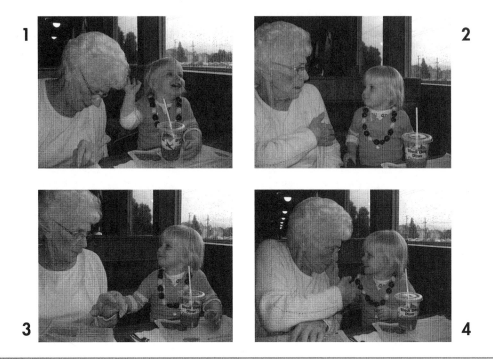

FIGURE 1–1.   A 7-second dyadic interaction between a 3-year-old girl and her great-grandmother.

In photo 1, the child throws her arm back while laughing after blowing bubbles through a straw into her tea, and she accidentally touches the hair of her great-grandmother. In photo 2, the great-grandmother's positive affect becomes negative, and the child's affect is likewise changing just milliseconds behind the change in her great-grandmother. In photo 3, the child makes a gestural bid for restoration of their harmonious state, a bid for repair, with a touch to the hand of her great-grandmother and presentation of her full face gaze with a positive affect. In photo 4, the harmonious state of positive matching affect is restored. Such experiences are the homeostatic pulse of the child's relational and somatosensory world and lay a foundation for lifelong interactional patterns.

blowing bubbles through a straw into her tea, and she accidentally touches the hair of her great-grandmother. In photo 2, the great-grandmother's positive affect becomes negative, and the child's affect is likewise changing just milliseconds behind the change in her great-grandmother. In photo 3, the child makes a gestural bid for restoration of their harmonious state, a bid for repair, with a touch to the hand of her great-grandmother and presentation of her full face gaze with a positive affect. In photo 4, the harmonious state of positive matching affect is restored. Such experiences are the homeostatic pulse of the child's relational and somatosensory world and lay a foundation for lifelong interactional patterns. The child's capacity for manipulating his or her environment contributes to a growing repertoire of schemata (Sander 1969) and relational archetypes, and the inability to restore the matching state can result in the child's "protective withdrawal and defensive reactions" (Sander 1969), with relational ramifications when these essential elements of interaction cannot be effectively negotiated. Such subtle relational impairment starting early in life and left unattended or therapeutically unaddressed can remain problematic throughout life (see Chapter 16, "Developmental Psychopathology").

Identifying the Patient in Infant-Parent Mental Health Work

Key to effective IMH practice is an understanding of who the "patient" is in clinical encounters. Shortly after the Napa Infant-Parent Mental Health Fellowship Program began, the transdisciplinary practice model for infant-parent mental health was created to forward both an understanding of the clinician's focus (who the patient is) and an awareness of the level at which the clinician is working in each case (Figure 1–2).

In this conceptualization, core infant mental health and well-being are seen as dependent on health and wellness in four component areas: 1) the child, 2) the parent, 3) the environment, and 4) the relationship. IMH clinicians working in component areas 1–3 would also be addressing the overall health of the fourth component: *the relationship.* For example, an occupational therapist working with a 3-month-old infant with brachial plexus would also be attending to the relationship in general, but would be particularly vigilant for any disruptions in the relationship associated with the infant's motor challenges and the related impacts on cueing and gesturing that play a key role in how the dyad partners relate to each other. Other perturbations could also manifest, such as vulnerable child syndrome (Scheiner et al. 1985) or a mother's grief or anger over her daughter's condition (McCaskill 1997). Likewise, both the obstetrician (or certified nurse-midwife) prescribing medication for the mother's postpartum depression and the psychotherapist providing psychotherapy for her depression would have the mother as their primary patient but the dyadic relationship as their shared concern; both practitioners would be attending to the relationship by promoting optimal dyadic functioning, taking appropriate therapeutic steps to prevent problems related to the relationship risks posed by maternal depression (Flykt et al. 2010), and providing various levels of direct treatment if the parent-child relationship showed evidence of problems. Such treatment might include therapeutic services provided either directly by the occupational therapist, obstetrician or certified nurse-midwife, or psychotherapist (depending on their IMH training and skills) or through referral of the dyad for particular therapy if this dyad might benefit from additional therapeutic work done by another clinician or program (e.g., Circle of Security, a therapeutic home visiting program, Video Intervention Therapy). Ideally, the occupational therapist, obstetrician or certified nurse-midwife, and psychotherapist would be meeting to discuss how best to support, safeguard, and foster the health and well-being of this dyad's relationship while each provided treatment for specific conditions within individuals in the dyad.

The concentric rings in Figure 1–2 delineate the various therapeutic levels in the field:

Promotion—Services focused on supporting the early development of safe, functional, nurturing, and loving relationships between infants, their parents, and other care-

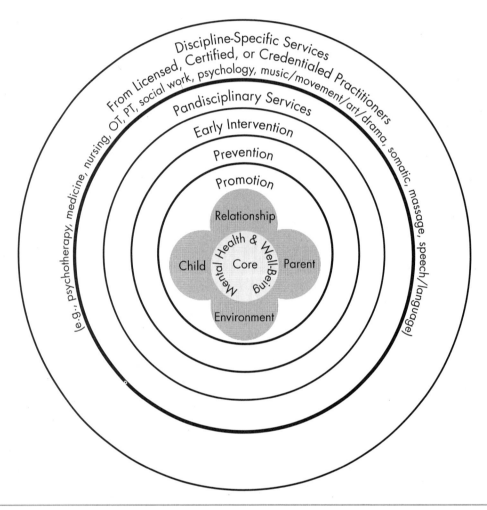

FIGURE 1–2. Transdisciplinary practice model for infant-parent mental health.

Note.   OP=occupational therapy; PT=physical therapy.
Source.   K. Brandt and E. Tronick 2003.

givers. Promotion services may occur at the policy level through public campaigns and training, be population based, or occur at a program level, but are most effective when delivered at the individual level. Mental health promotion is related to "improving the quality of life and potential for health rather than amelioration of symptoms and deficits" (World Health Organization 2002). With breastfeeding increasingly being shown to be associated with positive dyadic interactional patterns, maternal sensitivity, and attachment security, and with child advantages in cognitive, motor, and behavioral health and early neural development (Bernard 2013; Deonia et al. 2013; Herba et al. 2013; Oddly et al 2010; Tharner et al. 2012), IMH promotion strategies include programs that support initiation and continuation of breastfeeding to at least the duration recommended by the American Academy of Pediatrics (2012).

Prevention—Services that mitigate effects of risks and stress, and address potential early relationship challenges or vulnerabilities that impact early development. Intervention strategies are designed to nurture mutually satisfying parent-child relationships and prevent the progression of further difficulties (California's Infant, Preschool, and Family Mental Health Initiative 2003).

Early Intervention—Services that endeavor to clarify a concern about an infant and/or parent, observe for the emergence of infant-parent challenges, or provide initial services after a specific challenge or delay is suspected or has been identified (Zeanah et al. 2000, p. 551).

Pandisciplinary Services—Assessment, diagnosis, consultation, and/or therapy aimed at optimizing individual and/or parent-child dyadic functioning, as well as functioning within other important relationships, in the presence of serious health and mental health conditions, histories, and/or risks that are known or suspected. Providing therapy within this sphere requires practitioners to have specialized training, skills, and experience, but is not limited to a specific license, credential, or certificate. Examples of useful models include Developmental, Individual Difference, Relationship-based (DIR/Floortime), Circle of Security, Video Intervention Therapy, and Healthy Families America home visiting; although specialized training is required, training and use of these approaches are not limited to one discipline or classification of providers, and each approach can be used with fidelity across many disciplines.

Discipline-Specific Services—Assessment, diagnosis, consultation, and/or treatment aimed at optimizing overall individual and/or dyadic functioning, and functioning within other important relationships, in the presence of serious health and mental health conditions, histories, and/or risks that are known or suspected. Work within this sphere requires that practitioners have specialized training, skills, and experience, and *requires* the possession of a license, certificate, or credential to perform the discipline-specific scope of work necessary to address the needs of the infant, the parent, and/or the relationship. Examples include Trauma-Focused Cognitive Behavioral Therapy and Parent-Child Interaction Therapy, for which training and practice are limited to psychotherapists; Nurse-Family Partnership, for which training and service delivery are limited to registered nurses with a PHN certificate; and prescribing medication for disorders such as depression, attention-deficit/hyperactivity disorder, and anxiety, which is typically limited to physicians, nurse practitioners, nurse-midwives, and physician assistants.

Lifelong Impact of Infancy and Early Childhood

The enduring effects of the first 5 years are both astonishing and disquieting, yet somehow completely intuitive. The current state of science is sufficient to mark these early years as the most pivotal for human development in terms of lifelong health and well-being, learning, neural development, and healthy relationships throughout life. The Adverse Childhood Experiences Study has produced scores of publications demonstrating the range, nature, and lifelong impacts of adverse childhood experiences (ACEs) (Felitti et al. 1998). Experiencing six or more childhood ACEs has been correlated with 1) the development of a number of serious, even life-threatening, health conditions, behavioral health issues, and psychiatric disorders in childhood, adolescence, or adulthood; and 2) a lifespan shortened by an average of nearly 20 years relative to the life expectancy of individuals without ACEs (60.6 years vs. 79.1 years) (Felitti et al. 1998; Hillis et al. 2004).

The neuroscience and epigenetic literature has demonstrated the negative impacts on neuroanatomy and neurofunction resulting from early adversity, such as exposure to maternal stress in utero, child neglect, child maltreatment, and otherwise impoverished environments (Currie and Widom 2010; McCrory et al. 2011; also see Chapter 2, "The Neurosequential Model of Therapeutics," and Chapter 10, "Behavioral Epigenetics and the Developmental Origins of Child Mental Health Disorders"). Certain brain structures, including the corpus callosum, hippocampus, amygdala, and hypothalamus, as well as the related functions of memory and stress arousal regulation, are particularly sensitive to the caregiving environment (Teicher et al. 2003; Zhang et al. 2013). Longitudinal studies show the strong relationship of early childhood attachment to later development and functioning in areas that include adult attachment status, adult relational competence, communication styles, psychopathology, posttraumatic stress disorder, and reliance on the help of others when distressed (Grossmann et al. 2006; Sroufe 2005; Steele et al. 2008).

Multiple disciplines are contributing to an understanding of the lifelong impacts of this complex and susceptible period spanning from pregnancy through age 5 years, but these associations are not the sole basis for supporting children in thriving. Infants and young children deserve to be safe, loved, and happy regardless of later sequelae—they deserve it as human beings—so studies related to later poor outcomes from adversity in childhood do not become the basis for IMH work; they confirm the urgency.

Developmental Process and Context

In sub-Saharan Africa, a giraffe gives birth to a calf that falls 10 feet to the ground, lands on his back, and quickly sits up. Within minutes he will stand and within hours be able to run alongside his mother. A calf that is unable to accomplish the developmental motor tasks of standing, walking, and running so quickly after birth (something the typical human infant will not accomplish until age 10–14 months) will die by predation or starvation.

The human infant is born, breathes on his own, and is placed in his mother's arms. He, too, must accomplish a crucial developmental task or agenda, or he will not survive: the newborn must attract a caregiver who is competent and willing to invest in his survival. He must attract someone willing to keep him safe, feed him, and fall in love with him. Fortunately, he has come well equipped for this task, appearing vulnerable and small, but possessing myriad compelling capacities for undertaking the task at hand, such as the ability to move in rhythm to his mother's voice (Condon and Sander 1974); facial imitation abilities (Moore and Meltzoff 1999); attracting pheromones (Kaitz et al. 1987);

reflexes and capacities that can be interpreted by the parent as demonstrations of strength, health, connection, and so forth (Brazelton 1973; Klaus and Kennell 1976; Nugent et al. 2007); and countless other characteristics and abilities.

For both infant and parent, the nascent dyadic relationship is evolving within systems that are sensitized and/or destabilized by the bio-psycho-social valence of this period. These open systems are dynamically and inextricably interrelated and interacting and include the 1) Attachment System: safety, security, and love; 2) Meaning-Making System; 3) Behavioral System: cueing, gesturing, reflexes, and communicating; 4) Regulatory System: self and interactive regulation; 5) Relational System: engagement, responsivity, attunement, and contingency; 6) Somato-Sensory System: the body, affect, and senses; 7) Neurodevelopmental/Neuroendocrine System including hormonal, stress/arousal, and epigenetic elements; 8) Memory System: implicit, explicit, procedural, autobiographical; 9) Mentalizing System: reflection on the state of self and others; and 10) Intersubjective System of shared dyadic mental states and attention (Beebe and Lachmann 1998; Beebe and Stern 1977; Brazelton et al. 1974; Charles 2001; Bowlby 1953, 1958; Fonagy et al. 2004; Given 1978; The Human Memory 2013; Perry 1999; Stern 1985; Trevarthen 1979; Tronick 1989; see also the balance of chapters in this book). These open and activated systems expose the global system's core, and, whether rigid, flexible, or chaotic, the potential for change—functionally adaptive and maturational, or maladaptive and derailing—exists such that "intervention at this early stage is one of the best chances we have for prevention of child psychopathology" (Brazelton and Cramer 1990. p. xviii).

Starting at birth, and even to some extent in pregnancy, a series of thematic movements in the parent-child relationship and within the family constellation is now set in motion. Often viewed as the stepping-stones of development, *developmental milestones* might be conceptualized as hallmark events in the life of the child and family that are potent but brief rungs on a ladder of development. Each milestone is embedded in a transactional process of meaning making by the child, parents, family system, providers, and others. To illustrate this, I will briefly depart from our discussion of early childhood and use the metaphor of high school graduation, where receiving a diploma is the milestone, but as such it has implicit and explicit, emotional and concrete, real and imagined antecedents and reverberations within the life of the child and family. For both parent and child, hopes and dreams have been fused to this milestone, as have the processes of autonomy and individuation, independence and dependence, self-agency, grief, loss, separation, joy, pride, the "empty nest," and so forth. As a result, the *intra*personal or inner lives of the parent and the child have been destabilized, causing their *inter*personal interchanges to shift in ways that may range from barely perceptible to massively disruptive for the dyad. Perhaps parent and child are unaware of why something has shifted between them, and the "something" that has shifted now echoes within each person and their relationship. This process is embedded in their patterns of interaction and the representations held within themselves and within the relationship, and these in turn are embedded in family systems with their own gravitational pull. So the disequilibrium in the individuals and the relationship holds the potential for positive and negative impacts at all levels (individuals, relationships, and family system) and on the functional navigation through the developmental stage. Thus, the milestone, while symbolic, is embedded in and characterized by individuals, systems, relationships, and their past expectations, experiences, and meaning making—a complex and dynamic substrate in which the milestone rests, exerting its own multidirectional influence (e.g., advancing independence, loss of control, separation, success).

To appreciate the complexity of the individual, dyadic, and family experience in the child's first 5 years, one need only replace the above example of high school graduation with any number of developmental processes under way in early childhood, including sleeping through the night, thumb sucking, attachment, language acquisition, crawling, walking, toilet training, sibling rivalry, affect regulation, peer interaction, fine motor development, and problem-solving skills, to name just a few. Brazelton (1992) calls these thematic times *Touchpoints,* during which disorganization and functional regression can occur, relationships are pervious, systems may rigidify in their homeostatic pull or become chaotic when long-standing patterns are disrupted, and the potential exists for an optimal developmental trajectory or developmental derailment within the parent, child, dyad, or system (see Chapter 4, "Brazelton's Neurodevelopmental and Relational Touchpoints and Infant Mental Health"). In these thematic movements, IMH clinicians can not only observe and appreciate family dynamics and functioning but also find points in these processes for forging therapeutic alliances, entering into the family's system of care, and providing scaffolding in vulnerable periods.

Serve and Return

Babies develop a sense of themselves and a desire to reach the "other" through communicative exchanges that ideally are supported by delight on the part of each member of the dyad—the baby in seeing the parent's smile, warm affect, change in porosity of speech, gestures, and engagement, and the parent in hearing the baby's intonations and seeing and feeling the baby's engagement—and through inferring from this that each is important to the other. With time (again, ideally), these back-and-forth exchanges become more robust, expanding in duration, frequency, affect, and content. Before neuroscience could demonstrate much about such seemingly mundane relational moments, Bronfenbrenner (1994) wrote, "Human development takes place in the context of an escalating psychological ping-pong game between two people who are crazy about each other" (pp. 118–119). Described in many ways, including "mother-infant reciprocity" (Brazelton et al. 1975) and "two-way interchanges" (Greenspan and Greenspan 1989), this "serve and return" between a child and an important adult in his or her life is now considered fundamentally necessary for neural wiring and "the most essential experience in shaping the architecture of the developing brain" (Center on the Developing Child, Harvard University 2012). Assessment of the quality of a dyad's serve and return is within the purview of *all* providers working with a family, and it is vital to provide therapeutic support or an appropriate referral when this dyadic process appears to be impaired.

Transdisciplinary Practice

As discussed by Zeanah et al. (2000), Emde, Bingham, and Harmon described the field of IMH as having four basic characteristics: 1) multidisciplinary nature, 2) developmental orientation, 3) multigenerational perspective, and 4) preventive emphasis. However, moving beyond multidisciplinary to bona fide transdisciplinary work has challenges. To embrace transdisciplinary therapeutic approaches, providers are compelled to suspend their belief that their approach or disciplinary perspective is superior to others and to embrace the belief that coordinated and intersecting service delivery is coactive and synergistic. Providers working to preserve or restore health and well-being are all "therapists," with only the preceding adjective (e.g., *occupational* therapist, *psycho*therapist, *developmental* therapist) specifying the provider's perspective or expertise. Having a shared lexicon, philosophical approach, and core training supports transdisciplinary work. At a minimum, core training for all IMH providers, regardless of discipline or function, should include Touchpoints (Chapter 4), the Neurosequential Model of Therapeutics (Chapter 2), the NCAST Parent-Child Interaction Feeding and Teaching Scales (Barnard 1994), and the Newborn Behavioral Observations (NBO), the Neurorelational Framework (Chapter 5, "The Neurorelational Framework in Infant and Early Childhood Mental Health"), the Fussy Baby Network (Chapter 12, "Fussy Babies"), Video Intervention Therapy (Chapter 17), and Reflective Practice (see Chapter 19, "Transforming Clinical Practice Through Reflection Work"), and other core concepts found in the balance of this book that are categorically essential for all IMH providers, regardless of their discipline, primary therapeutic focus (e.g., cognitive-behavioral therapy, psychopharmacology, assessment, literacy, child health), or principal mode of service (e.g., home visiting, clinic-based work, private practice, early care setting). Baseline and shared fundamentals support providers in coordinating and expanding therapeutic work, and families in experiencing a seamless approach and perspective from service providers, agencies, and the community at large.

Therapeutic Approach Model

Consciously or unconsciously, therapeutic work emerges from the therapist's *theory of change*—operating to influence both micro and macro decisions, such as what is attended to, what is said, and what therapeutic strategies or directions are chosen—and is influenced by the clinician's conceptualization of the *process of change* (how someone changes). Ideally, therapeutic work is derived from and grounded in theoretical constructs, research evidence, and the logical construction of strategies or approaches where work is improvisational and contextual—and optimally this process is guided by an explicit therapeutic model. Some disciplines or approaches provide such conceptual guidance, but for those providers without a guiding framework, a basic therapeutic model is offered here (Figure 1–3). This model supports recognition of therapeutic gateways and pathways, in tandem with elements of the explicit, implicit, and plane of transformation (or zone of reflection) that are active in therapeutic work. From various disciplines, there may be different names for the parts of this model, but the elements remain constant.

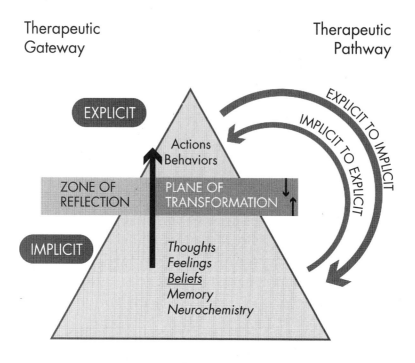

FIGURE 1–3. Therapeutic approach model.

Therapeutic Gateways: Implicit and Explicit

Clinicians are afforded opportunities for therapeutic work through explicit or implicit portals, when either the client offers an invitation (e.g., "I don't know why I get so angry when he acts like that. I just lose it!") or the clinician observes a portal of entry (e.g., during a home visit, a parent swats the child's hand when she reaches for a crayon on the table). The former invites the clinician through the *implicit gateway*, where work can begin with the exploration of thoughts and feelings, and the latter through the *explicit gateway*, where actions and behaviors can initiate the work. Brazelton often uses the explicit gateway as he holds the newborn infant and asks the parent to talk to the infant as he, too, talks to the infant. As the infant orients to the parent's voice and turns toward the caregiver, the parent may exclaim, "You know me already!" Brazelton nearly always asks about what meaning the parent makes of the infant's capacities. He enters the system through the explicit gateway by focusing on the baby's behavior, then skillfully moves to the implicit by asking about the parent's meaning making.

Effective clinicians are aware of the realm in which they are working with a client—in the implicit or the explicit—and whether the therapeutic goal is one that addresses the behavior and actions or addresses the underlying feelings, thoughts, meaning, and so forth. Some therapeutic work remains only in the explicit realm. For instance, home visiting programs that address early literacy and encourage nightly reading to the child, or work to ensure that the infant has home health care and attends well-child appointments, may remain exclusively in the explicit realm, because actions and behaviors are required of the parent (i.e., reading regularly to the child or taking the child to well-child pediatric appointments). Although it might be agreed that such efforts could be more efficacious if the implicit (e.g., thoughts, feeling, beliefs) was part of this work with the parent, as it very often is, such implicit work may not always be within the clinician's capacities or inclination, within the scope of the provider's work, or consistent with agency policies.

Therapeutic Pathway

Therapeutic work originating in either domain—explicit or implicit—inevitably influences the other. Video Intervention Therapy (Chapter 17) is a useful mode of using actions and behaviors to therapeutically influence the implicit.

The following case illustrates working from explicit to implicit.

An 18-year-old mother, Eva, has had her 6-month-old baby, Olivia, removed from the home for severe neglect. In supervised reunification visits, the clinician notes that Olivia is hypersensitive to sounds (auditory), movement (vestibular), and proximity. Eva swings the baby up to her face, close to her nose, saying loudly, "Oh, I missed you sooo much!" Olivia freezes, then turns her head laterally to gaze away from her mom. Eva jiggles Olivia, pleading stridently, "Olivia, look at your mommy. I missed you." As Olivia begins to scream and arch back in distress, the clinician reflects in action [see Chapter 19, "Transforming Clinical Practice Through Reflection Work"] on what portal of entry is being offered and the therapeutic pathway that may work in this moment. There are many choices, but in this recorded encounter, the clinician says, "What distance have you noticed works best for Olivia to be able to see your whole face? She's probably so excited by seeing you. I wonder what distance will work for her today." Eva moves her crying baby back several inches and shifts arms to better support Olivia, who stops crying but is only slightly turned toward Eva. Eva asks Olivia loudly if that is better, and the baby's face puckers into a cry face. The clinician says, "Looks like you found just the right distance for her today. I wonder if talking softly might help her deal with all her excitement in seeing you."

Skillfully, the clinician is working in the explicit domain to support mom and baby to interact, mom to help her baby regulate, mom to feel competent, and both to find some mutual delight in their time together—not only today but into the future. Notice, too, that the clinician used the word *excitement,* a word with complex meaning, in reference to the child's arousal level. The temptation for this clinician might be to launch into "telling" the mother information about regulation, sensory stimulation, signs of sensory overload or dysregulation, and so on, but "telling" has limited influence on deeply held beliefs, thoughts, and feelings. Eva may feel that a baby who loves her mother looks at her mother, and that turning away and crying means that Olivia does not love her or that Eva is not a good mother. Eva might believe that Olivia is a "bad" baby, irritable or hard to soothe. As Eva tries strategies to support Olivia, she is experiencing "something" and operating from a belief system. It is tempting to speculate on her experience and beliefs in the moment, but such speculation may tell clinicians more about their own projections than about Eva. The clinician can only know what is in the implicit if Eva shares that information. The clinician believed that providing didactic information on regulation, sensory stimulation, and so forth, in this high-arousal moment for Eva, would likely not be helpful or heard, and could even be further dysregulating for the mother, so the clinician chose behavioral observation and exploration as the path.

Plane of Transformation or Zone of Reflection

In IMH, clinicians encounter implicit thoughts, feelings, and beliefs that are underpinned by neurochemistry and memory and made manifest through behavioral patterns interlocked with procedural memories of infancy and early childhood. These can present as automatic or reflexive behaviors for which the origins may be wholly or partly out of awareness. Thoughts, feelings, and beliefs in the implicit manifest into actions and behaviors in a plane of transformation where strategies are chosen to carry out, align with, or achieve the implicit in a process that can be conscious or unconscious, deliberate or impulsive. Likewise, in this plane of transformation, actions and behaviors can be reflected on and sense or meaning made of the explicit, often with the surfacing of emotions evoked by the congruence between the implicit and the explicit, or the lack thereof—a mismatch between what one believes or thinks and what one does, or vice versa.

What Is Therapy?

Length constraints prevent much elaboration on therapeutic strategies in this chapter, but the balance of this book is directed at that purpose. As new research and scientific findings inform the field, both seasoned and novice clinicians may deliberate about how to translate these findings into clinical strategies. The chasms between and among researchers, theoreticians, and clinicians are worthy of discussion in another volume, and their related work has been compartmentalized and apportioned in ways that make transdisciplinary therapy challenging. Research and theoretical publications rarely include clinical implications, and clinicians caring to enhance their practice with new findings typically must derive and construct clinical inferences and strategies independently. To address this, the IMH field must identify strategies for more effectively moving research findings into clinical practice; for examining and disseminating clinically derived knowledge to other clinicians, researchers, and theoreticians; and for constructing new transdisciplinary therapeutic models to advance the field and better meet the needs of children and families.

After the obvious first objective of securing a safe passage for the mother and infant through the pregnancy and delivery (Rubin 1984), the next most important objective is to scaffold, support, and foster the process of the parent and child falling in love with one another (Brandt 2009). Bronfenbrenner's (2005) celebrated words should guide therapeutic work: "In order to develop intellectually, emotionally, socially, and morally—a child requires…progressively more complex reciprocal activities, on a regular basis over an extended period of time in the child's life, with one or more other persons with whom the child develops a strong, mutual, emotional attachment, and who are committed to the child's well-being and development, preferably for life" (p. 9). Following Bronfenbrenner's notion, therapeutic work should commence with identifying, securing, or reinforcing such a relationship for every child, and evaluating the child's attachment status within important relationships relative to presenting behaviors or concerns. To some, no doubt, this does not sound like therapy; however, no lasting improvement or conservation of wellness can be realized for a child in the absence of a relationship that provides the safety, protection, and nurturance of such a human connection.

IMH therapeutic work may be ascribed by some to certain disciplines (e.g., psychiatrists or psychotherapists) or limited to specific treatments (e.g., Parent-Child Interaction Therapy, Nurse-Family Partnership), but expansive transdisciplinary therapy is necessary to address the often complex and multifactorial challenges experienced and exhibited by clients, and to construct novel therapeutic approaches derived through evidence-based practice (see Chapter 18). The transdisciplinary cache of therapeutic approaches must be expansive enough to meet families where they are, literally and figuratively, and provide therapeutic work in a fashion tailored to address their needs, not the deliverables in a grant or the needs of an agency with only one approach to offer. Some families may be supported by working with a provider once a week, while comprehensive therapy addressing every hour of the day must be considered for children and families already exhibiting severe challenges. Mobius Care With a Tile and Grout Approach (Brandt 2011) is one such model that I developed in a blend of Brazelton's (1992) Touchpoints concepts (see Chapter 4) and Perry's (2006) Neurosequential Model of Therapeutics (see Chapter 2). This approach crafts hour-by-hour therapy for a child and parent that scaffolds their developmental progress within the context of the child's chronological, developmental, and functional age, through enlisting the unique resources their environment affords.

Therapeutic work must address the needs of the child and family, and come with a full measure of respect for families and passion for the work. Some forms of parental or dyadic therapy can be too slow to meet the needs of the rapidly developing child who, moment by moment, is making meaning of experiences, crafting internal representations and templates, shaping perception, and integrating new capacities, like layer upon layer of developmental "bricks being laid." A clinician's work with a parent must realize change in dyadic interactions quickly enough to support the child's development before the developmental sequences of multiple domains are delayed, derailed, or too significantly harmed. This compounding effect must motivate the clinician to approach therapy with a sense of urgency and fervor but also caution. Facilitating other safe and nurturing adults spending engaged time with the child can act as a buffer when parental or dyadic treatment is progressing too slowly to support the child's healthy developmental progress. Every provider at every contact with a young family should provide as much therapeutic support as possible to foster a strong parent-child relationship while also identifying and mobilizing resources in the environment to scaffold the child's specific developmental needs when these needs cannot be fully met by the caregiver(s) due to any of a variety of causes.

Conclusion

IMH is a dynamic and comprehensive transdisciplinary field that is on the leading edge of neuroscience. No longer are pregnancy and early childhood envisioned as a custodial phase before learning begins or before harm from impoverished caregiving occurs. Clinicians, however, are tasked with creating therapy that safeguards and leverages the capacities of the child and family while simultaneously addressing the vulnerabilities and risks—all within the rapidly advancing atmosphere of the developing child and family. Unlike any other field, IMH work reaches far into the future, touching the lives of the next generation or more with transgenerational transfer both through epigenetic mechanisms and through the awakening of procedural caregiving memories when the children served today embrace their own children.

William James (1890/1950) once described the infant's world as "one great blooming, buzzing confusion" (p. 462), but a contemporary view suggests that infancy is much more, and perhaps the most influential period of dyadic construction and neural development in one's life. IMH work endeavors to have all babies and young children experience safety, predictable patterns of caregiving from nurturing adults, mutual delight in the presence of their caregivers, and manageable and recoverable stress mediated by an attuned caregiver, all of which contribute to a lifetime of optimal development with healthy well-being, satisfying relationships, and unlimited opportunity.

KEY POINTS

- Every child must be provided with five essential ingredients for optimal mental health development: 1) a safe, healthy, and low-stress pregnancy; 2) the opportunity and ability to "fall in love" and "be in love" with a safe and nurturing adult; 3) support in learning to self-regulate; 4) support in learning to mutually regulate; and 5) nurturing, contingent, and developmentally appropriate care.
- The core of mental health and well-being is embedded in the nexus of what the child brings, what the parent brings, what the environment offers, and the quality of relationships. Mental health services can be generally organized into five levels: promotion, prevention, early intervention, pandisciplinary therapies, and discipline-specific treatment.
- The current state of science is sufficient to mark the first 5 years as the most pivotal for human development in terms of lifelong health and well-being, learning, neural development, and healthy relationships throughout life.
- Infants and young children have developmental tasks or agendas that create thematic shifts and disequilibrium in individuals, relationships, and family systems, holding the potential for positive and negative impacts at all levels and on navigation through the developmental stage.
- Each provider working to restore or maintain wellness is a therapist, and therapeutic work with parents is rooted in the clinician's theory of change (why people

change) and beliefs about the process of change (how people change). A therapeutic model can guide awareness of the therapeutic gateways for entering the work, pathways for change, strategies chosen, and congruence or alignment with beliefs and actions.

References

American Academy of Pediatrics: Policy statement: breastfeeding and the use of human milk. Pediatrics 129:3e827–e841, 2012 doi:10.1542/peds.2011-3552

Barnard KE: What the NCAST feeding scale measures, in NCAST Caregiver/Child Feeding Manual. Edited by Sumner G, Spietz A. Seattle, University of Washington School of Nursing, 1994

Barnard KE: Keys to developing early parent-child relationships, in Nurturing Children and Families: Building on the Legacy of T. Berry Brazelton. Edited by Lester B, Sparrow J. Hoboken, NJ, Wiley-Blackwell, 2010, pp 53–63

Beebe B, Lachmann FM: Co-constructing inner and relational processes: self and mutual regulation in infant research and adult treatment. Psychoanalytic Psychology 15(4):480–516, 1998

Beebe B, Stern D: Engagement-disengagement and early object experiences, in Communicative Structures and Psychic Structures. Edited by Freedman N, Grand S. New York, Plenum, 1977

Bernard JY, De Agostini M, Forhan A, et al: Breastfeeding duration and cognitive development at 2 and 3 years of age in the EDEN Mother–Child Cohort. J Pediatr 163:36–42, 2013

Birss SA: Transition to parenthood: promoting the parent-infant relationship, in Understanding Newborn Behavior and Early Relationships: The Newborn Behavioral Observations (NBO) System Handbook. Edited by Nugent JK, Keefer C, O'Brien S, et al. Baltimore, MD, Brooks Publishing, 2007, pp 27–49

Bohm D: Wholeness and the Implicit Order. London, Routledge & Kegan Paul, 1980

Bowlby J: Child Care and the Growth of Love. London, Penguin, 1953

Bowlby J: The nature of the child's tie to his mother. Int J Psychoanal 39:350–371, 1958

Brandt KA: Maternal-child and family nursing and preventive intervention: United States, in The Newborn as a Person: Enabling Healthy Infant Development Worldwide. Edited by Nugent JK, Brazelton TB, Petrauskas B. New York, Wiley, 2009, pp 141–146

Brandt KA: Translating concepts from neurobiology into therapeutic interventions for young children: use of mobius care with a tile and grout approach. Presentation at the Berry Street International Speaker Seminar "Changing Minds, Changing Behaviours: Supporting Therapeutic Relationships for Young Children," The Center Ivanhoe, Melbourne, Victoria, Australia, November 15, 2011

Brazelton TB: Neonatal Behavioral Assessment Scale (Clinics in Developmental Medicine, No. 50). Philadelphia, PA, JB Lippincott, 1973

Brazelton TB: Touchpoints: The Essential Reference—Your Child's Emotional and Behavioral Development. Boston, MA, Addison-Wesley, 1992

Brazelton TB, Cramer BG: The Earliest Relationship. Cambridge, MA, Perseus Publishing, 1990

Brazelton TB, Koslowski B, Main M: The origins of reciprocity: the early mother-infant interaction, in The Effect of the Infant on Its Caregiver. Edited by Lewis M, Roseblum LA. New York, Wiley, 1974, pp 49–76

Brazelton TB, Tronick E, Adamson L, et al: Early mother-infant reciprocity. Ciba Found Symp 33:137–154, 1975

Bronfenbrenner U: The Bioecological Theory of Human Development, in Making Human Beings Human: Bioecological Perspectives on Human Development. Edited by Bronfenbrenner U. Thousand Oaks, CA, Sage, 2005, pp 3–15

California's Infant, Preschool, and Family Mental Health Initiative: The delivery of infant-family and early mental health services: training guidelines and recommended personnel competencies. First 5 Children and Families Commission, 2003. Available at: http:\\www.wested.org/cpei/familyresource/personnelcomp.pdf. Accessed March 26, 2013.

Center on the Developing Child, Harvard University: Serve of return interaction shapes brain circuitry. 2012. Available at: http://developingchild.harvard.edu/topics/science_of_early_childhood/. Accessed March 25, 2013.

Charles M: Auto-sensuous shapes: prototypes for creative forms. Am J Psychoanal 61(3):239–269, 2001

Condon WS, Sander LW: Neonate movement is synchronized with adult speech: interactional participation and language acquisition. Science 183:90–101, 1974

Currie J, Widom CS: Long-term consequences of child abuse and neglect on adult economic well-being. Child Maltreat 12:111–120, 2010

Deonia SCL, Dean DC, Piryatinskya I, et al: Breastfeeding and early white matter development: a cross-sectional study. NeuroImage 82:77–86, 2013

Edwards VJ, Anda RF, Dube SR, et al: The wide-ranging health consequences of adverse childhood experiences, in Victimization of Children and Youth: Patterns of Abuse, Response Strategies. Edited by Kendall-Tackett K, Giacomoni S. Kingston, NJ, Civic Research Institute, 2005, pp 8-1–8-12

Felitti VJ, Anda RF, Nordenber D, et al: Relationship of childhood abuse and household dysfunction to many of the leading causes of death in adults. The Adverse Childhood Experiences (ACE) Study. Am J Prev Med 14:245–258, 1998

Fivush R, Haden CA (eds): Autobiographical Memory and the Construction of a Narrative Self: Developmental and Cultural Perspectives. Mahwah, NJ, Erlbaum, 2003

Flykt M, Kanninen K, Sinkkonen J, et al: Maternal depression and dyadic interaction: the role of maternal attachment style. Infant Child Dev 19:530–550, 2010

Fonagy P, Gergely G, Jurist E, Target M: Affect Regulation, Mentalization, and the Development of Self. London, Karnac Books, 2004

Fraiberg S: Clinical Studies in Infant Mental Health: The First Year of Life. New York, Basic Books, 1980

Given D: Social expressivity during the first year of life. Sign Language Studies 20:251–274, 1978

Greenspan SI: Overcoming Anxiety, Depression, and Other Mental Health Disorders in Children and Adults: A New Roadmap for Families and Professionals. Bethesda, MD, Interdisciplinary Council on Developmental and Learning Disorders, 2009

Greenspan SI, Greenspan NT: Life's First Feelings: Milestones in the Emotional Development of Your Baby and Child. New York, Penguin Books, 1989

Grossmann KE, Grossmann K, Waters E: Attachment From Infancy to Adulthood: The Major Longitudinal Studies. New York, Guilford, 2006

Herba CM, Roza S, Govaert P, et al: Breastfeeding and early brain development: the Generation R study. Matern Child Nutr 9:332–349, 2013

Hillis SD, Anda RF, Dube SR, et al: The association between adverse childhood experiences and adolescent pregnancy, long-term psychosocial consequences, and fetal death. Pediatrics 113:320–327, 2004

The Human Memory: What it is, how it works, and how it can go wrong. Available at: http://www.human-memory.net/types.html. Accessed January 12, 2013.

James W: The Principles of Psychology (1890), Vol 1. New York, Dover Publications, 1950, p 463

Kaitz M, Good A, Rokem AM, et al: Mothers' recognition of their newborns by olfactory cues. Dev Psychobiol 20:587–591, 1987

Klaus JH, Kennell MH: Impact of Early Separation or Loss on Family Development: Maternal-Infant Bonding. St Louis, MO, CV Mosby, 1976

McCaskill JW: Maternal grief reactions to their children's birth defects: factors influencing grief resolution. ETD Collection for Wayne State University. 1997. Paper AAI9815341. Available at: http://digitalcommons.wayne.edu/dissertations/AAI9815341. Accessed March 26, 2013.

McCrory E, De Brito SA, Viding E: The impact of childhood maltreatment: a review of neurobiological and genetic factors. Front Psychiatry 2:48, 2011

Moore MK, Meltzoff AN: New findings on object permanence: a developmental difference between two types of occlusion. Br J Dev Psychol 17:563–584, 1999

Nugent K, Keefer CH, Minear S, et al: Understanding Newborn Behavior and Early Relationships: The Newborn Behavioral Observations (NBO) System Handbook. Baltimore, MD, Brooks Publishing, 2007

Oddy WH, Kendall GE, Li J, et al: The long-term effects of breastfeeding on child and adolescent mental health: a pregnancy cohort study followed for 14 years. J Pediatr 156(4):568–574, 2010

Perry BD: Applying principles of neuroscience to clinical work with traumatized and maltreated children: the neurosequential model of therapeutics, in Working With Traumatized Youth in Child Welfare. Edited by Webb NB. New York, Guilford, 2006, pp 27–52

Radtke KM, Ruf M, Gunter HM, et al: Transgenerational impact of intimate partner violence on methylation in the promoter of the glucocorticoid receptor. Transl Psychiatry 1:e21, 2011

Perry BD: The memories of states: how the brain stores and retrieves traumatic experience, in Splintered Reflections: Images Of The Body In Trauma. Edited by Goodwin J, Attias R. Basic Books, 1999, pp 9–38

Rubin R: Maternal Identity and the Maternal Experience. New York, Springer, 1984

Sander L: The longitudinal course of early mother-child interaction: cross case comparison in a sample of mother-child pairs, in Determinants of Infant Behaviour IV, Based on the Proceedings of the Fourth Tavistock Study Group on Mother-Infant Interaction. Edited by Foss BM. London, Methuen, 1969, pp 189–228

Sander L: Reflections on developmental process: wholeness, specificity, and the organization of conscious experiencing, in Living Systems, Evolving Consciousness, and the Emerging Person. Edited by Amadei G, Bianchi I. Hoboken, NJ, Taylor & Francis, 2008, pp 195–204

Scheiner AP, Sexton ME, Rockwood J, et al: The vulnerable child syndrome: fact and theory. J Dev Behav Pediatr 6:298–301, 1985

Sroufe LA: Attachment and development: a prospective, longitudinal study from birth to adulthood. Attach Hum Dev 7:349–367, 2005

Steele M, Hodges J, Kaniuk J, et al: Forecasting outcomes in previously maltreated children: the use of the AAI in a longitudinal adoption study, in Clinical Applications of the Adult Attachment Interview. Edited by Steele H, Steele M. New York, Guilford, 2008, pp 427–451

Stern D: Affect attunement, in Frontiers of Infant Psychiatry, Vol. 2. Edited by Call JD, Galenson E, Tyson RL. New York, Basic Books, 1985, pp 3–14

Teicher MH, Andersen SL, Polcari A, et al: The neurobiological consequences of early stress and childhood maltreatment. Neurosci Biobehav Rev 27:33–44, 2003

Tharner A, Luijk MP, Raat H, et al: Breastfeeding and its relation to maternal sensitivity and infant attachment. J Dev Behav Pediatr 33(5):396–404, 2012

Trevarthen C: Communication and cooperation in early infancy: a description of primary intersubjectivity, in The Beginning of Interpersonal Communication Before Speech. Edited by Bullowa M. New York, Cambridge University Press, 1979, pp 321–347

Tronick EZ: Emotions and emotional communication in infants. Am Psychol 44:112–119, 1989

Tronick EZ: Of course all relationships are unique: how co-creative processes generate unique mother–infant and patient–therapist relationships and change other relationships. Psychological Inquiry 3:473–491, 2003

World Association for Infant Mental Health: WAIMH Handbook of Infant Mental Health, Vol 1, p 25. 2013. Available at: http:\\www.waimh.org/i4a/pages/index.cfm?pageid=1. Accessed March 26, 2013.

World Health Organization: Prevention and Promotion in Mental Health. Geneva, World Health Organization, 2002. Available at: www.who.int/mental_health/media/en/545.pdf. Accessed August 24, 2013.

Zeanah PD, Larrieu JA, Zeanah CH Jr: Training in infant mental health, in Handbook of Infant Mental Health, 2nd Edition. Edited by Zeanah CH Jr. New York, Guilford, 2000, pp 548–558

Zero to Three National Center for Infants, Toddlers, and Families: Early childhood mental health. 2012. Available at: http:\www.zerotothree.org/child-development/early-childhood-mental-health. Accessed March 26, 2013.

Zhang TY, Labonté B, Wen XL, et al: Epigenetic mechanisms for the early environmental regulation of hippocampal glucocorticoid receptor gene expression in rodents and humans. Neuropsychopharmacology 38:111–123, 2013

CHAPTER 2

The Neurosequential Model of Therapeutics

Application of a Developmentally Sensitive and Neurobiology-Informed Approach to Clinical Problem Solving in Maltreated Children

Bruce D. Perry, M.D., Ph.D.

Human brain development involves billions of complex, interactive biochemical processes, influenced by a myriad of factors (e.g., genetic, epigenetic, and developmental experiences). When these processes are disrupted or altered during development by intrauterine substance use, neglect, chaos, attachment disruptions, or traumatic stress, the development of the brain will be compromised (Perry 2001, 2002). The functional consequences will be complicated by the timing, severity, pattern, and nature of these developmental insults, resulting in a complex and heterogeneous clinical picture with increased risk of physical health, self-regulation, relational, cognitive, and other problems (e.g., Anda et al. 2006; Felitti et al. 1998). Perhaps no other group of individuals experiences a greater degree and duration of disruption in these developmental processes than maltreated children. The consequences are pervasive; the cost to these individuals is incalculable, and the economic cost to society is staggering, with an estimated lifetime economic burden of $585 billion for 1 year's worth of new cases of child maltreatment in the United States (Fang et al. 2012).

The complex and multidomain functional compromise associated with maltreatment poses several major challenges to the current clinical frameworks. This includes the inability of the new DSM-5 (American Psychiatric Association 2013)—and formerly the DSM-IV (American Psychiatric Association 1994)—neuropsychiatric labels to adequately describe this complexity. It is not unusual for maltreated children to accumulate multiple DSM diagnostic labels, assigned across multiple assessments. This heterogeneity has been a challenge for research, including outcomes research such as that required for the development of evidence-based treatments. The variability of developmental history and functional presentation impedes the creation of homogeneous "groups" required for quality neurophysiological, phenomenological or outcomes research (e.g., Jovanovic and Norrholm 2011).

The clinical and systemic issues posed by this complexity are even more challenging. A 10-year-old child, for example, may have the self-regulation capacity of a 3-year-old, the social skills of an infant, and the cognitive capabilities of a 5-year-old. Also, because of the unique genetic, epigenetic, and developmental history of each child, it is difficult—and ineffective—to apply a "one-size-fits-all" therapeutic intervention (Ungar and Perry 2012). The Neurosequential Model of Therapeutics (NMT) is an approach to clinical problem solving that attempts to incorporate this complexity into a practical assessment and treatment planning process (Perry 2006, 2009).

Overview of the Neurosequential Model of Therapeutics

The NMT is not a specific therapeutic technique; it is an approach that provides the clinician a "picture" of the client's developmental trajectory to his or her present set of strengths and vulnerabilities. This neurodevelopmental viewpoint, in turn, allows the clinical team to select and sequence a set of enrichment, educational, and therapeutic interventions to best match the individual's developmental needs in multiple domains of functioning. The splintered development seen following maltreatment makes it very difficult to select educational, therapeutic, and enrichment experiences that are appropriately matched to the client's development unless there is first some understanding of the child's current developmental picture. Selecting these experiences based on the child's chronological age is often a mistake. As well articulated by various developmental theories—for example, the zone of proximal development (Vygotsky 1978) and the Goldilocks Effect (Kidd et al. 2012)—optimal development in any domain (e.g., cognitive, social, motor, emotional) occurs when the child is given opportunities and expectations that are neither too familiar and simple nor too unfamiliar and complex. In other words, optimal caregiving, teaching, and therapeutics require awareness of the child's developmental capacity as well as his or her current internal "state" of arousal (Perry 2008). This means that developmental age, and not chronological age, in any given domain is the best indicator for where to target educational and therapeutic experiences; due to the complex developmental experiences of maltreated children, they often have wide variation in their developmental capabilities across domains of functioning.

To help address these challenges, the NMT draws on research from multiple disciplines (e.g., the neurosciences, anthropology, developmental psychology, public health) to create a semistructured, practical way for the clinical team to quantify elements of the client's developmental history and current functioning. These tools help the clinician practice in an evidence-based, developmentally sensitive, and trauma-informed manner (Brandt et al.

2012). The goal of this semistructured process is to "force" the clinician or clinical team to systematically consider key developmental factors that influence the client's current functioning. The NMT assessment elements are intended to complement but not replace other metrics or assessment elements; each organization and clinical team has developed some assessment process, and the NMT is designed to provide a neurodevelopmental framework for the data obtained in these various assessments. The functional data for a client gathered in either quantitative (e.g., Wechsler Intelligence Scale for Children, Wide Range Achievement Test, Child and Adolescent Functional Assessment Scale, Child and Adolescent Needs and Strengths, Child Behavior Checklist, Trauma Symptom Checklist for Children, Parent Stress Index) or qualitative ways are organized into a neuroscience-focused "map." This "brain map" provides the clinical team with an approximation of current functional organization of the client's brain (see Appendix 2–1; http://test.childtrauma.org/Appendix_BDP_2012_redact.pdf).

Manualized training elements have been developed for the NMT. These include the NMT Clinical Practice Tools (Table 2–1), an NMT Certification Process (90 hours of didactic and case-based training to ensure exposure to core concepts of traumatology, developmental psychology, neurobiology, and related areas relevant to a developmentally sensitive and trauma-informed approach), an ongoing NMT Fidelity process for certified users, NMT Psychoeducational Materials, and related caregiving and educational components (the Neurosequential Model in Education and Neurosequential Model in Caregiving) to facilitate the creation of a developmentally sensitive, trauma-informed clinic setting, home, school, or community (see www.ChildTrauma.org for information on these NMT elements).

The NMT is used with multiple clinical populations across the developmental spectrum (infants to adults), including maltreated children and youth (see, e.g., Barfield et al. 2012). Although the detailed theoretical background and rationale for the NMT have been reported previously (Kleim and Jones 2008; Ludy-Dobson and Perry 2010; Perry 2006, 2009), the best way to understand the NMT is to see it applied. The following clinical vignette (with names changed for confidentiality) provides an example of how a clinical team can use the NMT and the NMT metrics to develop and implement a developmentally informed treatment plan with a young maltreated girl.

> Suzy is a 5-year-old girl currently living in a preadoptive foster home. She has three older biological siblings, all living in other out-of-home settings after being removed from parental care at various ages. The preadoptive family includes two older biological children living in the home: a 9-year-old girl and a 15-year-old boy. The preadoptive parents are both employed, although the mother has flexibility that allows her to spend significant time at home when necessary. Suzy has been in this home for 14 months. This is the fifth foster/adoptive placement since final removal from her mother at age 3.
>
> Suzy's mother, Kay, was the third of eight children born to her mother. Kay was well known to child protective services (CPS) systems in three states and spent her youth in various foster and residential settings. She struggled with polysubstance abuse and dependence throughout her youth and young adulthood. Her first two children were born while Kay was

TABLE 2–1. **Key elements of the Neurosequential Model of Therapeutics Web-based Clinical Practice Tools (NMT Metrics)**

1. Demographics
2. Developmental history
   A. Genetic
   B. Epigenetic
   C. Part A. Adverse Events measure
   D. Part B. Relational Health measure
3. Current status
   A. Part C. Central Nervous System (CNS) Functional Status measure
      i. Brain stem
      ii. Diencephalon/cerebellum
      iii.Limbic
      iv. Cortex/frontal cortex
   B. Part D. Relational Health measure
4. Recommendations
   A. Therapeutic web
   B. Family
   C. Client
      i. Sensory integration
      ii. Self regulation
      iii.Relational
      iv. Cognitive

in the CPS system. Kay was involved in a series of abusive relationships characterized by transient living arrangements, substance use, and domestic violence. By the time she was pregnant with Suzy, her other children had been removed from her care due to multiple reports of neglectful supervision and suspected physical abuse by Kay's various boyfriends. Kay reports that she stopped drinking and using when she discovered she was pregnant with Suzy at the beginning of the second trimester. When Suzy's father learned that Kay was pregnant, he disappeared and has remained absent from her life. After Suzy's birth, Kay moved in with another man and resumed her chaotic, substance-using life. At 18 months, CPS removed Suzy from the home after reports from neighbors. Suzy was placed in temporary shelter care for 1 month and then in a foster home with six other foster children. She was described as lethargic, hypotonic, nonreactive, and severely malnourished, with multiple bruises, healed burns, and a large bald area on her scalp at the time of removal, and was below the fifth percentile in height, weight, and head circumference. In foster care she received no services or testing aside from routine pediatric care. She was reported as being "shy and compliant." She was an easy child to care for, but review of the minimal records available suggests that she was delayed in motor, social, and cognitive development; none of this triggered any additional assessment or services.

Because Kay complied with the parent training classes, met the 85% attendance requirement, and was present and compliant during supervised visitation, Suzy was returned to Kay's care when the child was 28 months old. At 42 months (3.5 years), Suzy was brought to the emergency room with multiple broken bones (in various stages of healing) in her arms and legs. Kay initially reported that Suzy fell out of bed. Kay's boyfriend at the time was charged. After 3 weeks in the hospital, Suzy was placed in foster care. She was described as extremely anxious, with extreme touch defensiveness (crying and flinching when anyone attempted to physically comfort her), sleep problems with short periods of sleep interrupted by nightmares, long periods of screaming during the day with no apparent precipitating event, delayed speech and language development, abnormal fine motor and large motor development (odd gait, stereotypies, tremor), head banging, rocking, and self-mutilatory scratching and picking at scabs. Suzy had no self-care capabilities; had enuresis, fecal smearing, and pica; and hoarded food. She showed no interest in engaging with other children in the foster home. She was profoundly undersocialized (e.g., she was unable to use silverware and ate with her hands) and motorically overactive alternating with lethargic. She was unable to focus on age-appropriate activities and seemed easily overwhelmed by loud noises, including television, group conversation, and raised voices. This challenging behavior led to a series of failed placements (four previous). At each placement, mental health or developmental pediatric specialists evaluated Suzy. She was given several diagnoses during this time, including autism spectrum disorder, pervasive developmental disorder, attention-deficit/hyperactivity disorder, and posttraumatic stress disorder. She was prescribed methylphenidate and risperidone, which were continued through the multiple placements. In one placement, two sessions of therapy were provided (play therapy was the primary modality). In the other placements, therapy was recommended but the placement disrupted prior to the onset. Kay ultimately agreed to relinquish parental rights, and Suzy was eligible for adoption and placed in a preadoptive foster home.

Within several weeks of placement at the current home, Suzy demonstrated several extreme behavioral outbursts a day, alternating with lethargic, nonresponsive periods lasting up to several hours. At night she was found wandering the house and occasionally would come into the carers' bedroom and lie on the floor of their room and rock herself back to sleep. Carer-initiated touch was always rejected, but within a month of placement Suzy would initiate physical contact and could sit with her foster mother while being rocked for extended periods of time. Efforts to leave Suzy in any child-care setting were met with extreme and prolonged tantrum-like behaviors, which were interpreted by the carers as anxiety related. Suzy was unable to tolerate minor transitions (such as leaving the house), new adults, or any shifts in daily routines without significant "meltdowns." After several "excruciating" weeks of attempting to leave Suzy at an early childhood therapeutic preschool, the foster mother stayed home and provided the primary caregiving for Suzy. When home alone with her foster mother, Suzy would explore the home, sometimes in a hyperactive and frenetic fashion. Conflict between the carers started when the foster father began to insist that Suzy was being spoiled, in that she was never leaving the foster mother's side, insisting on being fed by her foster mother, and having long periods of rocking and sleeping only with physical contact with the foster mother. At this point, the family consulted a local physician (a general practitioner who provided pediatric care for the family). He doubled the dosages of Risperdal and Ritalin and added clonidine at night. Even without the increase in Ritalin, Suzy's resting heart rate was 132. The physician recommended that the foster parents lock the bedroom door, suggested that the foster mother stop feeding and rocking Suzy, and insisted that Suzy be left at the therapeutic preschool (despite her meltdowns). There was an immediate deterioration in Suzy's behaviors. After a long "tantrum" she would sit "in a daze" at the preschool, rock herself, and gently bang her head. The therapeutic preschool program suggested that the family consider a consultation with a clinical team trained in the NMT.

Case Consultation

The initial NMT Metric Report for Suzy is shown in Appendix 2–1 (see also http://test.childtrauma.org/Appendix_BDP_2012_redact.pdf). The first portion of the report (pages 34–35) summarizes Suzy's developmental history; the NMT process asks the clinician to estimate the nature, timing, and severity of adverse experiences, as well as potential resilience-related factors (primarily related to relational health). These two scales are combined to create an overall estimate of developmental risk. Other commonly used metrics and inventories measuring so-called trauma do not have this developmental dimension and do not incorporate potential stress-attenuating factors such as relational buffers or connection to community.

As can be seen in the graphs on pages 34–35 of Appendix 2–1, estimates of developmental adversity and relational health for Suzy put her at high risk (the scoring strategy when there is incomplete historical information is to use clinical judgment to reconstruct the history but to be conservative so that the reconstruction is, if anything, an underestimate of developmental risk). The levels of developmental adversity (along with minimal relational or social buffers) that Suzy experienced would predictably alter her developing brain and lead to broad-based functional compromise. Complex and pervasive functional compromise was well documented in Suzy's history and was seen in her current presentation.

The second portion of this initial assessment (Appendix 2–1, pages 36–37) illustrates the organization of brain-mediated functioning into the NMT brain map. (See color plates near end of this book for all references to colors in discussion of the maps below.) This map readily illustrates Suzy's pervasive neurobiological compromise at the time of this assessment. The column on page 36 lists the specific functional areas that are scored, and the column on page 37 includes a series of "maps" that organize these functions into a heuristic construct that is reflective of the actual organization of the brain. The functional scores are color coded (see key in color plates near end of this book), with pink and red indicating either underdevelopment or severely impaired functioning, yellow shades indicating moderate compromise or precursor developmental functioning, and green shades indicating typical and appropriately emerging functioning (all in comparison to a young adult). Each client, therefore, is compared against a fully organized young adult (Mature) *and* age-typical peers. The report compares Suzy's brain map (the top map on page 37) against that of age-typical peers (ages 4–5; the second map on page 37). As can be readily seen, Suzy's map demonstrates significant and pervasive functional problems; there are multiple pink or red boxes (severe functional compromise) throughout her brain. This is a typical pattern scene for individuals with extreme and prolonged histories of developmental chaos, neglect, and trauma. As is obvious in the descriptions of her functioning at this time, Suzy has developmental capabilities in multiple domains that are more similar to those of an infant rather than a 4-year-old. The chart on page 38 indicates how far Suzy is behind her same-age peers in four main functional domains. Values in sensory integration, self-regulation, relational, and cognitive domains are derived by clustering the 32 items from the functional brain mapping process. Suzy is far behind her age-typical peers in every domain.

One of the most important items on this assessment report is the cortical modulation ratio (CMR), listed at the end of the graph on page 38. The CMR gives a crude indicator of the "strength" of cognitive regulatory capacity relative to the "dysregulation" (i.e., disorganization, underdevelopment, impairment) of lower networks in the brain; in essence, it is an estimate of how hard it is for an individual to use cortical (top-down, executive functioning) mechanisms to self-regulate. This factor is related to the executive function and self-control indicators known to be predictive of positive outcomes in high-risk children (Moffitt et al. 2012; Piquero et al. 2010). The higher the CMR value, the "stronger" the cortical mechanisms of self-control will be. A typical 4-year-old child would have a CMR of 2.42, whereas Suzy has a CMR of 0.42 (more typical of an infant—there is 1 millisecond between impulse and action). For an individual to function in any cognitive-predominant activity (e.g., following verbal commands from a caregiver, sitting and attending in the pre-K classroom), he or she needs the capacity for cortical (top-down) regulation; using this CMR construct, the value needs to be greater than 1.0. Even with a CMR of 1.0, the level of sustained attention will be very brief. The older a child gets, the more he or she is expected to be capable of listening, following directions, sitting for sustained periods of time, and "learning." These are all challenging tasks for many severely maltreated children. These children are often not biologically able to do the things that are expected of them based on their chronological age—the result can be a toxic negative feedback cycle of adults getting frustrated, angry, confused, and demoralized while the child feels stupid, inadequate, misunderstood, rejected, and unloved. This cycle just creates more threat, loss, rage, and chaos, and thereby reinforces and adds to the child's history of developmental adversity.

Recommendations

The rationale for the selection and sequencing of recommendations is provided on pages 38–39 of Appendix 2–1. The specific set of recommendations for Suzy following the initial assessment is provided in Appendix 2–2. A central element of NMT recommendations involves recognition of the importance of the therapeutic, educational, and enrichment opportunities provided in the broader community, especially school. The power of relationships and the mediation of therapeutic experiences in culturally respectful relational interactions are core parts of the NMT recommendations (Ludy-Dobson and Perry 2010). While not a formal wraparound, the NMT recommendation process starts with the therapeutic web, one of the most essential elements of successful intervention (Bruns et al. 2010; Mears et al. 2009). As seen on page 42 of Appendix 2–2, various elements of the community, culture, and school are considered as the clinical team attempts to increase and support healthy relational connections. Suzy was so developmentally immature that full engagement of the therapeutic web was not yet recommended. She was so easily overwhelmed by transitions and novelty that the recommendations for these resources were primarily psychoeducational and preparatory to the time when she would begin to venture into the broader community—primarily via her therapeutic preschool.

The next set of recommendations focuses on the family (Appendix 2–2, page 43). The family is often the key to the therapeutic approach. In many cases, the parents' history will mirror the child's developmental history if chaos, threat, trauma, or neglect is involved. When this is the case, the NMT will include the parents and provide recommendations to help address their multiple needs. Transgenerational aspects of vulnerability and strength in a family play important roles in the child's educational, enrichment, and therapeutic experiences. When the caregivers and parents are healthy and strong, their capacity to be present, patient, positive, and nurturing is enhanced. When the parents' needs are unmet, it is unrealistic to ask them to play a central role in the child's healing process. In Suzy's case, although the foster parents were experienced and nurturing, they were not accustomed to the level of dysregulation and dysfunction present in Suzy. Furthermore, the conflicting opinions and advice from family, physician, school, and each other contributed to confusion and frustration, all of which altered the relational and emotional atmosphere in the home. Suzy, being very sensitive to this, was further dysregulated by the family's growing confusion about how best to provide structure, predictability, and nurturing for her. Psychoeducation was recommended to help the parents understand her need for control, her "relational" sensitivity (i.e., sensitized to both intimacy and abandonment, making it difficult at times for the foster parents to find the "right" emotional distance), her developmental capabilities and needs, and the need for their own self-care. Also, the siblings needed to be included in psychoeducational efforts (see Appendix 2–2, page 43, for more detailed descriptions).

The last set of recommendations (Appendix 2–2, pp. 44–45) focuses directly on the individual client. These recommendations are based on the client's neurodevelopmental organization. As described on pages 38–39 of Appendix 2–1, the general direction for the selection and sequencing is based on selecting the lowest "level" of significant impairment and then moving up the neurodevelopmental ladder. The selection and timing of various enrichment, educational, and therapeutic experiences are guided by the child's developmental capabilities and vulnerabilities. The NMT consultation process suggests some, but not all, activities that can provide patterned, repetitive, and rewarding experiences. The goal is to help create therapeutic experiences that are sensitive both to developmental status in various domains and to state-regulation capacity. Again, because all functioning of the brain is state dependent, it is imperative, in order to find the "Goldilocks" point (i.e., the point where an expectation and experience is "just right" for optimal development; outside the child's comfort zone but not so far that it is impossible for the child to practice and, ultimately, master) for any given activity or experience, that the clinician, teacher, or caregiver know the stage and watch the state. As shown in the recommendations for Suzy, the clinical team targeted sensory integration and self-regulation domains. At this point in treatment, Suzy was not capable of benefiting from cognitive-predominant or even typical relational interactions; after all, her CMR was only 0.42, far below 1.0. She was too dysregulated. The individual recommendations (see Appendix 2–2, pages 44–45) suggest a variety of activities to provide rich somatosensory experiences, few transitions, and a limited variety of relational experiences to provide the necessary density of patterned rhythmic experiences required to help create bottom-up regulation and reorganization (see Kleim and Jones 2008; Perry 2008). The goal is to provide the bottom-up regulation that can allow other relational and cognitive experiences to succeed; the challenge in this case is to make sure that when Suzy is regulated, the relational and cognitive expectations and opportunities are developmentally appropriate for her (not selected by chronological age).

Reevaluation and Progress

The family and preschool staff responded well to the recommendations derived from the NMT assessment and sought frequent psychoeducational support and ongoing consultation. The school and foster family acted on the key initial recommendations (Appendix 2–2, pages 42–45); the foster father was very supportive and shifted from feeling that Suzy was being spoiled to guarding against moving her up the developmental ladder too fast. Suzy stayed home for the first 3 months following this initial assessment. Gradual introduction of novelty was successful in ultimately allowing transition back to school with no extreme behaviors (e.g., walking in the backyard; then walking in the front yard; walking down the block; and ultimately taking short drives to school, initially sitting in the car watching the children on the playground, then walking around the playground alone, and gradually starting to have brief visits to the school with the foster mother). An occupational therapy evaluation allowed the team to develop a more detailed sensory diet and range of activities used both at home and in school to focus on fine motor, large motor, and sensory integration issues. The therapeutic massage consultation and exercises resulted in a gradual tolerance of foster mother–initiated touch that ultimately led to a more generalized tolerance of touch. Suzy ultimately found touch very regulating and was described by siblings and teachers at the school as "warm and loving." A little over 1 year later, the team repeated the NMT metrics (see Appendix 2–3). The results of Suzy's multidimensional enrichment, educational, and therapeutic experiences are visible in the change in the brain map (Appendix 2–3, pages 50–51). Suzy was successfully tapered off all medications. Her resting heart rate dropped to 102. Her CMR doubled from 0.46 to 0.78, a level suggesting that she will soon be able to begin to tolerate and benefit from cognitive-predominant experiences such as more traditional educational experiences. Ongoing improvement seems likely, because no fundamental, nonresponsive domains of functioning have been seen.

Conclusion and Future Directions

The Neurosequential Model of Therapeutics offers a cost-effective way to integrate core concepts of developmental psychology and neurobiology into clinical practice. This approach can be used in public systems, thereby allowing the systematic assessment of large numbers of complex children with relatively high fidelity. This model will allow better studies of the complex clinical phenomenology and neurobiology associated with maltreatment.

The single case presented in this chapter is representative of hundreds of similar positive outcomes using this developmentally sensitive, neuroscience-informed approach. Ongoing studies of outcomes in several large clinical settings using the NMT will allow a more comprehensive evaluation of this approach in comparison with treatment as usual. Research needs to address which aspect(s) of this multidimensional approach resulted in the positive outcome: Was it the "in room" aide, therapeutic massage or occupational therapy–directed activities, psychoeducation for the foster family, and/or stopping the medications? The challenge of tracking outcomes and developing an "evidence base" and outcome studies for the clinical settings using the NMT will have to be dissected, to some degree, from the application of specific treatments (many of them evidence-based treatments) that end up being recommended by the NMT process. The NMT is a relatively new approach; however, the collection of data using the NMT Web-based metric is allowing a very rapid accumulation of data. The current data set includes information from more than 5,000 children, youth, and adults. The projected number of NMT-assessed individuals will approach 15,000 in the next 2 years. Over 50 organizations are using this approach in their standard clinical practice. More than 100 individuals and sites are currently being trained. As with any approach, there are shortcomings, primarily the time required to become trained to use the NMT metrics with fidelity and the challenge of having the resources and capacity to act on the NMT-derived recommendations. The developers of the NMT believe that these shortcomings are outweighed by the capacity to track outcomes, ensure acceptable fidelity, and help create a developmentally sensitive, trauma-informed lens through which to understand complex children and their families.

KEY POINTS

- Developmental trauma, chaos, and neglect can result in complex functional compromise in multiple domains, including physiological, motor, emotional, social, and cognitive.
- The specific nature and presentation of this multidomain functional compromise will vary depending on genetic and epigenetic factors, as well as the timing, nature, and pattern of both stressors and relational "buffers" in the child's life.
- A developmentally sensitive and neurobiology-informed clinical approach can aid the clinical team in understanding the impact of maltreatment and other developmental insults.
- The Neurosequential Model of Therapeutics is an evidence-based practice that can provide a practical and useful clinical framework to help clinicians identify the strengths and vulnerabilities of the maltreated child and implement developmentally appropriate therapeutic, educational, and enrichment services.

References

American Psychiatric Association: Diagnostic and Statistical Manual of Mental Disorders, 4th Edition. Washington, DC, American Psychiatric Association, 1994

American Psychiatric Association: Diagnostic and Statistical Manual of Mental Disorders, 5th Edition. Washington, DC, American Psychiatric Association, 2013

Anda RF, Felitti RF, Walker J, et al: The enduring effects of childhood abuse and related experiences: a convergence of evidence from neurobiology and epidemiology. Eur Arch Psychiatry Clin Neurosci 256:174–186, 2006

Barfield S, Gaskill R, Dobson C, et al: Neurosequential model of therapeutics in a therapeutic preschool: implications for work with children with complex neuropsychiatric problems. International Journal of Play Therapy 21:30–44, 2012

Brandt K, Diel J, Feder J, et al: A problem in our field: making distinctions between evidence-based treatment and evidence-based practice as a decision-making process. Zero Three 32:42–45, 2012

Bruns EJ, Walker JS, Zabel M, et al: Intervening in the lives of youth with complex behavioral health challenges and their families: the role of the wraparound process. Am J Community Psychol 46:314–331, 2010

Fang X, Brown DS, Florence CS, et al: The economic burden of maltreatment in the United States and implications for prevention. Child Abuse Negl 36:156–165, 2012

Felitti VJ, Anda RF, Nordenberg D, et al: Relationship of childhood abuse and household dysfunction to many of the leading causes of death in adults. The Adverse Childhood Experiences (ACE) Study. Am J Prev Med 14:245–258, 1998

Jovanovic T, Norrholm SD: Neural mechanisms in impaired fear inhibition in posttraumatic stress disorder. Front Behav Neurosci 5:44, 2011

Kidd C, Piantodosi ST, Aslin RN: The Goldilocks effect: human infants allocate attention to visual sequences that are neither too simple nor too complex. PLoS One 7:e36399, 2012

Kleim JA, Jones TA: Principles of experience-dependent neural plasticity: implications for rehabilitation after brain damage. J Speech Lang Hear Res 51:225–239, 2008

Ludy-Dobson C, Perry BD: The role of healthy relational interactions in buffering the impact of childhood trauma, in Working With Children to Heal Interpersonal Trauma. Edited by Gil E. New York, Guilford, 2010, pp 26–44

Mears SL, Yaffe J, Harris NJ: Evaluation of wraparound services for severely emotionally disturbed youths. Res Soc Work Pract 19:678–685, 2009

Moffitt TE, Arseneault L, Belsky D, et al: A gradient of childhood self-control predicts health, wealth and public safety. Proc Natl Acad Sci USA 108:2693–2698, 2011

Perry BD: The neuroarcheology of childhood maltreatment: the neurodevelopmental costs of adverse childhood events, in The Cost of Maltreatment: Who Pays? We All Do. Edited by Franey K, Geffner R, Falconer R. San Diego, CA, Family Violence and Sexual Assault Institute, 2001, pp 15–37

Perry BD: Childhood experience and the expression of genetic potential: what childhood neglect tells us about nature and nurture. Brain and Mind 3:79–100, 2002

Perry BD: The neurosequential model of therapeutics: applying principles of neuroscience to clinical work with traumatized and maltreated children, in Working With Traumatized Youth in Child Welfare. Edited by Webb NB. New York, Guilford, 2006, pp 27–52

Perry BD: Child maltreatment: the role of abuse and neglect in developmental psychopathology, in Textbook of Child and Adolescent Psychopathology. Edited by Beauchaine TP, Hinshaw SP. New York, Wiley, 2008, pp 93–128

Perry BD: Examining child maltreatment through a neurodevelopmental lens: clinical application of the neurosequential model of therapeutics. J Loss Trauma 14:240–255, 2009

Piquero AR, Jennings WG, Farrington DP: On the malleability of self-control: theoretical and policy implications regarding a general theory of crime. Justice Q 2:803–834, 2010

Ungar M, Perry BD: Trauma and resilience, in Cruel but Not Unusual: Violence in Canadian Families, 2nd Edition. Edited by Alaggia R, Vine C. Waterloo, ON, Canada, WLU Press, 2012, pp 119–143

Vygotsky L: Mind in Society: The Development of Higher Psychological Processes. Edited by Cole M, John-Steiner V, Scribner S, et al. Cambridge, MA, Harvard University Press, 1978

Additional Resources

www.ChildTrauma.org: The Web site of the ChildTrauma Academy includes a variety of resources about online training activities and other multimedia resources for clinicians and others. A monthly electronic newsletter is available with updates on research, promising clinical practices and programs, and ongoing training opportunities.

www.ChildTraumaAcademy.com: The ChildTrauma Academy's online classroom provides several free, self-paced teaching modules for parents, caregivers, educators, and other professionals on the brain, brain development, and the impact of maltreatment on children.

Perry BD, Szalavitz M: The Boy Who Was Raised as a Dog: And Other Stories From a Psychiatrist's Notebook—What Traumatized Children Can Teach Us About Loss, Love, and Healing. New York, Basic Books, 2006

Szalavitz M, Perry BD: Born for Love: Why Empathy Is Essential—and Endangered. New York, HarperCollins, 2010

Appendix 2–1

Excerpts of Initial Report for Suzy[1]

___

[1]See color plates near end of this book. For full report, see http://test.childtrauma.org/ Appendix_BDP_2012_redact.pdf.

Neurosequential Model of Therapeutics : Clinical Practice Tools

A Brief Introduction:

The Neurosequential Model of Therapeutics (NMT) is an approach to clinical work that incorporates key principles of neurodevelopment into the clinical problem-solving process. The NMT Metrics are tools which provide a semi-structured assessment of important developmental experiences, good and bad, and a current "picture" of brain organization and functioning. From these tools estimates of relative brain-mediated strengths and weaknesses can be derived. This information can aid the clinician in the ongoing therapeutic process.

The results from the NMT Metrics should not be viewed as a stand-alone psychological, neuropsychological, psychiatric or psychoeducational evaluation. These reports are intended to supplement the clinical problem solving process and provide broad direction for the selection and sequencing of developmentally appropriate enrichment, therapeutic and educational activities.

Client Data

Client: SuzySample
Age: 4 years, 1 month
Gender: Female
Case ID: CTA_Teach

Report Data

Clinician: Bruce Perry
Report Date: 8/28/2012
Time: 1
Site: CTA_Teach

Developmental History
A brief introduction

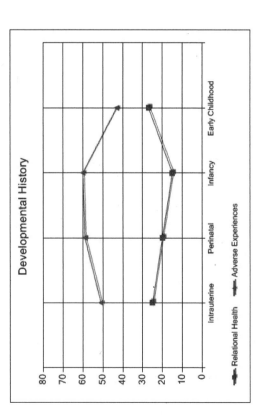

Developmental Risk

Legend:
- High Risk
- Moderate Risk
- Low Risk

Developmental History Values

	Adverse Events	Relational Health	Developmental Risk
Intrauterine	51	25	26
Perinatal	59	20	39
Infancy	60	15	45
Early Childhood	43	27	16

Adverse Experience Confidence: Moderate
Relational Health Confidence: Moderate

Current CNS Functionality

	Brainstem	Client	Typical
1	Cardiovascular/ANS	4	11
2	Autonomic Regulation	6	12
3	Temperature regulation/Metabolism	6	12
4	Extraocular Eye Movements	8	12
5	Suck/Swallow/Gag	6	11
6	Attention/Tracking	3	10

	DE/Cerebellum		
7	Feeding/Appetite	4	10
8	Sleep	3	10
9	Fine Motor Skills	5	8
10	Coordination/Large Motor Functioning	4	7
11	Dissociative Continuum	2	9
12	Arousal Continuum	3	9
13	Neuroendocrine/Hypothalamic	6	10
14	Primary Sensory Integration	4	9

	Limbic		
15	Reward	4	10
16	Affect Regulation/Mood	3	9
17	Attunement/Empathy	2	9
18	Psychosexual	5	7
19	Relational/Attachment	3	7
20	Short-term memory/Learning	6	9

	Cortex		
21	Somato/Motorsensory Integration	5	8
22	Sense Time/Delay Gratification	2	6
23	Communication Expressive/Receptive	5	9
24	Self Awareness/Self Image	4	6
25	Speech/Articulation	4	8
26	Concrete Cognition	4	7

	Frontal Cortex		
27	Non-verbal Cognition	5	6
28	Modulate Reactivity/Impulsivity	2	6
29	Math/Symbolic Cognition	1	6
30	Reading/Verbal	1	6
31	Abstract/Reflective Cognition	2	6
32	Values/Beliefs/Morality	2	6
	Total	**124**	**271**

Current CNS Confidence Level: Moderate

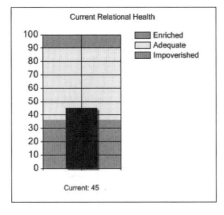

Current Relational Health Confidence Level: Moderate

Functional Brain Map(s) and Key

Client (4 years, 1 month)   **Report Date: 8/28/2012**

2	1	5	2	1	2
4	5	5	2	4	4
3	2	4	3	5	6
	6	2	3	4	
	5	4	3	4	
		6	3		
		6	8		
		4	6		

Age Typical - 4 to 5

6	6	6	6	6	6
8	9	8	6	6	7
7	9	10	9	7	9
	10	9	9	9	
	8	10	10	7	
		11	10		
		12	12		
		11	12		

Functional Item Key

ABST (31)	MATH (29)	PERF (27)	MOD (28)	VERB (30)	VAL (32)
SPEECH (25)	COMM (23)	SSI (21)	TIME (22)	SELF (24)	CCOG (26)
REL (19)	ATTU (17)	REW (15)	AFF (16)	SEX (18)	MEM (20)
	NE (13)	DISS (11)	ARS (12)	PSI (14)	
	FMS (9)	FEED (7)	SLP (8)	LMF (10)	
		SSG (5)	ATTN (6)		
		MET (3)	EEOM (4)		
		CV (1)	ANS (2)		

Functional Brain Map Value Key

DEVELOPMENTAL

Functional

12	DEVELOPED
11	TYPICAL RANGE
10	
9	EPISODIC/EMERGING
8	MILD Compromise
7	
6	PRECURSOR CAPACITY
5	MODERATE Dysfunction
4	
3	UNDEVELOPED
2	SEVERE Dysfunction
1	

Functional Domains

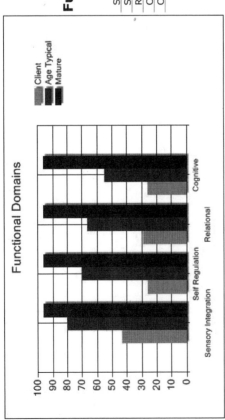

Legend: Client, Age Typical, Mature

Functional Domains Values

	Client Age	Age Typical	Mature	% Age Typical
Sensory Integration	43	80	96	53.75
Self Regulation	26	70	96	37.14
Relational	29	66	96	43.94
Cognitive	26	55	96	47.27
Cortical Modulation Ratio	0.42	2.42	49	17.35

General Summary

Recommendations are based upon data provided by the clinician when completing the NMT online metrics. Based upon the data provided, cut off scores are used to indicate whether activities in each of the 4 areas are considered essential, therapeutic or enrichment. Activities selected for each category should be age appropriate, positive and provided in the context of nurturing, safe relationships.

Essential refers to those activities that are crucial to the child's future growth in this particular area. In order to fall into the essential category the child's score must be below 65% of the age typical score. It is our belief that unless functioning in the essential area is increased the child will lack the foundation for future growth and development in this and other areas.

Therapeutic refers to those activities aimed at building in strength and growth in the particular area. Scores that fall within 65 to 85 percent of those typical for the child's age are considered appropriate for more focused treatment. Therapeutic activities are viewed as important for the child's continued growth and improvement in the area.

Enrichment refers to activities that provide positive, valuable experiences that continue to build capacity in the given area. Children who fall into the enrichment category are at or above 85 percent of age typical functioning. Activities recommended in this category are designed to enhance and reinforce strengths previously built into the particular area of focus.

The information below is designed to provide the clinician with broad recommendations based upon the NMT approach. These recommendations should be used as guidelines for the treating clinician when considering particular therapeutic activities. Final treatment decisions must be based upon the clinical judgement of the treatment provider. The CTA cannot be held responsible for any of the treatment decisions made by the clinician based upon their own interpretation of NMT principles or recommendations.

Sensory Integration

Client Score: 43   Age Typical: 80   Percentage: 53.75

Essential: (below 65%) – Scores below 65% of age typical functioning indicate poorly organized somatosensory systems in the brain. The introduction of patterned, repetitive somatosensory activities weaved throughout the day have been shown to lead to positive improvements. These activities should be provided multiple times each day for approximately 7-8 minutes at a time for essential reorganization to occur. Examples of somatosensory activities include massage (pressure point, Reiki touch), music, movement (swimming, walking/running, jumping, swinging, rocking), yoga/breathing and animal assisted therapy that includes patterned, repetitive activities such as grooming.

Self Regulation

Client Score: 26   Age Typical: 70   Percentage: 37.14

Essential: (below 65%) – Scores below 65% of age typical functioning suggest the child has poor self-regulatory capabilities. These children may have stress-response systems that are poorly organized and hyper-reactive. They are likely impulsive, have difficulties transitioning from one activity to another, and may overreact to even minor stressors or challenges. Children in this category require structure and predictability provided consistently by safe, nurturing adults across settings. Examples of essential activities in this category include: developing transitioning activity (using a song, words or other cues to help prepare the child for the change in activity), patterned, repetitive proprioceptive OT activities such as isometric exercises (chair push-ups, bear hugs while child tries to pull the adult's arms away, applying deep pressure), using weighted vests, blankets, ankle weights, various deep breathing techniques, building structure into bedtime rituals, music and movement activities, animal assisted therapy and EMDR.

Relational

Client Score: 29   Age Typical: 66   Percentage: 43.94

Essential: (below 65%) - Scores below 65% of age typical functioning suggest the child has poor relational functioning. Children who have a history of disrupted early caregiving, whose earliest experiences were characterized as chaotic, neglectful, and/or unpredictable, often have difficulties forming and maintaining relationships. In order to make sufficient gains in relational functioning, essential activities must include interactions with multiple positive healthy adults who are invested in the child's life and in their treatment. Examples of essential relational activities include: art therapy, individual play therapy, Parent-Child Interaction Therapy (PCIT), dyadic parallel play with an adult, and when mastered, dyadic parallel play with a peer. Once dyadic relationships have been mastered supervised small group activities may be added. Other examples of essential activities include animal assisted therapy and targeted psychotherapy.

Cognitive

Client Score: 26   Age Typical: 55   Percentage: 47.27

Essential: (below 65%) - Scores below 65% of age typical functioning suggest the child has poor cognitive functioning. As in other areas of focus, essential cognitive activities must take place in the context of safe, nurturing relationships with invested adults. It is in the context of safe, relationally enriched environments that essential healing and growth can occur. Examples of essential cognitive activities include: speech and language therapy, insight oriented psychodynamic treatment, cognitive behavioral therapy, and family therapy.

Cortical Modulation refers to the capacity of important cortical networks to regulate and modulate the activity and reactivity of some of the lower neural systems. As the brain organizes and matures, this capacity increases and the Cortical Modulation Ratio (CMR) increases. The CMR reflects both cortical "strength" and over-reactivity in lower neural systems involved in the stress response. Any Cortical Modulation Ratio below 1.0 suggests that the individual has minimal capacity to self-regulate. Ratios between 1.0 and 2.0 indicate emerging but episodic self-regulation capacity. This item can prove useful when determining whether a client is "ready" to benefit from traditional cognitive interventions.

Appendix 2-2

Initial Recommendations for Suzy

Initial Recommendations: Therapeutic Web

A central element of NMT recommendations includes recognition of the importance of the therapeutic, educational and enrichment opportunities provided in the broader community, especially school. In this section, samples of the sites, activities and relational opportunities that may be important in helping a child heal are listed. These sample listings may be helpful as the clinical team creates its reports and recommendations.

School/Childcare	Rating	Action	Notes
Psychoeducation	Essential	Discuss S. with school staff and provide ongoing consultation	key areas to cover: 1. State dependent functioning, 2. Relational sensitivity and the intimacy barrier, 3. reassurance re: pros/cons psychopharmacology
Special modifications	Essential	ignore traditional structure to day and minimize transitions	use in room aide as primary relational anchor
In room aide	Therapeutic	select one primary aide	remember present, parallel, patient and positive
Create somatosensory nest and opportunities	Therapeutic	depending upon OT eval, enrich OT/SS activities	pending report, however provide opportunities for motor vestibular and somatosensory exploration and regulation times

Extracurricular	Rating	Action	Notes
DEFER extracurricular at this time	Enriching	At present defer any extra transitions or out of home or school activities	S. is not yet able to manage this level of transition and novelty

Culture/Community of Faith	Rating	Action	Notes
Psychoeducation	Essential	provide psychoeducation to anticipate future engagement	At some point, Family will include S. in church and church-related activities; essential to prepare them to create gradual and positive transitions

Other	Rating	Action	Notes
DEFER additional relational complexity at this time	Essential	do not yet add complexity to S. life	help family understand the need for "simple" relational environment for S. right now. Ultimately all of these enriching activities can be added

Initial Recommendations: Family

The family is often the key to the therapeutic approach. In many cases, the parent's history will mirror the child's developmental history if chaos, threat, trauma or neglect is involved. Transgenerational aspects of vulnerability and strength in a family play important roles in the child's educational, enrichment and therapeutic experiences. When the caregivers and parents are healthy and strong, their capacity to be present, patient, positive and nurturing is enhanced and maintained. When the parent's needs are unmet it is unrealistic to ask them to play a central role in the child's healing process.

Mother/Female	Rating	Action	Notes
Psychoeducation	Essential	Go over NMT metrics and recommendations	focus on the "Rs" - developmentally relevant, rewarding, repetitive, rhythmic, relational, respectful
Respite	Essential	FM needs to create a regulatory map for herself	self care plan with opportunity to work and 'play' is essential - as is finding time for FM and FF to be alone
Physical hygiene	Therapeutic	FM needs to develop self-care plan	exercise, sleep, nutrition all essential to keep FM 'in the game'
Social Supports	Therapeutic	FM needs to resume her social activities	FM quit many of her activities when S. came and was so demanding. She needs to understand the importance of relational supports for herself
Father/Male	**Rating**	**Action**	**Notes**
Psychoeducation	Essential	As with FM, meet and go over recommendations	FF is likely harder sell but suspect he will be helped by NMT Map
Physical hygiene	Therapeutic	As with FM, same core recommendations	As FM above, Respite, self-care plan, focus on need for sleep, exercise and relational supports
Siblings	**Rating**	**Action**	**Notes**
Psychoeducation	Therapeutic	have family meeting to review impressions	Sibs can be great source of positive interactions for S. If they understand her, they will be more empathic, patient and positive.
Extended Family	**Rating**	**Action**	**Notes**
Engage and recruit	Therapeutic	try to get FF and FM extended family to help with respite and social support	there are multiple older cousins, aunties and uncles in the community who can be a positive presence for S.
Psychoeducation	Enriching	Hold large family meeting to share impressions and answer questions	find dates to hold meeting from FM

Initial Recommendations: Individual

The selection and timing of various enrichment, educational and therapeutic experiences should be guided by the developmental capabilities and vulnerabilities of the child. This listing suggests some, but not all, activities that can help the clinician select various activities and experiences that can provide patterned, repetitive and rewarding experiences as recommended by the NMT Metric. As the clinical team prepares final recommendations, use this listing (and related activities) to help create therapeutic experiences that are sensitive to developmental status in various domains, and to state regulation capacity.

Sensory Integration	Rating	Action	Notes
Healing touch/massage	Essential	refer to KB for therapeutic massage	KB to teach FM several simple techniques to be used during transition; focus on pattern - 4 to 5 minutes, multiple times/day
Primary somatosensory	Therapeutic	create SS schedule - and try to find S.'s preferences	use NMT Somatosensory mapping tool to figure out the timing
Rocking/Swing	Therapeutic	continue with rocking - but build in schedule	do not let S use rocking to "stay" in comfort zone. Slowly transition to scheduled and predictable rocking patterns during the day
Transitional plan to return to pre-school	Essential	pre-school is too overwhelming at this point	keep at home; and work with us to create a gradual transition plan with somatosensory regulatory "bridges" to help with transitions; after one or two months begin slow transitions to expose to PK - then add 15 min at PK etc.
Modify medications	Therapeutic	taper Risperdal and Ritalin off	no evidence that these are effective in this age-range with this set of problems. Slowly taper these off and closely observe for any behavioral effects.

Self Regulation	Rating	Action	Notes
OT directed activities	Essential	need sensory profile from OT assessment	schedule OT eval
Sleep hygiene	Therapeutic	build in sleep rituals	again - focus on slow and gradual transitions away from FM bed (X work on plan with FM)
Walk, run, exercise	Therapeutic	begin scheduled walks around the yard	as tolerated start to venture out of yard; parallel with FM, hand in hand; as tolerated, let her explore (do this at least 15 min 3x/day)
Music-⬚ movement	Therapeutic	let her use the headphones to listen to music	rather than trying to leverage this as reward or punishment view this as an important regulatory tool
Relational regulatory time	Therapeutic	continue to allow FM to be the relational anchor for her	over time sibs and FF wil be able to do this as well - but for now let FM be the primary relational regulator

Relational	Rating	Action	Notes
Parallel play - dyadic adult	Therapeutic	use FM as above and as tolerated, introduce others	S is very relationally 'sensitive' - for her, intimacy is an evocative cue - as is "abandonment" - so she is sensitized to both relational interactions that are intimate and perceived rejection - remember - present, attentive, attuned and responsive - and stay parallel - don't expect words to do too much
Psychotherapy (specify)	Enriching	not sure individual Tx is yet likely to be helpful	use therapeutic time to support and guide FM and school - at a later point, S will be ready for a therapeutic relationship - too dysregulated now to do much effective work
DO NOT push peer interactions	Essential	DO NOT overload S with peer relationships yet	S is not ready for dyadic relationships yet. This will come - remember she is more like an infant in this regard.
Cognitive	Rating	Action	Notes
Speech and Language Tx	Enriching	Needs S/L eval (but not yet)	S is too dysregulated to tolerate either an S/L evaluation or Tx
BE PATIENT about cognitive development	Essential	Do not expect too much from traditional cognitive interactions yet	S. is so dysregulated that she will not be able to either express her current cognitive capabilities nor easily internalize new cognitive experiences. Work on SS/SR domains - and the cognitive needs and strengths can be identified and addressed at a later point in the treatment process.

Appendix 2-3

Reevaluation Report for Suzy

Neurosequential Model of Therapeutics : Clinical Practice Tools

A Brief Introduction:

The Neurosequential Model of Therapeutics (NMT) is an approach to clinical work that incorporates key principles of neurodevelopment into the clinical problem-solving process. The NMT Metrics are tools which provide a semi-structured assessment of important developmental experiences, good and bad, and a current "picture" of brain organization and functioning. From these tools estimates of relative brain-mediated strengths and weaknesses can be derived. This information can aid the clinician in the ongoing therapeutic process.

The results from the NMT Metrics should not be viewed as a stand-alone psychological, neuropsychological, psychiatric or psychoeducational evaluation. These reports are intended to supplement the clinical problem solving process and provide broad direction for the selection and sequencing of developmentally appropriate enrichment, therapeutic and educational activities.

Client Data

Client: SuzySample

Age: 5 years, 5 months

Gender: Female

Report Data

Current Clinician: Bruce Perry

Report Date: Redacted

Developmental History

A brief introduction

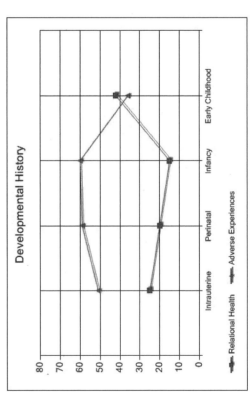

Developmental History Values

	Adverse Events	Relational Health	Developmental Risk
Intrauterine	51	25	26
Perinatal	59	20	39
Infancy	60	15	45
Early Childhood	36	42	–6

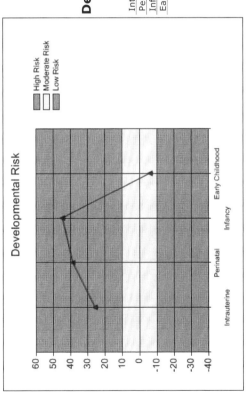

Developmental Risk

Adverse Experience Confidence: Moderate
Relational Health Confidence: Moderate

Current CNS Functionality

Brainstem		Time 1	Current	Typical
1	Cardiovascular/ANS	4	7	11
2	Autonomic Regulation	6	7	12
3	Temperature regulation/Metabolism	6	7	12
4	Extraocular Eye Movements	8	8	12
5	Suck/Swallow/Gag	6	6	11
6	Attention/Tracking	3	6	10

DE/Cerebellum				
7	Feeding/Appetite	4	6	10
8	Sleep	3	6	10
9	Fine Motor Skills	5	6	8
10	Coordination/Large Motor Functioning	4	5	7
11	Dissociative Continuum	2	6	9
12	Arousal Continuum	3	5	9
13	Neuroendocrine/Hypothalamic	6	6	10
14	Primary Sensory Integration	4	6	9

Limbic				
15	Reward	4	6	10
16	Affect Regulation/Mood	3	6	9
17	Attunement/Empathy	2	6	9
18	Psychosexual	5	6	7
19	Relational/Attachment	3	5	7
20	Short-term memory/Learning	6	7	9

Cortex				
21	Somato/Motorsensory Integration	5	6	8
22	Sense Time/Delay Gratification	2	4	6
23	Communication Expressive/Receptive	5	6	9
24	Self Awareness/Self Image	4	5	6
25	Speech/Articulation	4	4	8
26	Concrete Cognition	4	5	7

Frontal Cortex				
27	Non-verbal Cognition	5	5	6
28	Modulate Reactivity/Impulsivity	2	4	6
29	Math/Symbolic Cognition	1	3	6
30	Reading/Verbal	1	4	6
31	Abstract/Reflective Cognition	2	4	6
32	Values/Beliefs/Morality	2	4	6
	Total	**124**	**177**	**271**

Client (5 years, 5 months)   Report Date: 8/31/2012

4	3	5	4	4	4
4	6	6	4	5	5
5	6	6	6	6	7
	6	6	5	6	
	6	6	6	5	
		6	6		
		7	8		
		7	7		

Age Typical - 4 to 5

6	6	6	6	6	6
8	9	8	6	6	7
7	9	10	9	7	9
	10	9	9	9	
	8	10	10	7	
		11	10		
		12	12		
		11	12		

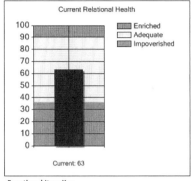

Current Relational Health

Enriched
Adequate
Impoverished

Current: 63

Functional Item Key

ABST (31)	MATH (29)	PERF (27)	MOD (28)	VERB (30)	VAL (32)
SPEECH (25)	COMM (23)	SSI (21)	TIME (22)	SELF (24)	CCOG (26)
REL (19)	ATTU (17)	REW (15)	AFF (16)	SEX (18)	MEM (20)
	NE (13)	DISS (11)	ARS (12)	PSI (14)	
	FMS (9)	FEED (7)	SLP (8)	LMF (10)	
		SSG (5)	ATTN (6)		
		MET (3)	EEOM (4)		
		CV (1)	ANS (2)		

Functional Brain Map Value Key

DEVELOPMENTAL
Functional

12	DEVELOPED
11	TYPICAL RANGE
10	
9	EPISODIC/EMERGING
8	MILD Compromise
7	
6	PRECURSOR CAPACITY
5	MODERATE Dysfunction
4	
3	UNDEVELOPED
2	SEVERE Dysfunction
1	

Client (4 years, 1 month)   Report Date: 8/28/2012

2	1	5	2	1	2
4	5	5	2	4	4
3	2	4	3	5	6
	6	2	3	4	
	5	4	3	4	
		6	3		
		6	8		
		4	6		

Age Typical - 4 to 5

6	6	6	6	6	6
8	9	8	6	6	7
7	9	10	9	7	9
	10	9	9	9	
	8	10	10	7	
		11	10		
		12	12		
		11	12		

Current Functional Domains Values

	Client Age	Age Typical	Mature	% Age Typical
Sensory Integration	51	80	96	63.75
Self Regulation	44	70	96	62.86
Relational	44	66	96	66.67
Cognitive	38	55	96	69.09
Cortical Modulation Ratio	0.78	2.42	49	32.27

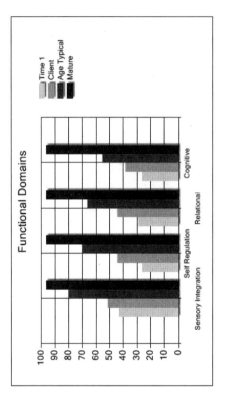

Functional Domains

General Summary

Recommendations are based upon data provided by the clinician when completing the NMT online metrics. Based upon the data provided, cut off scores are used to indicate whether activities in each of the 4 areas are considered essential, therapeutic or enrichment. Activities selected for each category should be age appropriate, positive and provided in the context of nurturing, safe relationships.

Essential refers to those activities that are crucial to the child's future growth in this particular area. In order to fall into the essential category the child's score must be below 65% of the age typical score. It is our belief that unless functioning in the essential area is increased the child will lack the foundation for future growth and development in this and other areas.

Therapeutic refers to those activities aimed at building in strength and growth in the particular area. Scores that fall within 65 to 85 percent of those typical for the child's age are considered appropriate for more focused treatment. Therapeutic activities are viewed as important for the child's continued growth and improvement in the area.

Enrichment refers to activities that provide positive, valuable experiences that continue to build capacity in the given area. Children who fall into the enrichment category are at or above 85 percent of age typical functioning. Activities recommended in this category are designed to enhance and reinforce strengths previously built into the particular area of focus.

The information below is designed to provide the clinician with broad recommendations based upon the NMT approach. These recommendations should be used as guidelines for the treating clinician when considering particular therapeutic activities. Final treatment decisions must be based upon the clinical judgement of the treatment provider. The CTA cannot be held responsible for any of the treatment decisions made by the clinician based upon their own interpretation of NMT principles or recommendations.

Sensory Integration

Client Score: 51   Age Typical: 80   Percentage: 63.75

Essential: (below 65%) – Scores below 65% of age typical functioning indicate poorly organized somatosensory systems in the brain. The introduction of patterned, repetitive somatosensory activities weaved throughout the day have been shown to lead to positive improvements. These activities should be provided multiple times each day for approximately 7-8 minutes at a time for essential reorganization to occur. Examples of somatosensory activities include massage (pressure point, Reiki touch), music, movement (swimming, walking/running, jumping, swinging, rocking), yoga/breathing and animal assisted therapy that includes patterned, repetitive activities such as grooming.

Self Regulation

Client Score: 44   Age Typical: 70   Percentage: 62.86

Essential: (below 65%) – Scores below 65% of age typical functioning suggest the child has poor self-regulatory capabilities. These children may have stress response systems that are poorly organized and hyper-reactive. They are likely impulsive, have difficulties transitioning from one activity to another, and may overreact to even minor stressors or challenges. Children in this category require structure and predictability provided consistently by safe, nurturing adults - across settings. Examples of essential activities in this category include: developing transitioning activity (using a song, words or other cues to help prepare the child for the change in activity), patterned, repetitive proprioceptive OT activities such as isometric exercises (chair push-ups, bear hugs while child tries to pull the adult's arms away, applying deep pressure), using weighted vests, blankets, ankle weights, various deep breathing techniques, building structure into bedtime rituals, music and movement activities, animal assisted therapy and EMDR.

Relational

Client Score: 44   Age Typical: 66   Percentage: 66.67

Therapeutic: (65% - 85%) – Scores between 65 and 85 percent suggest that the child has some difficulty with relational functioning. It is important to remember that unless and until re-organization takes place in the lower parts of the brain, specifically self-regulation, therapeutic efforts on more relationally related problems in the limbic system will likely be unsuccessful. In order to make sufficient gains in relational functioning, relational stability with multiple positive healthy adults who are invested in the child's life and in their treatment is required. Examples of relational therapeutic activities include: parallel play, first with an invested adult and/or therapist and when mastered, parallel play with a peer. Once dyadic relationships have been mastered, small group activities may be added. Other examples include animal assisted therapy.

Cognitive

Client Score: 38   Age Typical: 55   Percentage: 69.09

Therapeutic: (65% - 85%) – Scores between 65 and 85 percent suggest that the child has some difficulty with cognitive functioning. Once fundamental dyadic relational skills have improved, therapeutic techniques can focus on more verbal and insight oriented or cortical activities. Examples of therapeutic activities include: insight oriented treatment, cognitive behavioral therapy, reading enhancements, and structured storytelling.

Cortical Modulation refers to the capacity of important cortical networks to regulate and modulate the activity and reactivity of some of the lower neural systems. As the brain organizes and matures, this capacity increases and the Cortical Modulation Ratio (CMR) increases. The CMR reflects both cortical "strength" and over-reactivity in lower neural systems involved in the stress response. Any Cortical Modulation Ratio below 1.0 suggests that the individual has minimal capacity to self-regulate. Ratios between 1.0 and 2.0 indicate emerging but episodic self-regulation capacity. This item can prove useful when determining whether a client is "ready" to benefit from traditional cognitive interventions.

CHAPTER 3

Typical and Atypical Development

Peek-a-Boo and Blind Selection

Ed Tronick, Ph.D.

My work is driven by an attempt to understand the capacities that infants and children have for adapting to the world they are born into and how their engagement with it leads to typical or pathological development. Furthermore, as this understanding grows, I want to find pragmatic and clinically useful ways to prevent development along pathological pathways or to redirect developmental movement onto typical pathways. At a fundamental descriptive level, infants' and young children's social engagement with other people, along with myriad other processes (genetic, epigenetic, physiological, contextual, cultural, and more), is a primary force shaping children's normal as well as abnormal development. Normal social interaction leads to positive emotions, curiosity about the world of things, the capacity to cope with stress, and the development of close relationships during infancy, childhood, and even adulthood. Infants experiencing abnormal social interactions become sad or angry, hesitant and withdrawn, anxious and vigilant, and unengaged with people. The relationships they form lack emotional closeness, and these individuals have limited emotional range and empathy. They may also disengage from acting on the world of inanimate things. Whether the interactions are normal or pathological, social experience becomes the content of the brain and actually constitutes the brain. When social interaction is extremely and chronically distorted—emotionally neglectful or stressfully traumatic—infants' body and brain processes literally fail and they wither away and die. Thus, through interactions, the infant makes meaning about the nature of himor herself and his or her relations to other people and the world (Tronick 1989, 2005).

But how does social experience have these effects? What *is* normal social experience, and what *is* pathological social experience? What is the nature of infants that makes them reliant on social experience? Although the answers to these questions are not fully established, I would like to advance two linked models, the Mutual Regulation Model (MRM) and the Dyadic Expansion of Consciousness (DEC) hypothesis, as a framework for understanding these issues (Tronick 2007). Both rely on an open dynamic systems view of development and are linked through their focus on the meaning that individuals make of themselves in relation to the world of people and objects and the culturated (contextualized) nature of meaning made. The MRM focuses on the dynamic organization of the behavioral communicative system between a child and his or her adult interactant(s), which regulates behavior moment by moment and shapes development over ontogenetic time. The DEC hypothesis moves away from the behavioral account of the MRM to a more mindful phenomenological account of social-emotional development. Together, the MRM and the DEC hypothesis provide a thick understanding of the principles governing meaning making and its experiential consequences.

Peek-a-Boo and the Dynamics of Meaning Making

I begin this account with a mundane example—the game of peek-a-boo—and use it to instantiate my thinking. Peek-a-boo is a dynamic interplay of actions between an infant and an adult. The game is rule governed but flexible in its enactment, and the infant can play either role: the peeker-booer or the surprisee. Often there are unique variations. Although people say they play peek-a-boo with a 4-month-old, young infants do not actually play peek-a-boo. The game is typically played with an adult, who initially plays both sides of the game. Initially, infants make a large number and variety of behaviors, and have lots of varying intentions and apprehension of what is going on. Many of these actions are unrelated to the adult's game-playing actions. An infant may look away when he should be looking toward, or he may raise his shoe, or look at his hand. What he is doing is messy—variable, unstable, disorganized. With repetitions and development, the infant attends and begins to anticipate the coming "boo," and some of the messiness begins to subside. With still more repetitions and development, the infant begins to control some of the pace of the game and comes to signal the timing of the boo. The infant's reaction becomes more emotionally complex. As the game is acquired, the infant begins to learn pieces of how to be the surprisee and then the peeker-booer. Sequences and rhythms emerge. The adult continuously makes adjustments (e.g., holding positions longer) in relation to the infant's actions and apprehension of his intent. The selective assembling of the infant's self-organized actions and intentions *and* his apprehension of the adult's actions and intentions *and* the adult's reciprocal apprehension becomes incrementally more coherent. After endless repetitions, the game is fully "within" the child, and the way the infant and adult play it is fully within the dyad. Once this is accomplished, the infant begins to lose interest in the game.

A few points about the process of acquiring the game are important. The acquisition of a game depends on the infant's being with someone who knows the game, and that person must be willing to "teach" the child the game. Infants cannot teach themselves the game. At any age, the learning of the game is dependent on repetition of the game and the development of different capacities (cognitive, motor, emotional, and coping) that make acquisition of a game possible (infants cannot engage in pretend play; toddlers cannot engage in hide-and-seek). The game is individualized; the adult who is playing it with the infant does the game in a unique way, and the infant acquires that unique way. At the same time, the infant's way of doing things affects the adult shaping the ultimate form of the game. As such, the infant and adult co-create the game. The game, like all children's games, is arbitrary in the sense that it has a history in a cultural context. It is not built in by evolution. It is a unique cultural form played in the way it is played in a culture. Other cultures play other games in their own cultural form. Through playing these games, the infant is becoming human—learning to do something that is a "pure" cultural artifact in an individualized form.

More generally, the acquisition of a game by an infant is no different from the infant's learning any other cultural form of behavior and procedural knowing that involves spontaneous, natural interaction—that is, ways of being in the world. The infant learns the "game" of cuddling, the "game" of greeting a parent, and the "game" of greeting a stranger. The infant also learns the "game" of being demanding and the "games" (routines) of bathing, changing, nursing, and going to sleep. Each of these "games" is repeated dozens and hundreds of times a month, each has a form that is individualized and culturated, each changes with development, and each involves learning the "game" with another person. Furthermore, aberrant "games," such as interacting with a depressed parent or fear-inducing parent, are learned in the same manner (Reck et al. 2004).

Meaning Making and Open Systems

Keeping the process of acquiring peek-a-boo as canonical for acquiring ways of being in the world, my approach to understanding how ways of being in the world are acquired is to see infants and young children—indeed, all humans—as meaning-making systems (Tronick 2005; Tronick and Beeghly 2011). As meaning-making open systems, humans are governed by the operating principles of dynamic, open biological systems that fulfill those principles by making meaning with mutual regulatory communicative processes. More specifically, as open systems, children are made up of multiple subsystems (e.g., brain, physiological processes, and behavior) that are hierarchically organized and that continuously interact with each other and the external world in a circular causal fashion (Fogel 2006; Granic and Patterson 2006; Greenspan 2008; Prigogine and Stengers 1984; Seligman 2005; Smith and Thelen 2003). Playing a game like peek-a-boo requires organizing a myriad of subsystems in the moment and dynamically changing that organization over time. The subsystems include motor and emotional systems, memory, timing and contingency processes, perception, purposiveness, coping with arousal, and many others. These subsystems function to constantly gain resources, energy, and information from the world. Emergent from the interplay of the subsystems and their interplay with the world, the whole system—that is, the individual—develops a sense of self in the world that organizes and guides the individual's behavior as he or she engages with the world of people and things and with his or her own self.

States of Consciousness

I refer to this sense of oneself in the world as a psychobiological state of consciousness (SOC) (Tronick 2005; Tronick et al. 1998). An SOC is made up of the totality of meanings, purposes, intentions, and biological goals operating in every moment on every component and process at every level of the individual from molecules to awareness, such that "*All* of me is peek-a-booing with this person" or more generally "*All* of me is doing X in the world" (Tronick and Beeghly 2011). As Walter J. Freeman (2000) notes, an SOC is how individuals thrust themselves into the world. It organizes them in time as they move forward in time. To capture what I mean by an SOC, consider the multilevel cascade of meaning, both in and out of awareness—including emotions and thoughts, perceptions and actions, as well as feelings in your arms, feet, gut, and hands—as the wash of adrenaline flows through you when your plane is thwacked and shaken in flight by Mother Nature, who is punishing humans' hubris, because we all know it is impossible for something *so big* to fly. The multilayered totality of this SOC is not and could not be completely *in* awareness, even though adults are capable of such awareness.

It is harder to know the SOC of an infant, who is not capable of conscious awareness, while he or she plays an arousing game like peek-a-boo or has a robust bowel movement. Using the term *consciousness* can be misleading, however. In my usage the term does not imply that the individual is aware of the meaning. The infant or young child has awareness, but it is not a reflective awareness. Much of being in the world is *out* of awareness, including most of the processes that produce experience. Rather, the meaning is inherent in the organization of the flow of an individual's psychobiological state as he or she acts in the world. For example, put yourself in the shoes of a 1-year-old and try to experience the flow of her meanings as she watches her mother go toward the door, leaving her with an unknown stranger, only to see her mother stop, turn around, and come back; feel her mother pick her up; and hear her say, "You are coming with me!" The child's sense of this event (and perhaps yours, too) is *in* all of the 1-year-old's being.

Blind Selection of Information

A central question about states of consciousness is what information gets selected to be incorporated into it. Why would the infant and young child learn peek-a-boo and other "games" (Tronick and Beeghly 2011)? More specifically, what governs the selection of one way of being over another? Many processes have been suggested for governing selection. One can invoke ideas about reinforcement, but some of the "games" do not appear to be obviously reinforcing (changing, bathing, or peek-a-boo) and often elicit negative reactions. Modeling has been suggested, but it is at best a description. Importantly, it does not explain how children would learn "games" that have an alternating organization of complementary actions. Invoking mirror neurons as the mechanism of modeling simply displaces the issue to a different level and does not overcome the problems associated with reinforcement or modeling. Evolutionary preparedness is often invoked, but the way the "games" are enacted by different individuals in different cultures is highly variable and the particular "games" played with children ("this little piggy"; tossing up in the air; hide-and-seek) are culturally localized, making it unlikely that evolution actually "sees" and operates on games. Of course, capacities to learn are evolved (and develop), but they are broad and unlinked to specific conditions, in the service of flexibility in different contexts. The detecting of contingency, for example, likely evolved, but it is not limited to a narrow range of events (e.g., evolution did not prepare an infant to learn to "jump" in a bouncy sling). Other theorists invoke the idea that evolution prepared the child to seek out—be attached to—people in order to have a sense of safety and security. Such may be the case, but 1) there are many ways in which infants and children can find security, and 2) being securely attached does not explain how or why the infant would learn different games—ways of being—that have nothing to do with security but are simply social. Since largely giving up on drive theory (it would not help anyway), psychodynamic theorists might argue for a relational perspective, but, like attachment theory, it has little to offer about the processes that would lead a child to learn particular ways of being, just for fun. Behind many of these explanations is the idea that what is learned is adaptive, but that idea does not explain why a child learns ways of being that are pathological and damaging and why the child does not give up those ways of being when presented with a more adaptive alternative.

In my thinking, a principle of open dynamic systems comes into play as a selective force: the principle is that biological systems, such as humans, function to incorporate and integrate information into increasingly coherent and complex states (Prigogine and Stengers 1984; Sander 2008). Systems that are successful in gaining information grow and develop, whereas systems that fail to gain information dissipate and die. Dissipation has to be avoided at all costs. Simply think of an organism appropriating or failing to appropriate nutrients (food), and then think that the nutrient for the mind is information. An insidious feature of the principle of blind selection is that what gets selected is from the alternatives available in the moment. As a consequence, the selected alternative may fulfill the principle in the short term but have long-term damaging consequences. Think of a child choosing fatty foods instead of protein-rich foods, a choice that maximizes resource acquisition in the moment but has serious health consequences in the long run. Then think of a child becoming "attached" to an abusive parent. Staying with the abusive parent provides for more growth in the short term than the alternative of withdrawal and rigid detachment from the world, but choosing that alternative is blind to the long-term consequences of only learning "games" of abuse.

The Experiential Assumption

Dynamic systems theory is a "cold" theory in that it uses the metric of nonlinear equations to measure expansion and dissipation of any kind of system. However, infants and young children are not just any kind of system, and their mental life is "hot." How can systems theory be applied to children? My proposal to heat up dynamic systems theory for humans is to see it as having not only behavioral consequences (as it does for any biological system) but also *experiential* consequences—a radical phenomenology of dynamic systems for humans as a system that makes meaning about itself and its relations to the world of things and people (Tronick 2005). Figure 3–1 illustrates the experiential feature of the operation of humans as open systems.

Objectively, the system gains resources or not, resulting in an increase or decrease in its complexity and coherence (see Figure 3–1, top image). However, the success or failure is not simply objective, but also has experiential consequences (see Figure 3–1, bottom image). Success leads to an experience of pleasure and expansion and a seeking of more resources, whereas failure is associated with anxiety, shrinkage, fear, and withdrawal. These experiential products and ways of making meaning follow directly from the system principle. Success in gaining information is experienced as robust pleasure and expansion with little anxiety and fear, allowing the individual to tolerate a loss of coherence that comes with flexibility. An individual who is failing is already anxious and fearful and will attempt to preserve his or her current level of organization and avoid an even more intense experience of shrinkage, anxiety, and fear by rigidly maintaining the coherence already in place.

The process of gaining resources is often thought of as a self-generated characteristic of open systems. Certainly, the child is able to endogenously (self-) organize a coherent state of meaning about his or her self in the world (e.g., actions on objects; self-reflective thought). However, there are constraints on the complexity of this self-generated growth, determined by the limits of the infant's central nervous system (e.g., channel capacities of sensory modalities, motor control limitations) and developmental capacities. In humans, gaining resources is also a dyadic process—a process involving two minds, two brains, two individuals. As an open system, the complexity of the infant's state is expandable and some of the constraints can be overcome with input from an external source—an adult interactant. The adult interactant provides the infant with meaningful input that can expand the complexity and coherence of the infant's SOC. This expansion of consciousness is an emergent property of mutual regulatory processes.

Mutual Regulation

From the perspective of the MRM, during engagement with another interactant, the child conveys information about his or her SOC (e.g., intentions, affective states, arousal level) using behavioral and bodily configurations of face, gestures, postures, and vocalizations (Tronick 1989). The meanings of the configurations are apprehended by the adult interactant (caretaker), who, in response, provides additional input to scaffold the infant's

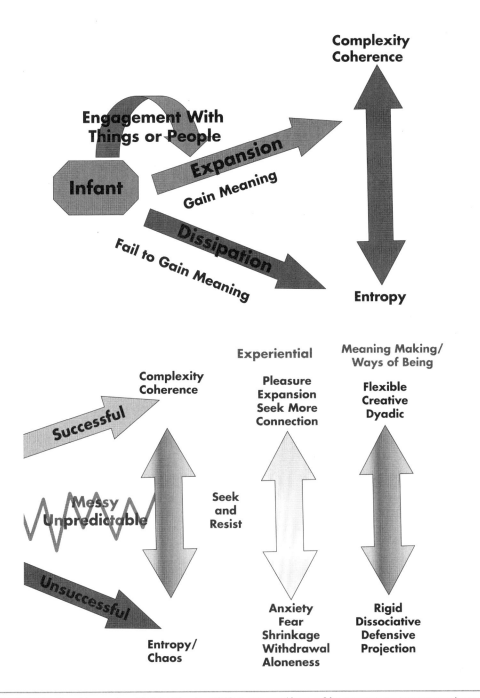

FIGURE 3–1. Experiential feature of the operation of humans as open systems.

Infants gain meaning by purposely acting to engage the world of things and the world of people and self. Objectively, the system gains resources or not, resulting in an increase or decrease in its complexity and coherence *(top image)*. However, the success or failure is not simply objective but also has experiential consequences *(bottom image)*.

actions to help the child achieve a more complex SOC. This regulatory communicative process is fast, taking place on a second-by-second basis between infant and adult. For example, Figure 3–2 shows an infant reacting to a spontaneous angry facial display by his mother as she attempts to get him to let go of her hair. The mother's angry facial expression and vocalization last less than half a second, but the infant makes meaning of it. He brings his hands up in front of his face, partially turns away in the chair, and looks at her from under his raised hands. Her angry face is not just interesting or novel. He makes meaning of it as a threat. Something dangerous is about to occur, and he organizes a defensive reaction to protect himself. The mother almost immediately realizes it too. She changes what she is doing and tries to overcome the rupture and to change the experience. At first the child stays behind his hands, but over the next 30–40 seconds, he begins to smile and then smiles and looks at his mother. The meaning changes over time as mother and infant engage with each other, and the experience of threat and its reparation is now part of their sense of the other and of themselves.

As in the example of peek-a-boo, this hair-pulling interaction demonstrates several features of the MRM. The infant and adult are active participants. The infant makes meaning of the mother's communicative displays. The mother's anger face means something like threat, and the infant reacts to the meaning. By implication, other displays mean something as well. Smiles might mean "this is fun," and the infant reacts with further engagement, whereas sad faces and vocalizations might mean "I don't know what to do" and cause the infant to withdraw.

Dyadic States of Consciousness

A critical and emergent property of successful mutual regulation is the co-creation of a dyadic state of consciousness (DSC) (Tronick et al. 1998). A principle governing the human dyadic system is that successful mutual regulation of social interactions requires a mutual mapping of elements of meaning from the SOC of the infant and adult into the other's SOC.

As Figure 3–3 illustrates, co-creation of this dyadic state necessitates that each interactant apprehend (take hold of) elements of meaning from the other's SOC. It is important to see the link between the formation of a DSC and the principle of maximizing coherence. When meanings from both interactants are in a DSC, it contains more information than the infant's or adult's own SOC. It contains unique information contributed by each. Once a DSC is formed, the infant and adult can incorporate—internalize, appropriate, and assimilate—information from the DSC into their own SOCs. As a consequence, there is a growth in complexity and coherence of their SOCs, with the attendant experiential effects of pleasure and expansion. A further consequence is that connections and relationships with others with whom DSCs are formed are sought out.

Successful mutual regulation does not always happen, and DSCs are not continually formed. The interactions between clinically normal mothers and infants are synchronous only a small proportion of the time. A more accurate characterization of mother-infant interaction is that there are periods of mismatching of emotions, intentions, and meaning,

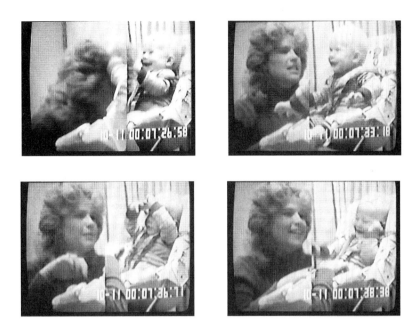

FIGURE 3–2. Infant's defensive reaction to maternal anger face after his mother disengaged his hands from her hair.

followed by periods of matching meanings (Gottman and Driver 2005). I think of this matching-mismatching as a kind of variability or messiness typical of the operation of dynamic systems. In well-functioning dyads, the messiness of interactions is quickly repaired from mismatching to matching states such that mismatching states are of short duration. Mismatches—the failure to mutually map meanings—make it impossible to form a DSC and lead to a loss of coherence and an experience, albeit only a microexperience, of anxiety and shrinkage. Thus, infants and mothers do not dance like Fred Astaire and Ginger Rogers, but they dance the way most people dance, with frequent stepping on toes, apologies, and the pleasure of then dancing a few coordinated steps together.

Effects of Reparation

The reparation of failed matching of meanings has important consequences. In interactions, reparation leads to a feeling in the infant (and the adult as well) of pleasure, expansion, trust, and security with *this* interactant, as well as an implicit knowing that "we can overcome problems." Furthermore, reparation leads to the learning of a critical lifelong lesson that negative affect (arising from a mismatch) can be transformed into positive affect (arising from achieving a match); one does not have to get stuck in a negative feeling state. With reiteration, effects accumulate and infants develop a sense of mastery and control over the world, a positive affective core, so that infants come to new situations with a hopeful

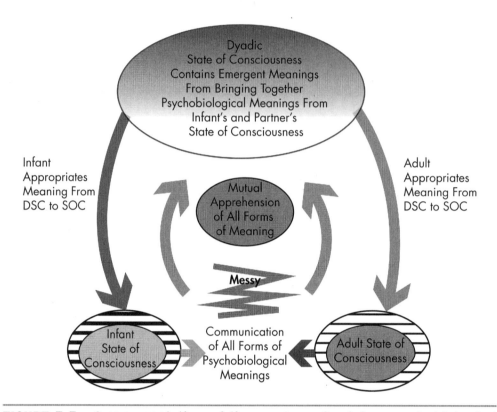

FIGURE 3–3. A representation of the process of gaining psychobiological meaning to form a dyadic state of consciousness.

Note.   DSC=dyadic state of consciousness; SOC=state of consciousness.

feeling. Most importantly, they develop an increasingly deep relationship with the adult. By contrast, when interactive mismatches are not repaired, the infant has repeated negative experiences that lead to accumulation of negative affect (depression, anger) and a sense of self as helpless. The infant carries this helpless mood state into new situations and is more likely to experience and react to them with anxiety. Negative mood states function to bias the infant's ongoing experience in the moment of an event (that in and of itself is not negative) as negative. In a sense, the infant's negative (or positive) mood is Janus-like. It brings something generated in the past into the present and alters the meaning of an event for ill or good.

Implications of the Mutual Regulation Model and Dyadic Expansion of Consciousness

What are some of the infant mental health implications of the MRM and the DSC and their phenomenology? Infants and young children have the opportunity to gain coherence and complexity in being with another person for at least two reasons that are deductions from the theory: engaging with the world of things and with the world of people. Given the unpredictability and messiness in being with another person, there is the potential for gaining more complexity and coherence by interacting with another person than by engaging with objects, which are governed by the laws of physics and contain less information. Thus, interacting with people is more likely to fulfill the systems principle of gaining coherence. However, when interacting with an adult is too messy, it generates anxiety, which will lead to a turning toward objects because engagement with objects is less likely to dissipate the child's level of coherence and less likely to generate more anxiety. Two implications are that child therapy with an adult is more likely to lead to growth and change but that the anxiety that is inherent to interacting has to be carefully managed. Failure to manage that anxiety will generate disengagement to objects and, if the anxiety is strong enough, withdrawal in the service of maintaining coherence and defending against the anxiety. Thus, relational therapy is a difficult and artful form of therapy.

Regardless of the potential benefits and problems of dyadic work, I do not fully agree with those who argue that infant therapy has to be in a relational context (Lieberman 2010). The picture is more complicated and nuanced. Dynamic systems theory and the MRM suggest that the child can gain complexity and coherence on his or her own. One nuance is that even when meanings are generated in interactions, the meanings have to be acted on by endogenous self-organized processes so that meanings "get in" the infant, thereby changing the infant's SOC. If the infant cannot apprehend and incorporate the information, it will have no growth-inducing effect. Indeed, it may even lead to shrinkage if the information stresses the child's meaning-making systems. Additionally, a system's self-organizing processes in and of themselves can lead to the emergence of new characteristics (Kaufman 1995; Modell 1993; Sander 2008). Infants, for example, have a positive affective core that carries the meaning of the world as safe and fun, which may lead to the enhancement and emergence of curiosity and exploration and consequently make it more likely that the infants will discover new meanings about themselves in the world, which may in turn further strengthen that core meaning and further amplify their tendency to explore (Emde 1983; Tronick 2005, 2007). In contrast, when these self-organized processes fail, infants may move into growth-limiting trajectories, and if such failures are chronic, their development can derail. While infants under stress may turn toward the world of objects as a defense against anxiety, it is also the obvious case that they can engage the world of objects (e.g., an infant playing with objects, a toddler exploring a sandbox) on their own. Although the child is dependent on an adult to set up these opportunities, when the child is interacting with the objects, the adult is not involved.

Furthermore, although I admit to this idea as being cryptic or sheer speculation, infants and young children can engage with their own SOC and make it more coherent and complex. The process is one of self-organization and is an inherent quality of states to dynamic open systems. It might be thought of as a kind of primordial self-reflective process, or perhaps it is a state that is something like the state of rapid eye movement sleep, during which experience is consolidated. Certainly, this process is observed when a toddler talks to him- or herself while going to sleep (Beeghly and Cicchetti 1994; Bruner 1990). The implication for therapy is that young children and even infants need time alone under their own agency as well as time in relationships. The ratio of time spent alone to time spent with others is unknown, as is the ideal context in which the infant should be alone; however, to always be with another may prove to be problematic for a child.

Not Everything Is Trauma

As contrasted with approaches that concentrate on trauma as a primary mechanism generating mental health problems, a dynamic systems perspective argues that a more intense focus on the life of infants and parents *as it is lived* in its most quotidian moment is warranted (DiCorcia and Tronick 2011). While not denying trauma's effects, my perspective views trauma as an interruption and distortion of meaning making in a way that forces the selection of meanings in the moment from only problematic options. Trauma creates fixed meanings that limit the expansion of complexity in dyadic open systems, and I believe it actually may impair meaning-making processes per se. Moreover, trauma's toxic effect on young children is to fix in place meanings (like moods) that limit and bias engagement with any and all interactions, even the ones that might be potentially growth enhancing. With time, these effects are amplified and further distort and preclude other, typical meaning-making processes that are foundational to positive developmental outcomes (Osofsky 1995; Pollak et al. 2000). The child comes to see the world as dangerous, whether or not it is in reality.

By focusing on the chronic, moment-to-moment social experiences of infants and caregivers, my approach demands that treatments for infants involve caregivers, because caregivers are chronically with the child. Caregivers too must change their ways of being together with their infants and may need therapy of their own in order to change. In interventions with infants, therefore, caregivers must actively scaffold their infants' intentions and meaning making and simultaneously make new meanings with them in order to induce change. This approach is more likely to succeed if it is begun early and reiterated often, because infants as developing systems are especially open to change (Gottlieb and Halpern 2008; Perry and Szalavitz 2006; Sander 2008). Anna Freud (1974) recognized this when she noted that the goal of therapy is to get children back on their normal developmental pathway. In some cases, having infants develop a therapeutic relationship with a person other than the disturbed caregiver may protect them because it enables them to develop ways of being with others that not only are generative for future relations with others but also, reciprocally, may help induce change in their caregiver(s). That is, infants as open systems can serve a therapeutic function with their caregivers (Field 1998), and the exchange can self-amplify into a virtuous (as opposed to vicious) therapeutic cycle. In other therapeutic contexts (with the exception of family therapy), a therapist who works with a couple and also individually with one or each of the members of the couple might be seen as engaging in a boundary violation, with its many attendant problems. However, in infant mental health work, such multipatient systems work may be extremely effective in scaffolding the process of change.

Multiple Levels of Meaning Making and Therapy

Meanings are biopsychological and come in a multitude of different (polymorphic) forms (Ogden et al. 2006; Tronick 2008). An implication is that infant mental health therapies that rely solely on one form of meaning making (e.g., dyadic, cognitive, or body therapies, be they focused on parent, or infant, or the relationship) may have only limited success because they may only be able to "remake" some of the forms of meaning made at other, untouched levels. The multifaceted nature of infants' meaning making suggests that a wide variety of infant therapies would be useful, such as touch, massage, holding, playing alone and with others, reverie, mindfulness and other states, and even psychophysiological interventions (Field 2003; Ham and Tronick 2009; Ogden 1997; Ogden et al. 2006; Siegel 2010). Multiple ways of working with infant-caregiver dyads are also needed, and perhaps the same holds true for adult therapy as well.

Moreover, clinicians working with at-risk infant-caregiver dyads need to recognize and tolerate the messiness around negative states that is generated in typical interactions, what Brazelton (1992) in his Touchpoints model has called "valuing disorganization." Such tolerance is not always easy or comfortable because it induces a loss of complexity in the system (dissipation). It may also increase anxiety, especially in the parent, as well as the therapist, perhaps resulting in problematic actions aimed at controlling their anxiety. However, when viewing the infant-caregiver dyad as an open system, therapists must allow for interactive disorganization (messiness) and sometimes even induce it in order to overcome rigid patterns. They then need to actively scaffold caregivers' and infants' attempts to co-create mutual strategies to modulate and repair their negative affective states during social interaction and to co-create new meanings. Then, as new and more complex meanings form, infants and caregivers (and therapists) can gain increasing confidence in their coping capacities and in others' reliability, which can amplify the possibility of change. Of course, the added difficulty in dealing with infants and children as opposed to adults is that their development is always moving forward, and too much disorganization may lead to derailment. Unfortunately, we do not know when the disorganization becomes too much.

Conclusion

Our focus on the dynamic moment-to-moment interchanges between infant and caregiver highlights the concept that every infant-caregiver relationship is unique. Therefore, treatment plans should not be overly formulaic or rigid but rather should focus on individual differences. Furthermore, an important advantage of this perspective is the recognition that the process of making sense out of the world is a lifelong transactional process, not a perspective in which early experience or genetics alone rigidly determines later outcomes (Kagan 1998). Rather, although the past does constrain the future, over the life span there is always the possibility of creating new SOCs—that is, new meanings of self in relation to the world. Even more vital is the need to recognize that no connection between individuals is perfect; however, out of all this imperfection, mutual regulatory processes generate unique meanings, and new relationships and ways of being emerge. Such is the dynamic wonder of the human condition: the ongoing emergence of new ways of experiencing the world, being together, and making new meanings in relation to the world and to one's self.

KEY POINTS

- All humans are meaning-making systems, attempting to make meaning about themselves in the world. Meaning is not made just by language and symbols but also by multiple systems—neurological processes, physiological processes, and behavior that continuously interact with each other and the external world. The meanings form a psychobiological state of consciousness made up of the totality of meanings, purposes, intentions, and biological goals operating in every moment on every component and process at every level of the individual from molecules to awareness.

- The process of meaning making is governed by principles from open systems theory. Humans as open dynamic systems must constantly engage the world to gain energy and information to grow and develop, and thereby to expand their state of consciousness. At any moment, the individual may make choices that maximize growth in the short term but the individual may be blind to the long-term consequences.

- The acquisition of a game such as peek-a-boo by an infant can be seen as the prototype for the infant as an open system learning any form of being in the world. The infant learns the "game" of cuddling, the "game" of greeting a parent, and the "game" of greeting a stranger. The infant learns the "game" of being demanding and the "games" (routines) of bathing, changing, nursing, and going to sleep. Each of these "games" is repeated dozens and hundreds of times a month, each has a form that is individualized and culturated, each changes with development, and each involves learning the "game" with another person.

- Normal development and abnormal development are governed by the same process. Aberrant "games" (i.e., ways of being in the world), such as interacting with a depressed parent or a fear-inducing parent, are learned in the same manner as the other "games." Both kinds of development are dependent on the individual's active engagement with the world of people and things available to him or her in the moment and his or her blind selection from what is available for good or ill in the long run.

- Therapy is a process of changing an individual's psychobiological state of consciousness, and it must operate at all the multiple levels of meaning making.

References

Beeghly M, Cicchetti D: Child maltreatment, attachment, and the self system: emergence of an internal state lexicon in toddlers at high social risk. Dev Psychopathol 6:5–30, 1994

Brazelton TB: Touchpoints: The Essential Reference—Your Child's Emotional and Behavioral Development. Boston, MA, Addison-Wesley, 1992

Bruner J: Acts of Meaning. Cambridge, MA, Harvard University Press, 1990

DiCorcia J, Tronick E: Quotidian resilience: exploring mechanisms that drive resilience from a perspective of everyday stress and coping. Neurosci Biobehav Rev 35:1593–1602, 2011

Emde RN: The prerepresentational self and its affective core, in The Psychoanalytic Study of the Child. Edited by Freud A, Hartmann H, Kris E. New Haven, CT, Yale University Press, 1983, pp 165–192

Field T: Maternal depression effects on infants and early intervention. Prev Med 27:200–203, 1998

Field T: Touch. New York, Bradford Books, 2003

Fogel A: Dynamic systems research on interindividual communication: the transformation of meaning-making. J Dev Process 1:7–30, 2006

Freeman WJ: How Brains Make Up Their Minds. New York, Columbia University Press, 2000

Freud A: Normality and Pathology in Childhood: Assessments of Development, Vol 6. New York, International Universities Press, 1974

Gottlieb G, Halpern CT: Individual development as a system of co-actions: implications for research and policy, in Human Development in the 21st Century: Visionary Ideas From Systems Scientists. Edited by Fogel A, King BJ, Shanker SG. New York, Cambridge University Press, 2008, pp 41–47

Gottman JM, Driver JL: Dysfunctional marital conflict and everyday marital interaction. J Divorce Remarriage 43:63–77, 2005

Granic I, Patterson GR: Toward a comprehensive model of antisocial development: a dynamic systems approach. Psychol Rev 113:101–131, 2006

Greenspan SI: A dynamic developmental model of mental health and mental illness, in Human Development in the 21st Century: Visionary Ideas From Systems Scientists. Edited by Fogel A, King BJ, Shanker SG. New York, Cambridge University Press, 2008, pp 157–175

Ham J, Tronick EZ: Relational psychophysiology: lessons from mother-infant physiology research on dyadically expanded states of consciousness. Psychother Res 19:619–632, 2009

Kagan J: Three Seductive Ideas. Cambridge, MA, Harvard University Press, 1998

Kaufman S: At Home in the Universe: The Search for the Laws of Self-Organization and Complexity. New York, Oxford University Press, 1995

Lieberman AF: Repairing the Effects of Trauma on Early Attachment. National Child Traumatic Stress Network, 2010. Available at: http://www1.extension.umn.edu/family/cyfc/our-programs/lessons-from-the-field/race-culture-and-childrens-mental-health/docs/Lieberman.pdf. Accessed March 27, 2013.

Modell A: The Private Self. Cambridge, MA, Harvard University Press, 1993

Ogden T: Reverie and Interpretation: Sensing Something Human. Lanham, MD, Rowman & Littlefield, 1997

Ogden P, Minton K, Pain C: Trauma and the Body: A Sensorimotor Approach to Psychotherapy. New York, WW Norton, 2006

Osofsky J: The effects of exposure to violence in young children. Am Psychol 50:782–786, 1995

Perry BD, Szalavitz M: The Boy Who Was Raised as a Dog: And Other Stories From a Psychiatrist's Notebook. New York, Basic Books, 2006

Pollak SD, Cicchetti D, Hornung K, et al: Recognizing emotion in faces: developmental effects of child abuse and neglect. Dev Psychol 36:679–688, 2000

Prigogine I, Stengers I: Order Out of Chaos: Man's New Dialogue With Nature. Toronto, ON, Canada, Bantam New Age Books, 1984

Reck C, Hunt A, Fuchs T, et al: Interactive regulation of affect in postpartum depressed mothers and their infants: an overview. Psychopathology 37:272–280, 2004

Sander L: Living Systems, Evolving Consciousness, and the Emerging Person: A Selection of Papers From the Life Work of Louis Sander. Edited by Amadei G, Bianchi I. New York, Analytic Press, 2008

Seligman S: Dynamic systems theories as a metaframework for psychoanalysis. Psychoanal Dialogues 15:285–319, 2005

Siegel D: Mindsight: The New Science of Transformation. New York, WW Norton, 2010

Smith LB, Thelen E: Development as a dynamic system. Trends Cogn Sci 7:343–348, 2003

Tronick EZ: Emotions and emotional communication in infants. Am Psychol 44:112–119, 1989

Tronick EZ: Why is connection with others so critical? The formation of dyadic states of consciousness and the expansion of individuals' states of consciousness: coherence governed selection and the co-creation of meaning out of messy meaning making, in Emotional Development: Recent Research Advances. Edited by Nadel J, Muir D. Oxford, England, Oxford University Press, 2005, pp 293–315

Tronick EZ: The Neurobehavioral and Social-Emotional Development of Infants and Children. New York, Norton, 2007

Tronick E: Multilevel meaning making and dyadic expansion of consciousness theory: the emotional and the polymorphic polysemic flow of meaning, in The Healing Power of Emotion: Affective Neuroscience, Development, and Clinical Practice. Edited by Fosha D, Siegel DJ, Solomon M. New York, WW Norton, 2008, pp 86–110

Tronick E, Beeghly M: Meaning making and infant mental health. Am Psychol 107–119, 2011

Tronick EZ, Als H, Adamson L, et al: Dyadically expanded states of consciousness and the process of therapeutic change. Infant Ment Health J 19:290–299, 1998

CHAPTER 4

Brazelton's Neurodevelopmental and Relational Touchpoints and Infant Mental Health

John Hornstein, Ed.D.

The Touchpoints approach is simultaneously a description of infant and child development and a method for working with families (Brazelton 1992; Brazelton et al. 1997; Stadtler and Hornstein 2009). The array of biological, environmental, and cultural forces that affect the process of a child's development is understood as a dynamic system that 1) is characterized by predictable points of disorganization and 2) is relational in nature. Professionals, in this view, join the system of care around the child by using specific strategies that acknowledge the complexity of these forces of development but are focused on the practical, day-to-day caregiving and educational practices of families and communities.

Each infant arrives with a unique physiology, into a unique family, and within a unique community. The child brings a range of individual physiological predispositions and capacities (Brazelton and Nugent 1995) to a particular culturally defined developmental niche (Super and Harkness 1986). Approaches to work with children and families in the fields of early education, health care, and mental health seldom integrate knowledge of the complex interaction of biological, environmental, and cultural influences in the process of forming relationships with families and structuring interventions. Touchpoints is a systematic and integrated approach that includes a view of children's development that acknowledges the complexity of various maturational and environmental forces affecting the child, the cultural nature of work with families, a set of relational assumptions and principles to guide the work, and a perspective on how this knowledge and practice relate to the organization of services and public policy.

Touchpoints in Development

> There is no such thing as a baby.... A baby cannot exist alone, but is essentially part of a relationship.
>
> D. W. Winnicott (1964, p. 88)

An infant or child's development is the result of a complex interplay between biological and environmental forces in dynamic interaction (Fogel 1999; Smith and Thelen 2003; Tronick 2007). Development is not simply guided by a genetically programmed maturational process triggered or influenced by environmental forces, but rather is an evolving and self-organizing system that results from the individually unique and particular combination of both biological and environmental influences. This is consistent with current neurodevelopmental study, which emphasizes experience-dependent aspects of brain development for many human functions (Nelson 1999; Shore 2010). A child's particular caregiving environment not only triggers the development of functions but also affects the neural circuitry that leads to the actual nature of many of those functions. Such a dynamic frame has been supported through empirical study of a variety of functions, including, among others, sleep patterns (Sander 1976), ambulation (Campos et al. 2000), emotional regulation (Lewis 2000), reaching (Smith and Thelen 2003), and parent-infant relationships (Tronick 2007).

In his first articulation of a view of development consistent with dynamic systems theory, T. Berry Brazelton (1992) described development as a discontinuous process marked, in typical development, by predictable periods of disorganization. Each of these points of development is shaped not only by neurological forces but also by the child's experience of those forces and by the caregiving environment. In this view, disorganization, or seeming regression, is not only characteristic of the process but is also a requirement of the system; it is a "touchpoint"—a key moment in development where the trajectory of development is particularly "sensitive" due to the nature of the disorganized and reorganizing system. As a system within a system, Touchpoints also provides others (professional help-givers) the opportunity to join the system.

Because development is a dynamic system, its course is affected by how these periods of disorganization and growth are experienced and managed by the child and family. For example, the predictable disorganization that accompanies ambulation for children ages 7–9 months may lead to a variety of disparate responses from parents, including anger and relational distancing (Campos et al. 2000). However, application of this developmental knowledge, particularly the understanding that disorganization is required by the system, may, according to Touchpoints practice, mediate negative consequences. As Smith and Thelen (2000) suggest, the dynamics of an individual's developmental trajectory is more important than the relative contribution of either nature or nurture. Physiological and environmental factors are important contributors, but only in the context of the meaning-making narrative about *this* child in *this* family. Because these individual trajectories are universally characterized by periodic regressions or, as Brazelton puts it, periods of disorganization, the meaning making of parents and families invariably includes narratives about the causes of such regression. Such narratives may include representations of the health of the child, competence of the parents, and historical influences such as "ghosts in the nursery" (Fraiberg et al. 1975).

As opposed to other, research-based articulations of dynamic systems, Brazelton's account is contextualized in day-to-day parenting. The data that support the approach come directly from the naturally occurring behavior of children and the accounts of parents (Brazelton 1992). Although the process is nonlinear and complex, it is described through the everyday child-rearing challenges faced by adults and other caregivers. Periods of disorganization that might be seen by researchers as prompted by a burst in cognitive development—for example, object permanence as described by Piaget (1952)—are seen as being expressed in parenting challenges, such as the 9-month-old calling for the parent when the parent is out of sight.

Development, in this view, is always understood as nested in relationships and in the context of everyday life in a family, community, and culture. Central to this understanding is the formative role of emotions. Whereas the approach—the descriptions of children's behavior and associated parental responses—includes all of the domains of development, it is particularly focused on the emotional development of the child in the context of family relationships. The challenges—for example, of sleep disruptions, toilet training, and discipline—all take place within the dynamics of the parent-child relationship. Because this relationship is fundamental to the child's developing capacity for self-regulation (Tronick 2010; Shonkoff and Phillips 2000), these challenges necessarily include capacities such as emotional expression (Malatesta 1988), the recognition of emotions (Eisenberg et al. 1992), and an emergent sense of self (Stern 1985). Emotions are the organizers of experience (Emde 1998), playing a constructive role in cognitive, social, and moral development (Greenspan 1997).

The Touchpoints described by Brazelton include various biobehavioral shifts throughout infancy and early childhood. The 13 outlined in the first 3 years of life are predominantly seen in relation to shifts in development associated with central nervous system maturation, such as the turning outward of a 4-month-old as he is more capable of attending to his broader environment or the verbal confrontations of a toddler as her language capacities explode. Those of the next 3 years may be largely the result of societal expectations (e.g., transition to formal schooling) but are also to some degree associated with neurological maturation. In the case of formal schooling, this maturation might include executive functions that are correlated with frontal lobe capacities (Diamond 2002). The child's capacity for self-regulation and the nature of the caregiving environment's support of developing capacities—including the regulation of states of consciousness of the newborn, the social referencing of the 9-month-old, the temper tantrums of the toddler, and the capacity for impulse control of the preschooler—are central themes of the developmental process addressed by the Touchpoints approach.

A corollary example of disorganization in development is provided by the research of a codeveloper of the Touchpoints training program. In a number of studies of parent-infant interaction, Tronick (2007) describes a natural process of connection, disconnection, and repair. Based on the microanalysis of parent-infant interactions via the still-face laboratory procedure, among others, Tronick suggests that the development of relationships is also marked by disorganization. However, in the case of these micro-events, which Tronick maintains occur thousands of times over the course of infancy, disconnections are also needed to support development. Disruptions are necessary, whether it is on the macro scale of child-rearing challenges—sleeping, feeding, dependence-independence—or in the intimate, second-by-second interactions between members of a dyad, so that members of the dyad learn how to maintain the relationship over time and to deal with future disruptions.

This focus on the dynamics of what happens between people is a critical element of the Touchpoints approach. The paradigm that defines formal systems of care for young children and families is based on medical, developmental, and educational models that emphasize individual functioning. However, human functioning, the result of both the evolution of the brain and the shaping of culture, is always social (Rogoff 2003). The establishment of pathways in the brain, as well as the corresponding development of the child, is experience dependent and can only be adequately understood in a relational context; "despite neurological maturation, new capacities require an interactive intersubjective environment to be optimally realized" (Tronick 2010, p. 422). Hence, in the Touchpoints view, self-regulation is not a discrete and emergent capacity of the child, but rather is understood in relation to how the family manages issues such as sleep, feeding, and behavior. A temper tantrum is not only a pivotal event in the development of emotional regulation but also a meaning-making opportunity for the child, the parent, and whomever the parent discusses the event with.

Touchpoints as a Cultural Activity

> Evolution has provided us with an arena in which caregiving *can* be learned, but it doesn't say *what* is to be learned.
>
> James McKenna (quoted in Small 1998, p. 230)

A child's development and behavior are not always predictable, given the variations in genetic contributions and early experience, as well as the interaction between them. Parents throughout history and across cultures have required others to help them understand how to raise children. The variations in children and the challenges presented in caregiving require culture as a means to make choices about how to manage development (Bruner 1990; Weisner 1996). As Small (1998) has demonstrated, child-rearing prescriptions vary a great deal among cultures. Furthermore, in modern American society, the messages about what to do, how to do it, and what is appropriate behavior vary tremendously. Co-sleeping is a good example: Parents throughout the world sleep with babies. Although the American Academy of Pediatrics (Task Force on Sudden Infant Death Syndrome and Moon 2011) warns against the practice, some sleep researchers recommend it (McKenna 1996).

Parents are often ambivalent. And those parents who want to get babies to sleep in their own beds are given advice from totally opposite points of view, from Ferberizing (Ferber 2006) the child to encouraging a family bed (Sears and Sears 2001). Cultural anthropologists maintain that the choice is based on implicit, culturally constructed goals for the child (Morelli et al. 1992). What are parents to do? There is no universal prescription for managing a child's sleep, and no one knows the child like the parent does.

Touchpoints is a cultural activity in that it provides a relational framework for the parent to make these types of choices. Rather than giving a prescription for child-rearing practices, it provides a scaffold for the parent to make decisions given 1) the cultural predispositions that the parent brings; 2) the knowledge of child development the practitioner brings; and, most importantly, 3) the unique behavior of the particular child.

From this perspective, conversations with parents take into account this complex and dynamic process. Indeed, the conversations themselves are seen as part of the dynamic process. A parent's representations of a child, and of parenting the child, are critical in the process. In vivo observations and recalled descriptions of the child's behavior, as well as the mutually constructed perspectives of the parent and the professional, become the currency of the intervention. Stern (1995) describes a systems approach in which various approaches to intervention in parent-child relationships use different entry points into the system, with behavioral pediatrics, as represented by Brazelton, using the actual behavior of the child. Stern concludes that no matter what the entry point—child behavior, parental representations, or therapeutic alliance between therapist and parent—the entire system is affected. Fundamental to the Touchpoints approach is the idea that the entry point is the child's behavior (e.g., thumb-sucking, waking at night, or aggressive behavior) but that the goals are systemic—an enhanced parent-child relationship, greater parental competence, and positive cognitive and emotional outcomes for the child. Throughout history and across cultures, parents have had someone with whom to discuss child-rearing challenges.

Touchpoints as Practice

> There the thing was, right in front of me. I could touch it, smell it. It was myself, naked, just as it was, without a lie telling itself to me in its own terms. Oh, I knew it wasn't for the most part giving me anything profound, but it was giving me terms, basic terms with which I could spell out matters as profound as I cared to think of.
>
> William Carlos Williams (1967, p. 357)

The automatic, seemingly intuitive practice of master clinicians includes "terms" through which they understand their work, and themselves in relation to their work. In the mid-1990s a group of researchers and clinicians—T. Berry Brazelton, E. Z. Tronick, Maureen O'Brien, Ann Stadtler, and John Hornstein—created a system of practice based on the developmental Touchpoints outlined by Brazelton. After an unsuccessful attempt to establish a system of practice by simply applying the developmental information, the group simulated actual practice with a family. Contextualized interactions were replicated and then deconstructed in building the approach. An inductive process was utilized in which the Touchpoints developmental material was used with a family and the method, principles, and assumptions—the "terms" of the work—were extracted qualitatively. As described by Benner (1984) in her examination of expert practice, master clinicians invent their own language to describe their work. The development team, by asking Brazelton to reveal the "terms" that W.C. Williams refers to, elaborated this language of practice so that others could apply it. Subsequently, thousands of practitioners have been trained in the method, and evaluation of the application of the approach has yielded positive outcomes for both practitioners and families (Brandt and Murphy 2010).

The Touchpoints principles and assumptions are a language for practice, basic terms through which practitioners can understand their work and themselves (Hornstein et al. 1997). These principles stand somewhere between broad philosophical statements and specific behavioral prescriptions. As tools of the mind, they guide practice as the person who uses them brings them into relationships with families. They act as guidelines for reflection-in-practice (Schon 1990) as well as means with which to prepare for or examine after an encounter. They actively guide professional practice, either individually or through supervision, in the service of a partnership with parents and in support of the parent-child relationship. Hence, they are not prescriptive, but rather they establish a means for joining a parent in consideration of the particular child and the unique culturally and personally driven challenges of parenting.

The fundamental principle upon which the entire approach rests is that of using the behavior of the child as the road to a partnership with the parent. The map of predictable regressions provided by Brazelton (1992), the unique temperament of the child, the dynamics of disorganization in development, and, most directly, the in vivo descriptions of what the child is actually doing provide the currency of the dialogue. Mutual observation of the child in action can yield a heightened sense of partnership between the practitioner and the parent when the attention and interest of both overlap. Skillful and selective description of the child's behavior by the practitioner elicits a process of meaning making that may be exclusively internal to the parent or, as demonstrated in Touchpoints practice, becomes public between the parent and the practitioner. As Stern (1995) describes, this can occur at the straightforward level of observations of the child's behavior, with the conversation focusing primarily on caregiving tasks related to that behavior—the currency of typical health care. Stern also maintains that the conversation may occur at the representational level, bringing into operation elements such as the parent's familial and cultural beliefs, his or her own adaptive childhood experiences, identification with his or her own parents, and "ghosts in the nursery" (Fraiberg et al. 1975). Hence, the Touchpoints principle *use the behavior of the child as your language* implicitly, but intentionally, acknowledges that behavior is an entry into the inner life of the parent (Figure 4–1).

Such opportunity is taken further with the principle *value passion wherever you find it*. As noted in the section "Touchpoints in Development" earlier in this chapter, emotions

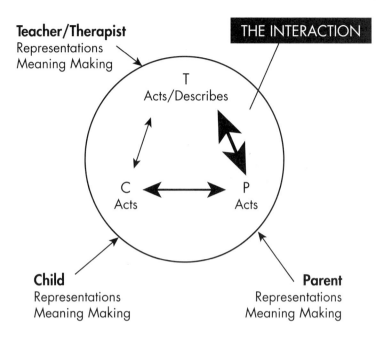

Teacher/Therapist
Representations
Meaning Making

THE INTERACTION

T
Acts/Describes

C
Acts

P
Acts

Child
Representations
Meaning Making

Parent
Representations
Meaning Making

FIGURE 4–1. Entry into child's system of care using Touchpoints.

The entry point into a child's system of care via the Touchpoints approach emphasizes the description of child behavior. Actions of the participants in the interaction are inside the circle; their representations influencing the interaction are on the outside. Parental representations are affected by the description of the teacher/therapist.

Source.   Adapted in part from Stern 1995.

play a fundamental and constructive role in child development; the parallel is acknowledged in adult development. The emotions of parents in considering the child are an essential ingredient in forming a partnership on behalf of the child. The emotions themselves provide deeper access to parental representations of the child, and of their role and corresponding behavior as parents. The anger of a parent who sees unfair treatment of her child by other children or adults, the fear of delays in his own child of a parent whose sibling has a disability, and the joy of a parent whose child surpasses expectations are all emotions that reflect both the commitment to the relationship with the child and the inner life of the parent. The emotions, both positive and negative, are forces that are to be worked with, rather than ignored or denied.

The principle *focus on the parent-child relationship* emphasizes that in addition to focusing attention on the child and attention on the parent, the clinician should focus attention on their relationship. Empirical study of children and families tends to bifurcate the elements of the system. Children are diagnosed and treated, and parents are diagnosed and treated. However, infant mental health, as a field, has changed this paradigm. The unit of analysis is neither the parent nor the child; it is the relationship. The Touchpoints approach adds to this perspective by informing the focus of a variety of practitioners and by articulating a language of observing relationships. The pediatrician not only notes the health of the child but also asks, "How are you doing together?" The child care provider sees the separation of the child from the parent in the morning as a measure of the relationship, not only as challenging behavior. Sleep, toileting, and discipline—indeed, all child-rearing tasks—are seen as nested in the relationship. Particularly, the child's developing capacity for self-regulation is seen as partly resulting from the nature and history of parent-child relationships.

Understanding the dynamics of the professional-parent relationship is also an essential component of the approach. The parallel between parent-child interaction—that is, the process of connection-disconnection-repair—and the knowledge that authentic connection leads to a greater ability to act (Miller and Stiver 1993) informs the professional-parent partnership. As a principle of Touchpoints practice, *supporting parental mastery* runs parallel to the support of self-regulation that the parent gives the child. Relationships throughout the system are seen in relation to the fundamental notion of a dynamic developmental process that occurs within the context of relationships and culture. In supporting parental mastery, the clinician not only praises the parent or the child, but also scaffolds a process in which the parent develops the capacity to manage the challenges a child presents as the child's growth and development bring in further regressions and new challenges. The emotional rejection of a parent by a toddler is foreshadowed by the crawling away of the 9-month-old. Parental mastery in addressing the toddler's behavior is, in part, built on how the earlier crawling away was understood. Professionals can be partners in building this understanding, as well as the associated mastery of parenting challenges.

Every conversation between a parent and a professional, whether it is about where a child sleeps, how to manage a tantrum, or how a child behaves in kindergarten, is based on often divergent, implicit cultural beliefs. Hence, the principle *recognize what you bring to the interaction* is fundamental to the reflective process. The predispositions that a practitioner brings to an interaction with a family not only influence what occurs but also offer reflective opportunities to realize, inform, and perhaps expand those views. Again, as a dynamic system, change in each element of the system affects the others, so the activity of the professional is seen not only as having an impact on the child and family, but also as empowering for the professional (Turnbull et al. 2000).

The developmental process and the corresponding dialogue between a parent and practitioner take place over time. Hence, the predictable periods of disorganization—that is, the Touchpoints described by Brazelton (1992)—offer opportunities to provide anticipatory guidance. By joining the parent in considering how regressions and bursts in development will be managed—for example, anticipating the negativity of a toddler—the practitioner supports parental mastery not by eliminating the disorganization that accompanies the developmental process, but rather by supporting the mastery of the system in managing it— that is, by scaffolding the learning within a self-organizing system.

Referring to Rosenthal and Fode's (1963) research with rats, Brazelton and Greenspan (2000) maintain that current systems of care apply a dumb rat model to work with families. What service providers bring to the interaction is a set of assumptions that the families are unable or unwilling to change or grow. Hence, in addition to the principles stated above, the Touchpoints approach also requires an intentional and positive stance toward parents. The parent assumptions—1) the parent is the expert on the child, 2) all parents have strengths, 3) all parents have something critical to share at each developmental stage, 4) all parents want to do well by their child, 5) all parents have ambivalent feelings, and 6) parenting is a process built on trial and error—help practitioners join the system of care in a manner that helps establish mutuality and depth in the partnership (Brandt et al. 1997). When the expertise and strengths of the parent are fully acknowledged, mutuality in the relationship evolves. When what the parent has to share in the context of a conversation about the authentic challenges he or she faces is heard, then his or her mastery can be supported.

In sum, the Touchpoints principles and assumptions allow practitioners both to apply specific reflective techniques to their work and to establish a particular stance that enables a genuine partnership on behalf of the child. Rather than offering prescriptions or advice, the approach encourages professionals to come alongside parents so that the capacities that exist within the system of care around the child can be utilized along with what the formal system of care has to offer. Service providers throughout the country currently use the Touchpoints approach, both individually and through supervision, as a means to reflect on their practice (www.brazeltontouchpoints.org). The principles and assumptions are the tools with which practitioners apply the developmental understanding of the approach in dynamic interaction with a family. The process, then, involves change not only for the child and parent, but also for the practitioner and the system of care in which the practitioner operates.

Touchpoints and the Support of Practice: Parallel Process

> You need to have an experience with someone first—then you can reproduce it.
>
> Sue Gerhardt (2004, p. 110)

A relational approach with families, according to the Touchpoints approach, is supported by a relational approach within a service delivery system. The essential skills involved in work with families, as represented in the Touchpoints principles and assumptions—the capacity to reflect, to listen, to have empathy, and to understand the nature of the relationship—can also be applied to the supervision of staff and the organization of services (Gilkerson and Ritzler 2005; Moore 2006).

The fundamental neurological and interpersonal model of a relationship, and a developing relationship, is that between parent and infant. The dynamic relationship between the genetic and epigenetic characteristics of the child as actualized in the child's behavior and the caregiving environment is, as described by Tronick (2010), goal directed—for example, feeding, state-regulation, or play—and, in part, dependent on the parent's responsiveness.

Similarly, the interaction between a practitioner and a parent is goal directed—for example, managing caregiving and behavior, or school readiness—and, in part, dependent on the practitioner's relational strategies. The capacity of the practitioner, in turn, to establish such relationships is dependent on the relational capacities of the practitioner, and the quality of that work is similarly both goal directed and supported by relationships among professionals and within the organization.

In particular, reflective practice, as required by the Touchpoints view of development in tandem with the principles and assumptions, supports the intentional use of the approach within an organization. The practitioner is held, both emotionally and intellectually, through the intentional application of the Touchpoints principles and assumptions within the supervisor-supervisee relationship and among members of an organization, and in turn within the larger service delivery system.

An effective learning organization, as described by Senge (1990), is one in which "people continually expand their capacity to create the results they truly desire, where new and expansive patterns of thinking are nurtured" (p. 3). The Touchpoints approach can be seen as a type of "mental model" (Senge 1990) that can guide the delivery and organization of services to families. Indeed, several of the Touchpoints principles have correlates in Senge's five disciplines (systems thinking, personal mastery, mental models, shared vision, team learning). The view of a discontinuous developmental process within the context of relationships is not a formal guide for managing an organization; however, it can provide a shared vision about working with families to guide the growth of an organization.

This dynamic mental model can inform both public awareness and public policy. Brazelton and Greenspan (2000) present an argument for a public policy that supports the nurturance of children as the most fundamental element of a society. Application of the Touchpoints approach represents one part of such a perspective as it guides change at both the interpersonal and organizational level. This approach acknowledges the true complexity of dynamic systems and cultural influences while at the same time providing guidance on how to intervene to support the capacity of these systems (i.e., parent-child, professional-family, service organizations) to support healthy growth and development of members of the system. Furthermore, it is driven by the imperative that the irreducible needs of children receive "the highest international priority, alongside human rights, as a 'right' for all" (Brazelton and Greenspan 2000, p. 182).

KEY POINTS

- Child development is a complex and dynamic process influenced by biological and environmental forces over time and characterized by predictable periods of disorganization.
- Such periods of disorganization in development can lead to a derailment of the parent-child relationship and of the child's overall developmental trajectory.
- Clinicians can use these disruptions in the developmental process to join parents in making meaning of children's behavior.

- The meaning making in clinician-parent interactions is always guided by the implicit cultural beliefs of both the parent and the clinician.
- A privileged entry into the parent's meaning-making process about the child is a description of the child's behavior as a means of communication.

References

Benner P: From Novice to Expert: Excellence and Power in Clinical Nursing Practice. Menlo Park, CA, Addison-Wesley, 1984

Brandt K, Murphy M: Touchpoints in a nurse home visiting program, in Nurturing Children and Families: Building on the Legacy of T Berry Brazelton. Edited by Lester B, Sparrow J. New York, Blackwell Scientific, 2010, pp 177–191

Brazelton TB: Touchpoints: The Essential Reference—Your Child's Emotional and Behavioral Development. Boston, MA, Addison-Wesley, 1992

Brazelton TB, Greenspan S: The Irreducible Needs of Children: What Every Child Must Have to Grow, Learn, and Flourish. Cambridge, MA, Da Capo Press, 2000

Brazelton TB, Nugent K: Neonatal Behavioral Assessment Scale. 3rd Edition. London, Mac Keith Press, 1995

Brazelton TB, O'Brien M, Brandt K: Combining relationships and development: applying Touchpoints to individual and community practices. Infants and Young Children: An Interdisciplinary Journal of Special Care Practices 10:74–84, 1997

Bruner J: Acts of Meaning. Cambridge MA, Harvard University Press, 1990

Campos J, Anderson D, Barbu-Roth M, et al: Travel broadens the mind. Infancy 1:149–220. 2000

Diamond A: Normal development of prefrontal cortex from birth to young adulthood: cognitive functions, anatomy, and biochemistry, in Principles of Frontal Lobe Function. Edited by Stuss D, Knight R. New York, Oxford University Press, 2002, pp 466–503

Eisenberg N, Fabes R, Carlo G, et al: Emotional responsivity to others: behavioral correlates and socialization antecedents, in Emotion and Its Regulation in Early Development. Edited by Eisenberg N, Fabes R. San Francisco, CA, Jossey-Bass, 1992, pp 57–73

Emde R: Early emotional development: new modes of thinking for research and intervention, in New Perspectives in Early Emotional Development. Edited by Warhol J. New York, Johnson & Johnson Pediatric Institute, 1998, pp 29–45

Ferber R: Solve Your Child's Sleep Problems. New York, Touchstone Press, 2006

Fogel A: Systems, cycles, and developmental pathways. Hum Dev 42:213–216, 1999

Fraiberg S, Adelson E, Shapiro V: Ghosts in the nursery: a psychoanalytic approach to the problems of impaired infant-parent relationships. J Am Acad Child Adolesc Psychiatry 14:387–421, 1975

Gerhardt S: Why Love Matters: How Affection Shapes a Baby's Brain. London, Brunner-Routledge, 2004

Gilkerson L, Ritzler TT: The role of reflective process in infusing relationship-based practice into an early intervention system, in The Handbook of Training and Practice in Infant and Preschool Mental Health. Edited by Finello KM. New York, Jossey-Bass, 2005, pp 427–452

Greenspan S: The Growth of the Mind: And the Endangered Origins of Intelligence. Reading, MA, Addison-Wesley, 1997

Hornstein J, O'Brien M, Stadtler A: Touchpoints practice: lessons learned from training and implementation. Zero to Three 17(6):26–33, 1997

Lewis M: The emergence of human emotions, in Handbook of Emotions, 2nd Edition. Edited by Lewis M, Haviland-Jones J. New York, Guilford, 2000, pp 265–280

Malatesta CZ: The role of emotions in the development and organization of personality, in Socio-emotional Development. Edited by Thompson R. Lincoln, University of Nebraska Press, 1988, pp 1–56

McKenna J: Sudden infant death syndrome in cross-cultural perspective: is infant-parent sleeping proactive? Annu Rev Anthropol 25:201–216, 1996

Miller JB, Stiver IP: A relational approach to understanding women's lives and problems. Psychiatr Ann 23:424–431, 1993

Morelli GA, Rogoff B, Oppenheim D, et al: Cultural variation in infants' sleeping arrangements: questions of independence. Dev Psychol 28:604–613, 1992

Moore T: Parallel processes: common features of effective parenting, human services, management and government. Presentation at the Early Childhood Intervention Australia Annual Conference, 2006

Nelson C: How important are the first 3 years of life? Applied Developmental Science 3:235–238, 1999

Piaget J: The Origins of Intelligence in Children. New York, International Universities Press, 1952

Rogoff B: The Cultural Nature of Human Development. New York, Oxford University Press, 2003

Rosenthal R, Fode K: The effect of experimenter bias on the performance of the albino rat. Behavioral Science 8:183–189, 1963

Sander L: Issues in early mother-infant interaction, in Infant Psychiatry: A New Synthesis. Edited by Rexford L, Sander W, Shapiro T. New Haven, CT, Yale University Press, 1976, pp 127–147

Schon D: Educating the Reflective Practitioner: Toward a New Design for Teaching and Learning in the Professions. San Francisco, CA, Jossey-Bass, 1990

Schore A: A neurobiological perspective of the work of Berry Brazelton, in Nurturing Children and Families: Building on the Legacy of T. Berry Brazelton. Edited by Lester B, Sparrow J. New York, Blackwell Scientific, 2010, pp 141–153

Sears W, Sears M: Attachment Parenting Book: A Commonsense Guide to Understanding and Nurturing Your Baby. New York, Little, Brown, 2001

Senge P: The Fifth Discipline: The Art and Practice of the Learning Organization, London, Random House, 1990

Shonkoff J, Phillips D (eds): From Neurons to Neighborhoods. Washington, DC, National Academies Press, 2000

Small M: Our Babies, Ourselves: How Biology and Culture Shape the Way We Parent. New York, Anchor Books, 1998

Stadtler A, Hornstein J: The Touchpoints approach, in The Newborn as a Person: Enabling Healthy Infant Development Worldwide. Edited by Nugent K, Petrauskas B, Brazelton TB. New York, Wiley, 2009, pp 159–170

Stern D: The Interpersonal World of the Human Infant. New York, Basic Books, 1985

Stern D: The Motherhood Constellation: A Unified View of Parent-Infant Psychotherapy. New York, Basic Books, 1995

Super CM, Harkness S: The developmental niche: a conceptualization at the interface of child and culture. Int J Behav Dev 9:545–569, 1986

Task Force on Sudden Infant Death Syndrome, Moon RY: SIDS and other sleep-related infant deaths: expansion of recommendations for a safe infant sleeping environment. Pediatrics 128:1030–1039, 2011

Tronick E: The Neurobehavioral and Social-Emotional Development of Infants and Children. New York, WW Norton, 2007

Tronick E: Infants and mothers: self and mutual regulation and meaning-making, in Nurturing Children and Families, Building on the Legacy of T. Berry Brazelton. Edited by Lester B, Sparrow J. New York, Blackwell Scientific, 2010, pp 83–94

Turnbull A, Turbiville V, Turnbull HR: Evolution of family professional relationships: collective empowerment as the model for the early twenty-first century, in Handbook of Early Childhood Intervention, 2nd Edition. Edited by Shonkoff J, Meisels S. New York, Cambridge University Press, 2000, pp 630–650

Weisner T: Why ethnography should be the most important method in the study of human development, in Ethnography and Human Development: Context and Meaning in Social Inquiry. Edited by Jessor R, Colby A, Shweder R. Chicago, IL, University of Chicago Press, 1996, pp 305–324

Williams WC: The Autobiography of William Carlos Williams. New York, New Directions, 1967

Winnicott D: The Child, the Family, and the Outside World. Harmondsworth, UK, Penguin Books, 1964

CHAPTER 5

The Neurorelational Framework in Infant and Early Childhood Mental Health

Connie Lillas, Ph.D., M.F.T., R.N.

Everyone lives in a very busy world. Infant, child, adolescent, and family practitioners are increasingly pressured with paper trails, the application of evidence-based treatments, and higher productivity levels. Infant and child psychiatrists are typically asked to quickly assess and then prescribe. In this context of whirlwind diagnoses and treatments lie problems all practitioners have inherited due to issues arising from *fragmentation, isolation, hierarchy,* and *specialization.*

The purpose of the Neurorelational Framework (NRF; Lillas and Turnbull 2009) is to provide a conceptual framework that addresses these four common problems. Turning to principles of brain development and functioning for guidance and organization, the NRF uses brain functioning as a template for 1) understanding the meaning of behavior by holding multiple dimensions at the "micro" individual level in mind at the same time, 2) neutralizing disciplinary competition, and 3) providing a common language for team collaboration at the "macro" community level where a part-to-whole perspective underscores all assessment, diagnostic, and intervention processes. Using this template, the NRF offers an integrated core curriculum of cross-sector knowledge that is germane to all pediatric disciplines and supplies a part-to-whole clinical view that helps clinicians find distinctions from as well as intersections with other disciplines within this complex, multidisciplinary workforce.

In the current age of evidence-based treatments, the NRF aligns itself with evidence-based *practice* (as distinct from *treatment*) as a decision-making process that holds the tension between the best available research, the best of clinical expertise, and the family's cultural values (see Chapter 18, "Evidence-Based Treatments and Evidence-Based Practices in the Infant-Parent Mental Health Field," for a thorough exploration of this topic). The NRF is not meant to supplant what practitioners already know; rather, it is intended to enhance and highlight the biopsychosocial components of cases. By following the sequence and structure of the NRF, one gains neurodevelopmental organization of a case that can save time and money and can help allocate resources with more precision. In this sense, the NRF holds potential for being its own evidence-based treatment.

A Brief Overview of the NRF

The two overarching goals in the NRF are to assess the infant's or child's and the parent's *individual neurodevelopmental differences* and to assess the *quality of engagement* between parent and child: 1) individual differences are assessed according to the constructs included within the four brain systems (regulation, sensory, relevance, and executive; described in later sections of this chapter), each of which reflects a set of related brain functions (referred to as "functional capacities") that are associated with various brain regions, and 2) the quality of engagement is assessed using the social-emotional milestones (Chapter 3 in Lillas and Turnbull 2009; see also Greenspan 1985; Greenspan and Wieder 1998; Zero to Three 2005). The baseline evaluation of both the individual and the parent-child dyad is considered in terms of stress and stress recovery patterns. Identifying these patterns provides an initial "hit" as to the degree of health and/or toxicity. *Toxicity* is defined in terms of four allostatic load, or stress, patterns, which are discussed in the next section, "The NRF Assessment Process." A basic assumption of the NRF is that one or more allostatic load patterns underlie medical and mental health diagnoses (McEwen 2002). Once a load pattern is identified, the clinician then evaluates each brain system's functional capacities in terms of the degree of strengths and preferences versus the degree of triggers and concerns to gain a precise overview of which system or systems are contributing to the load pattern(s) and what factors facilitate stress recovery.

The development of the NRF was influenced primarily by four complementary neuroscience theories that reflect the global and dynamic functions of the brain and its intimate connectedness to the body and the environment (Chapter 2 in Lillas and Turnbull 2009). With the emphasis on function, the NRF has identified each of the four brain systems as having certain functional capacities that serve as markers for assessment and intervention decisions.

The NRF Assessment Process
Step 1: Document Baseline Health Benchmarks (Allostasis)

The first step of the NRF assessment process is to document baseline health benchmarks, which are organized around a broad, dynamic construct of health known as *allostasis* (Berntson and Cacioppo 2007; Sterling and Eyer 1988). Allostasis holds the tension between flexibility (*allo*) with stability (*stasis*). The *flexible* side of allostasis, and one of the baseline health benchmarks, is represented by a nervous system's ability to adapt to stress, to shift into a variety of stress responses that are contextually warranted, and to recover from them. An analogy that holds the balance between flexibility and stability, which allostasis represents, is a healthy rubber band. When stressed, the rubber band stretches and can get tight, yet it can always bounce back to its stable state of elasticity. The three normative responses to stress, documented from infant research on states of arousal, are *flooded* (a continuum from agitated to screaming behavior), *hypoalert* (a continuum from dampened/depressed to dissociative behavior), and *hyperalert* (a continuum from anxious to vigilant behavior) (Als 1984, 2002; Barnard 1999; Brazelton 1973, 1984; Sander 1988; Tronick 2007). The *stable* side of allostasis is represented by two predominant states of arousal that characterize self-regulation, one during the sleep cycle and one during the awake cycle. During the *sleep* cycle, stability is shown by cycling into deep sleep, along with adequate sleep cycles—a critical benchmark for baseline health that provides background support to smooth daytime state-of-arousal functions. Deep sleep is restorative; it resets one's thresholds for optimal arousal regulation the next day. During the *awake* cycle, stability is shown via stress recovery back to a stable awake state, with the ability to get into, and stay in, what is referred to as an *alert processing state* (Als 2002). This baseline health benchmark means that when awake, an individual can be calm, alert, present, and engaged with learning and relationships.

The coordination of flexible expressions of all three stress responses (the rubber band gets tight), along with stress recovery (the rubber band bounces back), supported by a stable alert processing state and deep sleep cycling, is one way to operationalize allostasis into parameters that are clinically relevant and observable.

Step 2: Assess for Individual or Dyadic Allostatic Load

When any of the baseline health benchmarks are missing, assessment for individual or dyadic allostatic load, or stress patterns, is indicated. When the *duration* of any of the three primary stress responses is too long, or the *intensity* goes too high, or the *rhythm* is too fast, stress shifts from adaptive to maladaptive parameters—from allostasis to allostatic load. The term *allostatic load* means that there is long-term wear and tear occurring on bodily organs (for elaboration of these associated disease processes, see Lillas and Turnbull 2009, pp. 121–122; see also McEwen 2002). The following are the four *toxic* load patterns:

1. *Over Reactivity to Stress:* Too quick and too frequent stress responses to real or perceived stressors (e.g., poverty, child abuse, caregiver for someone with a chronic illness)
2. *Repeated Reactivity to Stress:* Inability to adjust (habituate) to initial challenges that, over time, should no longer be threatening (e.g., *for child:* transitions to preschool, transitions to divorced parents' home; *for adult:* daily commute, job performance reviews)
3. *Extended Reactivity to Stress:* Prolonged stress response after stressor is removed (e.g., remaining agitated long after an argument, elevated blood pressure hours following a test, staying depressed after losing a game)

4. *Chronic Reactivity:* Chronic stress response, with inadequate stress recovery back to baseline health (e.g., chronic conditions of agitation/hostility, depression, hypervigilance, and/or disrupted sleep cycling)

In summary, *over reactive stress responses* to life experiences that do not adjust, but *repeat* and/ or become *long and drawn out,* result in a condition of *chronic reactivity to stress.*

Step 3: Assess Each Brain System's Functional Capacities

With any toxic stress pattern, the process is to assess each brain system's functional capacities for both sources of resilience and triggers that can then guide treatment implications and recommendations. The case study in the following section illustrates each brain system and its pertinent functional capacities, as well as the assessment of stress, or load, patterns and the corresponding development of treatment interventions. Individualized risk factors associated within each brain system are also described: medical issues are referenced in the regulation system; sensory concerns include developmental delays and disabilities; relevance issues encompass mental health concerns; and motor, attentional, and learning weaknesses are considered in the executive system.

Case Study Illustrating Application of the NRF

Adam's parents came to me when he was 3 years old due to baffling behaviors that had stretched their parenting skills beyond their perceived capacities and had them spinning in professional circles, with no one able to identify what ailed him. In the early phase of assessment, before meeting Adam, I "mapped" him and his parents, using the four brain systems.

It quickly became apparent that Adam was suffering from the first three stress (load) patterns. Adam quickly and frequently went into a flooded state of arousal, manifesting in very loud, high-pitched screaming. Later, when he came to my office, which was in a quiet neighborhood, his intensity and volume were so high that one could hear his screaming nearly a block away.

Adam was not habituating (adjusting) to normal transitions, which is the second load pattern. Even when the transitions were to familiar places, such as to the grocery store or to a therapy office he frequented two or three times a week, Adam could not acclimate. Furthermore, Adam's flooded reactions lasted after the provocative event was over. For example, if a toy train that fell off the track was quickly put back on the track, Adam nonetheless remained in a flooded stress response for 10 minutes or more.

The abruptness and frequency of these screaming episodes would likely tax anyone's nervous system, creating a hypervigilant state in defense against the next spontaneous outbreak. Sadly, James, Adam's father, was doubly stretched due to his own traumatic history of having had a father who would quickly and suddenly go into loud rages. James would react to Adam's sudden flooded state with a startle response that amounted to a flashback of his own father's rages. As a consequence, James was in the fourth load pattern: his sleep cycle was disrupted with disturbing dreams at night, and James was chronically hypervigilant during the day. This made James vulnerable to his chronic reactivity to Adam's screaming (Kaltsas and Chrousos 2007).

Evaluating the Brain Systems

More of this story unfolded as I looked at salient risk factors that pertain to Adam's regulation system, strengths that support the balanced functioning of the regulation system, and any triggers that might be contributing to load conditions.

Regulation System

The *regulation system* influences all developmental domains, providing the basis for all learning and engagement in relationships. *Regulation* refers to the use of energy across the 24-hour sleep-awake cycle, which was introduced as baseline health in Step 1. A *state of arousal* is defined as a cluster of physiological and behavioral signals that regularly occur together (Barnard 1999), with the focus on assessing the flexibility of stress responses (flooded, hypoalert, and hyperalert) in the context of stress recovery (deep sleep and alert processing state).

As described in Table 5–1, both mother and child had a rough start: mother (Eliza) with preeclampsia (gestational maternal high blood pressure), and Adam with a traumatic birth. Adam's nervous system showed signs of vulnerability when his heart rate dropped in response to his umbilical cord being wrapped around his neck. The fact that there was thick meconium (the first stool of the fetus) in Adam's amniotic fluid is evidence of Adam's intense stress over time in utero. Meconium, when inhaled at birth, causes respiratory distress. The degree of distress depends on the amount of inhalation, and Adam had a mild version of respiratory distress.

Although Adam's vulnerability continued to be expressed via frequent respiratory illnesses, his overall development was reported as "normal" until he turned 2. This was another stressful time for this family. His father's work, in construction, became slim to none. Eliza was forced to return to her career in the banking industry, requiring a move. With transitions like these, stress responses in young children are typical. However, Adam's intensity level, frequency, and duration of screaming were not typical, and the behavior continued beyond the 3–6 months that would account for an adjustment disorder. The parents began a rigorous search for answers. As shown in Table 5–1, Adam's strength was his robust sleep cycle. In addition, he was a healthy eater. However, already established through the load patterns, his awake arousal pattern had too little alert processing with inefficient stress recovery. Because of Adam's traumatic birth and the inherent vulnerability in his autonomic nervous system, likely with poor vagal tone (Porges 2001), the other brain systems needed to be assessed for more information. (Table 5–1 is an example of mapping out an individual's risk factors, functional capacities, and subsequent treatment im-

TABLE 5–1. **Regulation system risk factors, functional capacities, and treatment implications**

Child: Adam, male, age 3   Parents: Eliza and James

Regulation system history and risk factors

- Maternal preeclampsia
- Full-term pregnancy with severe fetal distress during labor
- Cord wrapped around neck three times during delivery
- Heavy meconium-stained fluid at birth; Apgar scores of 6 and 8; to the neonatal intensive care unit for 3–4 days with oxygen for mild respiratory distress
- Frequent respiratory illnesses as young child
- When age 2 years, father's work stopped; mother was able to find work out of town; family moved, and father is now primary caretaker
- At age 2 years, Adam began expressing himself through a flooded state of arousal, primarily screaming; this triggered father's traumatic history and dysregulation

Functional capacities	Preferences and strengths	Triggers and concerns
Capacity for deep sleep cycling	• Sleeps well; goes to sleep easily and stays asleep for 12 hours	• Some days he stays awake during afternoon naptime; he is more irritable on these days
Capacity for alert processing	• Limited, but does have periods of stability, especially in very safe environments, such as home	• Very narrow window and vulnerable to staying in this window
Capacity for adaptive use of and efficient recovery from all stress responses		• Primary stress response is flooded, lasting 10–30 minutes
		• Hypervigilance is also dominant; Adam seems very anxious to please others
		• No sign of hypoalert state

Treatment implications

- Due to a vulnerable immune system, protect from too much exposure to other children who are ill at preschool.
- Because Adam is beginning to "lose" his afternoon naptime, be aware that on days he does not sleep, he is more vulnerable to stress.
- Anticipate the need for food and snacks; bring snacks and drink in the car.
- Keep regular sleep routine to support his sleep cycle.
- Begin to anticipate the context for his hypervigilance, providing gentle support for transitions and experiences that cause his stress levels to rise (e.g., fine motor activities such as art, gross motor activities during recess, preschool teacher's somber face and firm tone of voice in dealing with a disruptive classroom).

plications emanating from the regulation system. This can be used as a template for mapping out each brain system.)

Sensory System

The *sensory system* translates various forms of energy into sensory information. Receptor sites in the body (e.g., skin, ears, tongue, eyes) are specialized to pick up specific types of energy (thermal, mechanical, chemical, and electromagnetic). The progression of sensory messages from their elemental features (e.g., perception of motion, contrast, phonemes, volume) to the level where multiple senses cohere as a whole (e.g., a football game, music) is achieved via *sensory processing* capacities, which are the first functional capacity of this brain system. For the sensory system to represent sensory information fully, it must also translate the more dynamic dimensions of the sensory message, such as intensity, rhythm, and volume, across all sensory modalities. This second functional capacity of this brain system is called *sensory modulation*. This is the capacity to balance the flow of sensory signals in a way that is appropriate to the situation: how long or short the duration, how high or low the intensity, and how fast or slow the rhythm of the sensations.

Examination of Adam's sensory system shed light on what triggered many of Adam's toxic load patterns. Although he was a fast sensory processer of visual and auditory information, he was overly reactive to stimuli as well. The NRF emphasizes the relational aspects of sensory information. Muscle output in the form of eye contact, facial expressions, tone of voice, and body posture or gestures (all signals for arousal states) is a source of sensory stimulation for an infant, child, or adult. It became clear that Adam was quickly stressed, becoming hypervigilant or flooded by others whose "output" included fast rhythms, high intensity, and long durations. As a clinician gains information on a child's preferences within each brain system, treatment strategies can be devised. In Adam's case, slowing down all transitions, reworking his schedule so that it was calm and relaxed, and using low-intensity vocal, facial, and gestural rhythms were beginning intervention strategies that matched his sensory preferences. Eliza's calmer, slower rhythm was a natural fit for Adam. This helped James see that if he could become calmer as well, Adam might be able to get better, faster. This possibility became an incentive for James's personal growth.

As described in a later section on the executive system, Adam's fast sensory processing speed was in a serious mismatch with his very slow and poor motor output. These disparities made it difficult to understand him. At first glance, a serious speech delay, sensory modulation difficulties, and poor motor control began to suggest pervasive developmental delays. Adding his intellectual brightness might lead one to conclude that he has high-functioning autism. This was indeed the first assumption as to what was driving Adam's difficulties, and it was revisited many times by many professionals.

The relevance and executive systems are important to understanding the quality of Adam's engagement. Does he avoid eye contact? Can he read others' emotional cues?

Relevance System

The *relevance system* is concerned with what is relevant and meaningful to each individual. What holds personal significance is guided by what strikes a person in a positive or negative manner. The first functional capacity of this brain system is to flexibly experience, express, and modulate a full range of positively *and* negatively experienced, or *appraised,* emotions in ways that are contextually appropriate. Furthermore, memories shape what becomes relevant to an individual. The second functional capacity of the relevance system is to learn from experience by having access to a full range of positive and negative memories that are appropriate to the context. As emotions and memories combine, meanings emerge. Based on the appropriate balance of positively and negatively valenced emotions and memories, the third functional capacity is to create meanings and appraisals that accurately reflect self and others.

Adam's social-emotional milestones and range of emotions were contingent on his state of arousal. When in an alert processing state, Adam was able to make full eye contact, share joy, have a back-and-forth flow of communication, and use his gestures and words to express what he wanted. He could be funny and had a sense of humor. With enough self-regulation in a familiar environment, when it was not overly stimulating, Adam played with his friends, had play dates with them, and, recently, could be found hugging and kissing his friends good-bye. These were all signs that he was not autistic. In fact, Adam's hypervigilance toward reading others' cues and his own intense desire to please others moved him away from autism and shifted him toward an anxiety disorder. Adam's hypervigilance was fueled by feedback from adults in his environment, including his parents, who now quickly labeled his behavior as "bad."

James's own trauma history left him with negative *appraisals* of his own, so it was all too easy for him to transfer those appraisals to a son whom he could not quite understand, and about whom professionals disagreed as to the origins of his difficulties. Working individually with parents whose appraisal systems are too negatively experienced is critical. In private sessions with James, it was decided that the best route toward providing him with the immediate help he needed was to find proper medical support for his chronic sleep and awake regulation instability. A judicious medication regimen began to help James calm down so that he could better care for Adam. At the same time, neither parent was open to medicating Adam at age 3 years, even though the professional team was suggesting it as an option. Given the resources available through the regional center, the school district, and private insurance, Adam was able to have a full-scope team. Other children in poverty are often not as fortunate. A sad reality is that often such children are quickly medicated but are not paired with intervention services.

Executive System

The *executive system* relies on all the other brain systems to provide information in real time. Ultimately, the executive system is about *movement*—whether initiating or inhibiting behavior is the best choice to promote the accomplishment of one's goals in light of the context. For infants and toddlers, the qualities of motor stability, control, and output are the central aspects of the executive system. For young children on up, the first functional capacity is to express spontaneous, automatic, and consciously controlled behaviors in a flexible and purposeful manner; the second functional capacity is to integrate bottom-up influences of emotion with top-down control of thoughts; and the third functional capacity allows the individual to integrate his or her own needs in relation to another's needs according to the context—in essence, to be consciously considerate of others.

Adam's motor system was delayed on multiple levels, including fine motor, gross motor, and speech delays. These delays were huge contributing triggers to Adam's load patterns. A crisis ensued when the school district's psychologist diagnosed Adam with autism and offered a placement in the special education classroom. However, because Adam was already reading and doing math at age 3, placing him with young children with serious intellectual disabilities would have created a serious mismatch. Adam did not fit any of the school district's categories of attention-deficit/hyperactivity disorder, autism, or even socioemotional disturbance. A neuropsychologist and I helped the parents to successfully advocate for Adam to be recognized as a "twice-exceptional child" (i.e., a gifted child with learning disabilities, behavior disorders, and/or communication disorders; Nielsen 1994), allowing Adam to remain at his academic preschool (the most natural environment for him) with the help of an aide for coregulation. With special training, his aide and his teachers now understood Adam's profile and knew how to help him with transitions, guide him through his anxiety during art, and calmly yet firmly redirect him to other activities if the current ones were overly stimulating.

Current Status

As time has passed, Adam has made great gains and is thriving. At age 4 years, he functions academically at first- and second-grade levels. Adam still receives occupational therapy, physical therapy, speech and language therapy, and parent-child dyadic treatments. Due to fiscal constraints, Adam's parent-child sessions alternate with parent and/or individual sessions for James on an every-other-week basis. Adam's top-down gains with his use of words for regulatory modulation ("I'm hungry, Dad"; "I'm tired and want to go to bed") as well as emotional regulation ("I'm scared, I want to leave now") are helping him regulate himself. He no longer has to scream out his words all the time; he can speak in a modulated tone. Visual and verbal prompts avert many an outbreak on the front end. When Adam does scream, he can recover within a few short minutes, albeit still too long for James. Adam is still at risk for respiratory illnesses, and Adam's parents feel very alone in this journey. In all of their circles, from family to professionals to friendships, no one has heard of "twice-exceptional children." Although they sometimes slip, they usually can catch themselves when labeling his behavior as "bad." Adam remains a very anxious child. On a recent field trip to a fire station, even with many executive prompts to prepare, Adam was hypervigilant in anticipation of sudden movement or a loud sound. His hands were sweating as he held his dad's hand; when James picked Adam up to hold him for more support, James could feel Adam's heart pounding and racing. Even though Adam has primarily recovered from his first and third load patterns, he still has trouble adjusting to what others would consider "normal" transitions and experiences (load pattern 2). His parents have a written medication prescription for anxiety ready to go, and they talk about filling it almost every week. (Although medication was considered a last resort for Adam, it might need to be tried first for other families.) With all of his supports in place, will Adam continue to mature developmentally to the degree that he will not need medication? Only time will tell.

The NRF's construct of the four brain systems has been useful in mapping the complex case of Adam and in serving as a template to clarify what services Adam needed, why he needed them, and how his parents could advocate for receiving the services in a much more timely and efficient manner than is often the norm. Following identification of both his strengths and triggers, Adam could be "seen" and begin to thrive, rather than being left to languish. At the same time, his parents could get help for themselves. As James became an advocate for Adam with the school district, he could reflect, with sadness, on how he had not previously understood his son. Learning to understand Adam and to speak up for him was a turning point in James's journey of healing as well. By first mapping the load pattern and then systematically mapping the strengths and triggers of the functional capacities in each brain system, treatment could be organized with clarity.

Conclusion

The case example presented in this chapter illustrates the comprehensiveness of the NRF for assessing the presenting problems of children and their families across multiple domains—regulatory, sensory, emotional, and executive systems—and for identifying multiple interventions across many different disciplines in a cohesive manner. If stress (load) patterns become a common language for assessment across disciplines, are understood as drivers of multiple disease processes, and are addressed via intervention through multiple sources of triggers and resilience, at an early level, public health prevention could occur on a larger scale than is presently practiced. This is both the challenge and the promise of the NRF approach.

KEY POINTS

- The multiple layers of fragmentation across disciplines include breakdowns on a "macro" community level where funding resources are tied to isolated, and often competing, diagnostic categories. The breakdowns on a "micro" individual level are where individual differences across multiple dimensions for both the child and the parent are not integrated into a comprehensive whole.
- The Neurorelational Framework (NRF) is a comprehensive and wholistic approach to assessment, diagnosis, and intervention for any age, from infancy throughout the life cycle.
- Stress response patterns include over reactivity, repeated reactivity, prolonged reactivity, and chronic reactivity from early life stress and, over time, become toxic, supporting long-term wear and tear on the body and brain, often leading to both medical and mental health disorders at later stages of life.

- The three primary steps elucidated in this chapter can be followed by any practitioner from any discipline to assess and therapeutically address stress and toxic stress. Once a stress response becomes part of a toxic stress pattern, four brain systems are used to map out both neurodevelopmental triggers and sources of resilience for each individual.
- The four NRF brain systems—regulation, sensory, relevance, and executive—mirror the complexity of families' presenting problems, as well as the multiplicity of approaches across disciplines, and provide the comprehensive map for providing wholistic assessment and intervention for children and families.

References

Als H: Manual for the Naturalistic Observation of Newborn Behavior (Preterm and Full Term). Boston, MA, Children's Hospital, 1984

Als H: Program Guide—Newborn Individualized Developmental Care and Assessment Program (NIDCAP): An Education and Training Program for Health Care Professionals, Revised Edition. Boston, MA, Children's Medical Center, 2002

Barnard KE: Beginning Rhythms: The Emerging Process of Sleep-Wake Behavior and Self-Regulation. Seattle, Nursing Child Assessment Satellite Training, University of Washington, 1999

Berntson GG, Cacioppo JT: Integrative physiology: homeostasis, allostasis, and the orchestration of systemic physiology, in Handbook of Psychophysiology, 3rd Edition. Edited by Cacioppo JT, Tassinary LG, Berntson GG. New York, Cambridge University Press, 2007, pp 433–452

Brazelton TB: Neonatal Behavioral Assessment Scale (Clinics in Developmental Medicine, No 50). Philadelphia, PA, JB Lippincott, 1973

Brazelton TB: Neonatal Behavioral Assessment Scale, 2nd Edition. Philadelphia, PA, JB Lippincott, 1984

Greenspan SI: First Feelings: Milestones in the Emotional Development of Your Baby and Child. New York, Viking Penguin, 1985

Greenspan SI, Wieder S: The Child With Special Needs: Encouraging Intellectual and Emotional Growth. Reading, MA, Addison-Wesley, 1998

Kaltsas GA, Chrousos GP: The neuroendocrinology of stress, in Handbook of Psychophysiology, 3rd Edition. Edited by Cacioppo JT, Tassinary LG, Berntson GG. New York, Cambridge University Press, 2007, pp 303–318

Lillas C, Turnbull J: Infant/Child Mental Health, Early Intervention, and Relationship-Based Therapies: A Neurorelational Framework for Interdisciplinary Practice. New York, WW Norton, 2009

McEwen B: The End of Stress as We Know It. Washington, DC, Joseph Henry Press, 2002

Nielsen ME: Helping twice-exceptional students to succeed in high school: a program description. Journal of Secondary Gifted Education 5:35–39, 1994

Porges SW: The polyvagal theory: phylogenetic substrates of a social nervous system. Int J Psychophysiol 42:123–146, 2001

Sander LW: The event-structure of regulation in the neonate-caregiver system. Progress in Self Psychology 3:64–77, 1988

Sterling P, Eyer J: Allostasis: a new paradigm to explain arousal pathology, in Handbook of Life Stress, Cognition, and Health. Edited by Fisher S, Reason J. New York, Wiley, 1988, pp 629–649

Tronick E: The Neurobehavioral and Social–Emotional Development of Infants and Children. New York, WW Norton, 2007

Zero to Three: Diagnostic Classification of Mental Health and Developmental Disorders of Infancy and Early Childhood, Revised (DC:0-3R). Washington, DC, Zero to Three, 2005

CHAPTER 6

Attachment Theory

Implications for Young Children and Their Parents

Carol George, Ph.D.

Attachment is an evolutionary-based concept that identifies a specific human social relationship and influences development across the life span (Bowlby 1969/1982). Some professionals are quite satisfied with their knowledge about attachment and see little utility in clarifying or extending it. One study reported that infant mental health practitioners prefer to focus on children's difficult behavior and adaption problems (Hadadian et al. 2005) and fail to understand that attachment insecurity likely contributed to the very problems they are trying to help parents manage.

In this chapter I discuss the concepts that are instrumental in integrating attachment theory successfully in the field of infant mental health, including the biological roots of attachment and its development across the life span, individual differences in patterns of attachment and the ways these patterns are maintained, the main attachment assessment procedures for both children and adults, and an illustration of how child-parent attachment and caregiving assessments can be helpful tools in family evaluation procedures.

Attachment

The term *attachment* is shorthand for a complex set of interrelated behavior and thought patterns directed toward a protective parent figure. Attachment behavior is guided by a biologically based behavioral system that evolved to ensure protection and safety (Bowlby 1969/1982). Attachment organizes human motivational, emotional, cognitive, and memory processes. The attachment relationship begins in infancy and affects development, behavior in other relationships, risk taking, and mental health throughout the life span (Bowlby 1969/1982, 1973, 1980; Cassidy and Shaver 2008). Attachment is characterized by the following constellation of behaviors and processes: 1) proximity seeking; 2) distress when separation is not understandable; 3) happiness at reunion; 4) grief/sadness at loss; 5) secure base behavior—capacity to explore when attachment figure is present (Ainsworth 1989); 6) confidence that the attachment figure has an enduring commitment to the relationship; and 7) capacity for mutual enjoyment or vicarious joy (Bowlby 1969/1982; George and Solomon 2008; Kobak et al. 2004). Children develop preferred attachment relationships with parents and a finite number of other caring adults (e.g., foster parents and day care providers); the quality of these relationships contributes to an integrated self, confidence in self and others, and developmental resilience (George and West 2012; Lyons-Ruth and Jacobvitz 2008; Sroufe et al. 2005).

Attachment behavior is adaptive. Selected by human evolution as a protection strategy, it increases a child's chance for survival. Attachment is guided by a neurologically based system; it has specific biological substrates that influence physiological homeostasis (Bowlby 1973; Cassidy and Shaver 2008). This system, formally termed the *attachment behavioral system,* is activated by stress or threat, which creates the desire for physical or psychological contact or proximity with attachment figures (Bowlby 1969/1982, 1973). Internal cues (illness, fatigue, hunger, pain) and external cues (frightening and stressful events) activate attachment behavior. Some activating events are universal to humans and shared by nonhuman primates (peripheral movement; darkness), whereas others are learned or taught by parents (Bowlby 1973).

Understanding the evolutionary foundation of attachment is especially useful when thinking about young children and their parents. Attachment behaviors signal distress and the need for care and comfort in many situations that are programmed by human biology (being left alone, separation). This programming is so fundamental that young children, and even sometimes adults, have little control over the distress or fear they experience. Attachment behavior in early childhood is a form of communication, not a dependency problem (Bowlby 1973). Attachment needs are based on genuine feelings caused by real experiences; therefore, a perspective that views attachment behavior as irrational or infantile is not useful (Bowlby 1973).

The feelings of closeness and love in attachment relationships are linked to neural and biochemical substrates. These feelings regulate the child's response to parent proximity, soothing, and protection, as well as the parent's attunement to the child's goals for protection (Bowlby 1969/1982; Cassidy and Shaver 2008; George and Solomon 2008). These feelings also foster the intimacy and shared enjoyment that are essential in deepening attachment relationships (Bowlby 1969/1982). Relationships that lack mutual enjoyment, and in which the parent does not share the child's attachment goals and respond to the child's real attachment needs, foster a chronic and intense negative affect. As a result, negative feelings—anger, sadness, depression, anxiety, and fear—compromise emotion regulation, exploration, cognitive competence, and, ultimately, mental health (Bowlby 1973, 1980; Lyons-Ruth and Jacobvitz 2008; see also Cassidy and Shaver 2008).

Developmental Course of Attachment in Childhood

Infants develop unique and qualitatively different attachments with each of their primary caregivers. These relationships emerge gradually over the first 3 years of life. Early preferences for human relationships—the human face and voice, the sweet taste of mother's milk—are hardwired (Bowlby 1969/1982; Fogel 2009). Implicit memory processes facilitate recognition and recall memory for events and people (especially when infants perceive they can control interesting events); by age 5 months, an infant shows a full range of emotion expressions and ties to relationship-guided emotion regulation and communication (Fogel 2009).

Between ages 6 and 9 months, the infant clearly discriminates among different attachment figures, a developmental shift that is marked by clear demonstration of the need to be close, and by separation and stranger anxiety. The infant at this age has "person permanence" (object permanence for people), as well as locomotion and communication competence, and therefore is viewed as truly "attached," even though organized and predictable attachment behavior is not consolidated until around the first birthday (Ainsworth et al. 1978; Marvin and Britner 2008). There is little variation in attachment behavior or conditions that activate the attachment system between ages 1 and 3 years. A 3-year-old may experience more separation anxiety and be more susceptible to attachment distress than an infant (Bowlby 1969/1982; Marvin and Britner 2008).

By age 4 years, attachment is marked by cognitive-affective representational models of relationships. These internal working models produce a shift in attachment behavior and processes; they permit the child to anticipate, appraise, and make plans with parents, rather than simply react to their presence (Bowlby 1969/1982; Marvin and Britner 2008). This shift marks an important transition, the beginning of an attachment-caregiving partnership. The child has some basic understanding of a parent's needs, and his or her own attachment needs are guided by the established trust of parent availability and responsiveness (Bowlby 1969/1982; Marvin and Britner 2008).

Childhood Attachment Patterns

Individual differences in attachment patterns are referred to as "quality of attachment" or "attachment status" (Ainsworth et al. 1978). *Attachment status* captures the full constellation (range and kind) of attachment experiences (Ainsworth et al. 1978). Attachment is typically described in terms of *four* major patterns, three of which are organized and one disorganized. Professionals in the field have developed a number of different child assessments, conceived following the well-validated separation-reunion Strange Situation procedure for infants (Ainsworth et al. 1978). Methods with well-established construct validity are shown in Table 6–1 (see also Solomon and George 2008).

The three patterns of attachment conceived as *organized* are *secure, insecure-avoidant,* and *insecure-ambivalent-resistant* (Ainsworth et al. 1978; Main and Solomon 1990). Children

TABLE 6–1. Examples of child and adult attachment assessments

Age	Measure/procedure	Classification groups	Description
Child-parent behavior			
Infant/toddler (under age 3)	Strange Situation (Ainsworth et al. 1978; Main and Solomon 1990)	• Secure; organized insecure (avoidant, ambivalent-resistant); disorganized	• Videotaped 21-minute separation-reunion sequence in laboratory or office setting. • Requires modest training to administer. • Reliable classification judges available for analysis.
Preschool (ages 3–5 years)	Strange Situation (see Marvin and Britner 2008)	• Secure; organized insecure (avoidant, ambivalent-resistant); disorganized • Parallel parent patterns	• Videotaped 21-minute separation-reunion sequence in laboratory or office setting. • Requires modest training to administer. • Reliable classification judges available for analysis.
Child naturalistic behavior			
Ages 12 months to 5 years	Attachment Q-Sort (Waters and Deane 1985)	• Descriptive statements sorted into a fixed distribution for secure-insecure scored as a continuous variable	• Distilled record of naturalistic behavior in the home and other locations. 2–3 observations of 60 to 90 minutes each. • Trained observer–produced Q-sort is best. • Requires modest training to administer. • Instruction available to do Q-sort analysis.
Adult attachment representation			
Age 13+ years	Adult Attachment Interview (George et al. 1984; see Hesse 2008 for details)	• Adult attachment groups (parallel to child groups) • Secure; organized insecure; unresolved	• 60- to 75-minute recorded interview of childhood experiences. Analyzed from transcript (typically 25–40 pages); 8- to 10-hour transcription time. • Requires training seminar to administer and classify. • Judges available for analysis.

TABLE 6–1. Examples of child and adult attachment assessments *(continued)*

Age	Measure/procedure	Classification groups	Description
Adult attachment representation *(continued)*			
Age 13+ years	Adult Attachment Projective Picture System (George and West 2012)	• Adult attachment groups (parallel to child groups) • Secure; organized insecure; unresolved • Attachment defensive processes	• 20- to 30-minute recorded "interview" responses to standardized attachment situations (picture stimuli). Analyzed from transcript (typically 3–4 pages); 1- to 2-hour transcription time. • Easy to administer. Requires some training. • Requires training seminar to analyze. Judges available for analysis.
Caregiving representation			
Parents (including adolescent parents)	Caregiving Interview (George and Solomon 2008)	• Caregiving groups that parallel child attachment groups • Secure, organized insecure (rejecting, uncertain), dysregulated/helpless • Caregiving defensive processes	• 60-minute recorded interview describing a particular child. Analyzed from transcript (typically 20 pages); 6–8 hour transcription time. • Requires training to administer. • Requires training seminar to analyze. Judges available for analysis.
Parents of children ages 3–12 years	Caregiving Helplessness Questionnaire (George and Solomon 2011)	• Assesses dysregulated caregiving • Not intended to differentiate caregiving groups	• 10-minute, 26-item questionnaire. • Screening tool for disorganized caregiving.

Source. Adapted from George et al. 2011.

with organized attachments signal their need and get close to their parents when distressed, and being together contributes to connectedness and enjoyment.

The *secure* child signals his or her needs promptly and clearly and prefers the parents' care above all others'. The secure child is confident that the parent is accessible, sensitive, and responsive, and that the parent will follow through as promptly and completely as possible. The quality of their interactions when the child is not distressed is punctuated by mutual enjoyment and the parent's vicarious joy in the child's development (George and Solomon 2008). Security fosters competence, cooperation, and the child's desire to explore and achieve mastery. The parents of the secure child view him or her as deserving care and work hard to meet their child's attachment needs as well as their own needs in a developmentally and contextually appropriate manner (George and Solomon 2008). As a result, the secure attachment-caregiving relationship is balanced, mutually satisfying, comfortable, and characterized by emotional sharing and the co-construction of plans and activities—a true working partnership (Bowlby 1969/1982; George and Solomon 2008; Marvin and Britner 2008).

Two patterns of *organized* attachment are considered *insecure*. These develop when parental accessibility and sensitivity are compromised but the child maintains some confidence that the parent can or will provide basic care or protection. The *organized, insecure* child is anxious and uses defensive processes to manage distress (exclusion, transformation of attachment experience, and affect) and to maintain successful physical and psychological proximity to the parent.

Insecure-avoidant attachment is characterized by distance in the relationship, which helps the child diffuse anxiety and anger by maintaining an independent façade (Main 1990; George and Solomon 2008). Deactivation, the goal of which is to cool down negative affect, is the primary form of defense associated with avoidant attachment (Solomon et al. 1995). Deactivation is not always fully effective, however, and distress does leak through (e.g., as strong separation anxiety when the child is separated from the parent). The parent contributes to relationship distance with mild rejection and behavior that shifts the child's attention away from attachment needs. Attachment-caregiving balance is compromised by mutual emphasis away from comfort and intimacy and toward exploration, achievement, and activity.

When attachment is *insecure-ambivalent-resistant,* the child is chronically and overtly anxious, immature, and clingy. The primary form of defense is cognitive disconnection, a regulating maneuver that separates negative affect from its source in an effort to maintain an overall positive, happy state (Solomon et al. 1995). Disconnecting compromises the affective integrative synchrony (Tronick 1989) that is needed for security. As a result, the ambivalent child's attachment signals are often confusing and contradictory. Moods and affective states are intense because of compromised capacity for regulation of affect, especially anger (Ainsworth et al. 1978). The parent contributes to the child's ambivalence by being an inconsistent and contradictory caregiver, as well as being confused, distracted, frustrated, and guilty (George and Solomon 2008). The attachment-caregiving balance is compromised by the parent and child's mutual emphasis on intimacy and having fun despite the fact that the caregiver lacks sensitivity and tends to become overinvolved (thus stifling the child's exploration and autonomy).

Disorganized attachment is conceived as *insecure;* however, the behaviors and underlying processes associated with disorganization are quite different from those associated with avoidant and ambivalent-resistant patterns. This form of attachment is termed disorganized because defensive processes literally break down organized strategies to signal and gain proximity to attachment figures, leaving the child overwhelmed by attachment distress and helpless to seek and find the kind of protection and care needed for even minimal feelings of safety (Solomon and George 2011a). The disorganization terminology stems from observations of infants' reunions with parents following separation (Main and Solomon 1990). The disorganized infant appears disoriented (in a trancelike state), frightened (freezing, apprehensive), conflicted about proximity (head uncomfortably averted), and hostile (aggressive without apparent cause) (Main and Solomon 1990). Typically by age 5 years, disorganized children have developed *controlling* strategies that organize and direct the parent's behavior (Main and Cassidy 1988). Disorganized/controlling relationships are completely out of balance. Children under age 3 act frightened and helpless to get their needs met; children age 3 and older resort to punitive (rude, vindictive) or precociously caregiving (overly solicitous) behavior to get their needs met (George and Solomon 2008).

Disorganized/controlling attachment patterns reflect dysregulation of the attachment system at the behavioral, representational, and biological levels (Solomon and George 2011a). The child's natural desire to seek and maintain proximity to the parent is blocked by parental abdication and failure to provide care and comfort at the very moment the child needs them (George and Solomon 2008). The attachment relationship is characterized by intense conflict (associated with punitive attachment behavior) or merging and child glorification (George and Solomon 2008). The etiology of the disorganized/controlling relationship appears to be a complex interaction of the parent's current experience with past attachment trauma, which contributes to 1) extreme parental psychological or physical withdrawal and "invisibility" (dissociative behavior); 2) unresolved, contradictory, or unpredictable frightening experiences (rage, hostile-intrusive interaction) sometimes associated with certain forms of psychopathology (anxiety disorder, borderline personality disorder, depression), abuse, alcoholism, or parental conflict; 3) helplessness; 4) child empowerment/deference (glorification—the child viewed as more capable of caring for others than the parent); and 5) dissolution of parent-child boundaries (parent merged with child and/or acts like a child, and/or treats child like a spouse) (Lyons-Ruth and Jacobvitz 2008; Solomon and George 2011b). The single underlying thread in this list is the fear generated by feelings of helplessness and isolation in both the parent and the child.

Secure attachment is the most common form of attachment for children around the world (van IJzendoorn and Sagi-Schwartz 2008). Insecure attachment patterns vary culturally, influenced by the degree to which families and cultures emphasize closeness. Avoidant patterns are more predominant in groups that value independence; ambivalent-resistant patterns are more predominant in groups that value closeness and enmeshment. The proportion of dysregulated forms of attachment ranges from 13% to 90%, depending on the presence of family risk factors (maltreatment, chemical dependency, poverty, war/neighborhood terror) (Lyons-Ruth and Jacobvitz 2008).

Attachment security is a buffer factor, whereas insecurity is a risk factor, for social, cognitive, and emotional development—autonomy, confidence, self-esteem, emotion regulation and stress, problem solving, abstract reasoning, mastery, ego resilience, sociability, peer and leadership skills, and the development of conscience (see Cassidy and Shaver 2008). Security with the father contributes to play and exploratory competence (Grossmann et al. 2008). Dysregulated (disorganized/controlling) attachment is associated with developmental risk, including internalizing and externalizing problems; peer aggression; defiance; coercion; poor academic achievement and self-esteem; poor social competence; poor math and deductive reasoning skills; and fantasies of helplessness, destruction, and death (Lyons-Ruth and Jacobvitz 2008). Disorganized attachment in infancy predicts dissociative symptoms and high psychopathology ratings in adolescence (Lyons-Ruth and Jacobvitz 2008).

Continuity and Stability of Attachment

Attachment patterns become increasingly stable and resistant to change during early childhood (infancy through age 5 years) as relationships become internalized through the development of representational skills. Continuity and discontinuity, however, are connected to experiences with parents. Changes in attachment status occur when there are significant changes in parental sensitivity and responsiveness due to life events that can stabilize (infant mental health intervention) or threaten (loss of a parent) attachment security (McConnell and Moss 2011).

Attachment as a Component of Family Evaluations

Infant mental health practitioners, in particular, need precise information about patterns of attachment and caregiving when family dynamics involve abuse and/or when the practitioners' recommendations have legal implications (McIntosh 2011). The following case summarizes an example of a comprehensive attachment evaluation completed as part of a high-conflict divorce custody dispute involving 2-year-old Emily and her siblings (see George et al. 2011 for the complete case description).

Emily, the youngest of three children, had two older brothers, ages 7 and 9. Her father had had affairs regularly before Emily was born. Her parents separated after 9 years of marriage and several years of failed marriage counseling. A year and a half later, they filed for divorce because of irreconcilable differences. Emily's father was by then involved in a new romantic relationship. The children visited back and forth with both parents for several days at a time, with overnights. Parental conflict escalated and led to police involvement.

The custody evaluation was performed because Emily's father wanted full physical custody of the children, alleging that the mother was uncooperative, had mental health problems, and was alienating him from his children. Emily's mother alleged that the father was insensitive and unavailable to his children because of his heavy work schedule. The evaluation was done for Emily because she was the youngest and considered the most vulnerable to the custody decision.

The attachment evaluation included three attachment assessments. The Strange Situation (Ainsworth et al. 1978; Main and Solomon 1990) was conducted with Emily and each parent, with an added cleanup session. These structured observations provided behavioral information about the balance between attachment distress and exploration, as well as insights about behavior management and affect management not readily observable in other settings (at home using the Attachment Q-sort [Ahnert et al. 2006], for example). The Caregiving Interview (George and Solomon 2008) was used to assess caregiving representation. The Adult Attachment Projective Picture System (AAP; George and West 2012) was used to assess each parent's adult attachment representation. These assessments are described in Table 6–1.

The two adult assessments also provide information about defensive processing patterns (indicators of stress and coping potential). The caregiving assessment evaluates each parent's current subjective evaluation of his or her relationship with the child. The adult attachment assessment also detects continuing effects of past childhood attachment trauma on the current relationship and provides information about parents' expectations for adult attachment figures (prediction of future interaction between parents). The results are summarized in Table 6–2.

None of the assessment results indicated obvious developmental risk. Both mother-daughter and father-daughter relationships were organized and generally within normal developmental range. The next step in the evaluation was to examine more closely the individual patterns within each relationship to help understand how interactive patterns of behavior were associated with representational evaluations.

The interaction and representational assessments for Emily and her mother were consistent, although somewhat out of sync. Emily's mother's representational assessments (Caregiving Interview, AAP) demonstrated a clear capacity for security. The strongest features of the mother's caregiving assessment were her capacity for reflection, her dedication to protecting and supporting Emily's developmental competence, and her view of their relationship as mutually enjoyable. (Her mother valued and demonstrated the representational capacity for sensitive caregiving, suggesting that her mother could provide security for Emily and expected attachment figures to do the same for her. The AAP demonstrated similar results. It also demonstrated the mother's use of deactivating defenses to cool down attachment distress, sometimes to the extent of pushing others away [rejecting them]. It was this "push" that was evident at first in the Strange Situation.) In terms of caregiving, parents create distance from their children when they push competence and exploration over intimacy and attachment (George and Solomon 2008). The interactive observation suggested, however, that once Emily's mother warmed up to the situation, defensive deactivation processes no longer guided her parenting behavior. All of the assessments demonstrated the mother's capacity for security and balance.

TABLE 6–2.　**Summary of Emily and her parents' attachment and caregiving assessments**

Mother		Father	
Strange Situation+cleanup			
Emily's attachment	**Caregiving behavior**	**Emily's attachment**	**Caregiving behavior**
Avoidant: Some tension during separation → cool response to mother's return; comfortable engagement in play and delighted with mother's contribution. Cooperative during cleanup.	Avoidant/secure (on border): Competence was a higher priority at first than autonomy and enjoyment → balanced. No problem taking executive role during cleanup, too directive at first → balanced.	Ambivalent-resistant+ dysregulated undercurrent: Dependent, worried, anxious+frozen/constricted. Refused to cooperate during cleanup.	Secure/ambivalent-resistant (on border)+ dysregulated undercurrent: Some balanced support for comfort/play, but became confused, passive+frozen/helpless. Unable to take executive role during cleanup.
Caregiving			
Secure: Thoughtful, balanced, mutually enjoyable relationship with Emily. Committed to Emily's protection and buffering her from distressing situations, especially her own problems with Father and separation distress during visitation. Developmentally and context sensitive.		Confused+dysregulated undercurrent: Enjoys being a father. Overly sentimental; confused, frustrated, and sometimes oblivious to Emily's developmental needs or the contextual demands of a situation. Overwhelmed, helpless, and failed to take action if he believed his response to Emily's need would fuel Mother's incriminations.	
Adult attachment			
Secure: Values attachment figures and relationships. Portrayed self as receiving and providing sensitive care. Thinks carefully when distressed and values problem solving. Deactivates distress and can be rejecting when feels personally threatened.		Preoccupied+dysregulated undercurrent: Portrayed attachment figures as not noticing, not concerned with, or not responding to his attachment needs. Confused about accessibility and presence of attachment figures+frightened, isolated.	

The assessments with Emily's father demonstrated a more worrisome picture. Although he showed some capacity to be engaged and responsive to Emily during the Strange Situation, this observation was not confirmed by Emily's response to him or by the results of adult assessments. Emily and her father shared an ambivalent-resistant attachment, which was consistent with his assessed patterns of confused caregiving and preoccupied adult attachment. The father's prominent defensive strategy was cognitive disconnection, which explained his confusion, passivity, and sentimental attempts to maintain a positive attitude at the expense of taking a realistic look at what was going on. More distressing was a strong undercurrent of relationship dysregulation. Emily's father could become so incapacitated by his own distress that he became frozen and helpless. The Strange Situation demonstrated that Emily could become captured by her father's frozen state. The AAP demonstrated that the father suppressed his own attachment fears, rather than face them; he camouflaged fear with sentimentality, expressing hopes that things would turn out (but without his having a plan or taking action). He seemed incapable of understanding that his own feelings of fear and isolation, rooted in childhood, undermined his relationships with both his daughter and his wife.

Even though attachment and caregiving were within normal range, the imbalances elucidated by these assessments indicated the kind of risk associated with strong parent conflict (McIntosh 2011; Solomon and George 1999). The main recommendations regarding custody and visitation—parent participation in conflict management counseling, joint custody, and limited overnight visits with her father until Emily was older—focused on the ways in which parent conflict could continue to undermine Emily's attachment and create increased developmental risk. Although this evaluation was not part of a more extended infant mental health evaluation, the results were useful in making specific recommendations for intervention and treatment. The Strange Situation assessment did not demonstrate an immediate need for parent-child intervention. Emily's mother appeared to have benefited from two brief periods of psychological counseling in the past (the form of counseling was not documented) and would likely continue to benefit from individual psychotherapy to help manage her feelings of frustration and anger, sense of betrayal by Emily's father, and grief over the divorce. Assessment results indicated that trauma from the father's past had leaked into current relationships and that he would benefit from long-term psychotherapy.

The Value of Attachment Observations and Assessments

Observing the quality and characteristics of attachment can provide a key perspective in understanding the roles of both distress and mutual enjoyment in child-parent relationships. Through the lens of attachment observations, behavior that might otherwise be interpreted as dependence or manipulative is viewed as fundamental to achieving the physical and psychological proximity required to feel safe and foster development. Individual differences in attachment are broadly categorized into child and adult patterns termed secure (flexible), avoidant (dismissing), ambivalent–resistant (preoccupied), and disorganized (unresolved). Attachment status in children and adults is maintained by measurable defensive processes.

Disorganized, unresolved attachment is best understood as dysregulation of the protective function seen in organized attachment relationships; such dysregulation renders the individual frightened and helpless. Although there is a tendency for childhood attachment problems to be carried forward to adult relationships (and parenting), adults have a unique capacity to earn security and develop balanced internal working models of attachment in spite of compromised or abusive childhoods.

Valid attachment assessments used systematically can be tremendously important for making recommendations, especially in the context of trauma or custody, because formal child attachment, parent caregiving, and adult attachment assessments provide a rich picture of the relationship factors that either foster or challenge the young child's development.

KEY POINTS

- Attachment is an evolutionary-based concept that identifies a specific human social relationship that influences development across the life span. According to one study, some infant mental health practitioners may prefer to focus on children's difficult behavior, failing to understand that attachment insecurity likely contributed to the very problems they are trying to help parents manage.
- Attachment behaviors signal distress and the need for care and comfort in many situations that are programmed by human biology. Such behaviors are forms of communication, not a dependency or misbehavior problem.
- The feelings of closeness and love in attachment relationships are linked to neural and biochemical substrates. These feelings coregulate parent and child proximity and synchrony—the child's response to parent proximity, soothing, and protection, as well as the parent's attunement to the child's goals for protection.
- Attachment is typically described in terms of four major patterns, three organized and one disorganized. The three organized patterns of attachment are secure, insecure-avoidant, and insecure-ambivalent-resistant. Disorganized/controlling attachment patterns reflect dysregulation of the attachment-caregiving systems at the behavior, representational, and biological levels.
- Attachment patterns become increasingly stable and resistant to change during early childhood (infancy through age 5) as relationships become internalized through the development of representational skills.
- Infant mental health practitioners need precise information about patterns of attachment and caregiving as a foundation for their work, and this is especially true when family dynamics involve abuse and/or when practitioners' recommendations have legal implications.

References

Ahnert L, Pinquart M, Lamb ME: Security of children's relationships with non-parental care providers: a meta-analysis. Child Dev 74:664–679, 2006

Ainsworth MD: Attachment beyond infancy. Am Psychol 44:709–716, 1989

Ainsworth M, Blehar M, Waters E, et al: Patterns of Attachment: A Psychological Study of the Strange Situation. Hillsdale, NJ, Erlbaum, 1978

Bowlby J: Attachment and Loss, Vol 1: Attachment (1969). New York, Basic Books, 1982

Bowlby J: Attachment and Loss, Vol. 2: Separation. New York, Basic Books, 1973

Bowlby J: Attachment and Loss, Vol. 3: Loss. New York, Basic Books, 1980

Cassidy J, Shaver PR (eds): Handbook of Attachment: Theory, Research, and Clinical Applications, 2nd Edition. New York, Guilford, 2008

Fogel A: Infancy, 5th Edition. Cornwall-on-Hudson, NY, Sloan, 2009

George C, Solomon J: The caregiving system, in Handbook of Attachment: Theory, Research, and Clinical Applications, 2nd Edition. Edited by Cassidy J, Shaver PR. New York, Guilford, 2008, pp 833–856

George C, Solomon J: Caregiving helplessness: the development of a screening measure for disorganized maternal caregiving, in Disorganized Attachment and Caregiving. Edited by Solomon J, George C. New York, Guilford, 2011, pp 133–163

George C, West M: The Adult Attachment Projective Picture System. New York, Guilford, 2012

George C, Kaplan N, Main M: The Adult Attachment Interview (unpublished interview). Berkeley, University of California, Berkeley, 1984

George C, Isaacs M, Marvin RS: Incorporating attachment into custody evaluations. Fam Court Rev 49:483–500, 2011

Grossmann K, Grossmann KE, Kindler H, et al: A wider view of attachment and exploration, in Handbook of Attachment: Theory, Research, and Clinical Applications, 2nd Edition. Edited by Cassidy J, Shaver PR. New York, Guilford, 2008, pp 857–879

Hadadian A, Tomlin AM, Sherwood-Puzzello CM: Early intervention service providers. Early Child Dev Care 175:431–444, 2005

Hesse E: The Adult Attachment Interview, in Handbook of Attachment: Theory, Research, and Clinical Applications, 2nd Edition. Edited by Cassidy J, Shaver PR. New York, Guilford, 2008, pp 552–598

Kobak R, Cassidy J, Ziv Y: Attachment-related trauma and posttraumatic stress disorder, in Adult Attachment: Theory, Research, and Clinical Implications. Edited by Rholes WS, Simpson JA. New York, Guilford, 2004, pp 388–407

Lyons-Ruth K, Jacobvitz D: Attachment disorganization, in Handbook of Attachment: Theory, Research, and Clinical Applications, 2nd Edition. Edited by Cassidy J, Shaver PR. New York, Guilford, 2008, pp 666–697

Main M: Cross-cultural studies of attachment organization. Hum Dev 33:48–61, 1990

Main M, Cassidy J: Categories of response to reunion with the parent at age 6. Dev Psychol 24:1–12, 1988

Main M, Solomon J: Procedures for identifying infants as disorganized/disoriented during the Ainsworth Strange Situation, in Attachment in the Preschool Years: Theory, Research, and Intervention. Edited by Greenberg MT, Cicchetti D, Cummings EM. Chicago, IL, University of Chicago Press, 1990, pp 121–160

Marvin RS, Britner P: Normative development, in Handbook of Attachment: Theory, Research, and Clinical Applications, 2nd Edition. Edited by Cassidy J, Shaver PR. New York, Guilford, 2008, pp 269–294

McConnell M, Moss E: Attachment across the life span. Australian Journal of Educational and Developmental Psychology 11:60–77, 2011

McIntosh J: Attachment theory, separation and divorce: forging coherent understandings for family law. Guest editor's introduction. Fam Court Rev 49:418–425, 2011

Solomon J, George C: The development of attachment in separated and divorced families: effects of overnight visitation, parent and couple variables. Attach Hum Dev 1:2–33, 1999

Solomon J, George C: The measurement of attachment security in infancy and childhood, in Handbook of Attachment: Theory, Research, and Clinical Applications, 2nd Edition. Edited by Cassidy J, Shaver PR. New York, Guilford, 2008, pp 383–416

Solomon J, George C: The disorganized attachment-caregiving system, in Disorganization of Attachment and Caregiving. Edited by Solomon J, George C. New York, Guilford, 2011a, pp 3–24

Solomon J, George C: Dysregulation of maternal caregiving across two generations, in Disorganization of Attachment and Caregiving. Edited by Solomon J, George C. New York, Guilford, 2011b, pp 25–51

Solomon J, George C, De Jong A: Children classified as controlling at age six. Dev Psychopathol 7:447–463, 1995

Sroufe LA, Egeland B, Carlson EA, Collins AW: The Development of the Person. New York, Guilford, 2005

Tronick EZ: Emotions and emotional communication in infants. Am Psychol 44:112–119, 1989

van IJzendoorn MH, Sagi-Schwartz A: Cross-cultural patterns of attachment, in Handbook of Attachment: Theory, Research, and Clinical Applications, 2nd Edition. Edited by Cassidy J, Shaver PR. New York, Guilford, 2008, pp 880–905

Waters E, Deane KE: Defining and assessing individual differences in attachment relationships: Q-methodology and the organization of behavior in infancy and early childhood. Monogr Soc Res Child Dev 50:41–65, 1985

CHAPTER 7

Psychoanalytic and Psychodynamic Theory

Play Therapy for Young Children

Alexandra Murray Harrison, M.D.

My goal in this chapter is to set forth the basic foundation of psychodynamic play therapy for young children. I begin with Freud's psychoanalytic theory and the work of the early child analysts, and progress to the present, when child psychiatrists frequently work as part of a team that includes not only the parents but also other professionals treating children. I include descriptions of a psychodynamic clinical model for evaluating young children and of a theoretical model for integrating a contemporary developmental theory with psychodynamic theory. Finally, throughout the chapter, I use clinical examples to illustrate my points.

Psychoanalysis Theory and Practice: Sigmund Freud

At the turn of the twentieth century, Sigmund Freud developed his model of the unconscious mind and presented it in his essay "The Interpretation of Dreams" (S. Freud 1900/ 1953). In his writings, Freud introduced the idea that the unconscious mind has a powerful influence on the individual's experience and behavior. Freud shocked Viennese society with his paper "Three Essays on the Theory of Sexuality," in which he proposed that young children were sexual beings and had sexual fantasies and desires (S. Freud 1905b/ 1953). In a theory derived from reconstructions of the childhoods of his adult patients, Freud postulated that human behavior was driven by instincts, starting in infancy. At first, the infant's instincts aimed at the gratification of basic needs for nurturance, but later the child's ambitions became grander and focused on the attributes of the parent of the same sex—in the case of the little boy, his father. Freud took the name of this developmental stage from the classical myth of Oedipus. Freud's understanding of the language of unconscious symbolism of young children finds support in the play and speech of young children even today, at least in Western cultures. "Might we not say that every child at play behaves like a creative writer, in that he arranges a world of his own, or, rather, rearranges the things of his world in a new way which pleases him?" (Freud 1908/1959, pp. 133–134). Freud also had remarkable insight into the characteristics of play in childhood: "It is not to be wondered at that these pleasurable effects [during play] encourage children in the pursuit of play and cause them to continue it without regard for the meaning of words or the coherence of sentences" (S. Freud 1905a/1953, p. 157). He described his grandson's game of throwing a spindle out of his crib and pulling it back again ("fort, da") as a reparative attempt of the toddler to manage separation from his mother (S. Freud 1920/1955, pp. 5–7). In 1909, Freud published "Analysis of a Phobia in a Five-Year-Old Boy" (S. Freud 1909/1955), an account of the psychoanalytic treatment of a 5-year-old boy, "Little Hans," treated by his father, who was coached by Freud.

Early Child Analysts

During the early years of psychoanalysis in Vienna, a number of educated women—principal among them Hermine Hug-Hellmuth—began to practice psychoanalysis of children in their homes. Hug-Hellmuth and her colleagues had trained as teachers, which may explain the emphasis on moral education in their psychoanalytic technique. Later, Anna Freud, practicing first in Vienna and then in London, became an important innovator in the theory and technique of psychoanalysis, especially with children. Around her gathered some of the greatest contributors to psychoanalysis, including Erik Erikson and Margaret Mahler, among others. I merely mention Erikson and Mahler here, without attempting to do justice to the contributions of these great early psychoanalytic thinkers (see Erikson 1950, 1977; Mahler 1975).

Anna Freud modified classical analytic technique to accommodate children's developmental capacities, including their inability to free-associate and the vulnerability of their defenses (A. Freud 1965, 1974). One of her most important contributions to the psychoanalytic literature, "The Ego and the Mechanisms of Defense" (A. Freud 1936/1966), is useful for the understanding of adults as well as children. Anna Freud was an astute observer of young children; this was evidenced in her work in the war nurseries she founded in World War II. Under the influence of her father's drive theory, but also informed by her own observations, Anna Freud developed the idea of defenses against inner conflict. She elaborated a theory that emphasized defense interpretation and aimed at freeing the child's spontaneous energies toward progressive development.

The controversy between Melanie Klein and Anna Freud is one of the most colorful stories in psychoanalytic history, of which there are many. Referred to as the "Controversial Discussions," the dispute involved not only Klein and Anna Freud but also their followers, and resulted in a mediation in the British Psycho-Analytical Society from which three groups emerged: the "Freudians," the "Kleinians," and the "Independents." The theoretical differences between Anna Freud and Melanie Klein revolved around Klein's views on maintaining the analytic setting from the beginning, the primacy of aggression as a focus of analytic intervention, the importance of the analysis of negative transference from the outset of the analysis, and the analyzability of young children. In contrast, Anna Freud advised an initial period of "education" to prepare for analysis; this preparatory period included supporting the development of the positive transference for the sake of building the therapeutic alliance. Also, Anna Freud at first did not recommend analyzing children younger than 7 years. Although these discussions were primarily theoretical, the hostility between the two analysts was legendary and was also reflected in the attitude of their followers toward those in the other group. Mrs. Klein moved from Berlin to London before Miss Freud moved with her family from Austria to London, and they both worked in Hampstead, London, only blocks apart: Klein at the Tavistock Clinic and Freud at the Hampstead Clinic. Whereas Freud focused on conflicts and defenses, Klein believed that the meaning of any experience, even at an instinctual level, is represented in unconscious fantasy, comprising all of the anxieties and details of a person's inner world of object relations (Klein 1955; Klein et al. 1952). It was Klein who initially developed the technique of play therapy, in which the analyst responds to a child's activities with toys, just as an adult analyst responds to the free association of an adult. An important follower of Klein, Wilfred Bion, expanded on and further developed Klein's concepts in many areas, including that of projective identification (Bion 1962, 1972), a theory even further developed in child analysis by Ferro (1999).

The next generation of child analysts included Donald Winnicott, who, although following Klein in the thematic content of his interpretations, placed particular value on the process of play. Winnicott pointed out that play requires trust and that playing involves the body (differentiating it from adult and adolescent talk therapy). He noted that play is "essentially satisfying" but also "exciting and precarious" (Winnicott 1971/1977, p. 52). He noted that the play of his patients became more organized in response to his interpretive interventions, and he remarked, "The psychoanalyst has been too busy using play content to look at the playing child, and to write about playing as a thing in itself" (Winnicott 1971/1977, p. 40). Winnicott's theoretical contributions related to play, including an understanding of creativity, transitional objects (immortalized in Linus's blanket), and the "good enough mother" (Winnicott 1960/1982), have continued to influence both adult and child psychoanalysis and psychotherapy (Modell 1976). In addition, his writings include rare examples of the analyst as a collaborator in the child's creative play, such as in the Squiggle Game and The Piggle (Winnicott 1971/1977, pp. 119–137). This participation of the analyst in the child's play was clearly ahead of its time; however, because Winnicott did not formulate a theory about how he played with children, he did not provide a clear indication of how child analysts (and therapists) should think about their role in the play.

Disagreements and New Developments in Psychodynamic Psychotherapy for Children

There have been ongoing disagreements about the technique of play in child treatment. Some therapists have emphasized decoding the content of the play (Fraiberg 1951, 1966), whereas others have felt it better to leave the symbolic content in displacement (Ablon 1996; Yanof and Harrison 2012). A therapist in the first group might say to a child, "When you throw the baby doll away under the couch, it helps us understand how you feel toward your little sister when she gets all your mom's attention." A therapist in the latter group might just remark about the baby doll always getting thrown away, smashed, or eaten by monsters, or even make the voice of the doll complain about these terrible events, without making an explicit connection to the child in the room.

Thinkers outside the field of psychiatry have influenced the theory and technique of dynamic play therapy. Lev Vygotsky, a learning theorist at the time of the Bolshevik Revolution, emphasized the relationship between a child and an adult partner in the learning process (Vygotsky 1978). His concept of the "zone of proximal development" guides the child therapist to stay close to the child's agenda in the play, using adult capacities to help the child achieve his or her goal (Vygotsky 1967).

The reciprocity between the child's competence in pretend play and features of mature psychosocial development, such as intersubjectivity, empathy, and autonomy, has become a recent topic of interest and research (Fonagy et al. 2002; Greenspan 1995; Greenspan and Shaker 2006; Slade and Wolf 1994). In line with Winnicott's admonition that if the child is unable to play, it is the job of the child therapist to help the child learn how to play, these more recent writers emphasize the crucial developmental achievement of pretend play. This issue is particularly relevant in the case of children with developmental disorders such as autistic spectrum disorders, for whom "play" is often stereotypic, repetitive, and without a narrative content. Even children with the capacity to play imaginatively may need the therapist's help to increase the range of the play and help it move forward toward greater complexity. For example, a therapist was playing "bad guys and good guys" with an impulsive little boy on the autistic spectrum when she noted that the story line was limited to the bad guys and good guys fighting each other and the bad guys dying, over and over again, without any narrative. The therapist wondered aloud about the reason for the fight. At first, the child just insisted that the good guys were fighting the bad guys because they were bad. The therapist then wondered what the bad guys did to make them bad. It took more patient "wondering" on her part, as well as hesitancy to proceed with the play, before the boy explained that the bad guys did not have enough food and were stealing food from the good guys, and that was why they were fighting. This led bit by bit to further elaboration of the story of these starving bad guys (now more complex characters and easier to link with the boy's subjective experience in his family), which finally concluded with the bad guys being punished with a time-out on the sun, where they "sizzled" and became good guys. The possibility of a transformation from bad guy to good guy was, of course, hopeful, and led therapist and child on an interesting and productive path.

Dyadic Treatment for Infants and Preschool Children

In the 1970s, Selma Fraiberg, a social worker and psychoanalyst, began to work with mother-infant dyads using a psychoanalytic model. Alicia Lieberman is the most direct follower of Fraiberg in her dyadic treatment model, but others have elaborated models of dyadic work with mothers and infants, although not all with a psychodynamic theoretical base (Fraiberg et al. 1975; Lieberman 2004, 2007; Osofsky 1995). In most dyadic treatment techniques, the therapist chooses remarks that address simultaneously both caregiver and child. To do that, the therapist identifies themes that preoccupy both, such as the threat of loss. For example, when the therapist says, "When Susie thought she broke the toy, she looked worried. Lots of times people are afraid that if they break something, they can never come back to play," she is thinking that both caregiver and child are afraid that destructive aggression could break apart the relationship with the therapist, and—in displacement—their relationship with each other.

Dyadic treatment that uses video recording as a therapeutic tool has special advantages. One is that the subtle patterns of behavioral and affective exchange between child and caregiver are more easily identified in videotape than in any one live session (Downing 2005). Another is that review of the video recording with the caregiver following the session allows the therapist to take a "side-by-side" position with the caregiver, reinforcing an empathic and nonjudgmental connection.

For example, the mother of an adopted boy from Central America had always suffered from a painful lack of self-esteem that she related in part to her distant and critical mother and also to her chronic social anxiety and a tendency to withdraw when hurt or disappointed. Early on in the relationship with her son, whom she adopted when he was a toddler, she began to feel like a failure as a mother. Although discussion of the issue in her own psychotherapy led to intellectual understanding, her feelings did not change. The boy began to have difficulties with impulse control and peer relationships in preschool, and the mother entered treatment with a child psychiatrist, who video recorded the dyadic play sessions.

Examination of the videos revealed a recurring pattern in which the child would make a demand of the mother (e.g., the request for a particular toy or that she "come here"), but immediately after she accommodated him, he would say, "No." Each time, the "no" would be followed by a different rationalization as to why what she had just done was not quite right, drawing attention away from the original rejection, so the basic pattern was disguised and hard to identify in the moment. In response to the boy's rejection, the mother would make a subtle affective and bodily withdrawal, again not easily recognizable without the videotape. The withdrawal, however, was effective in validating the child's sense of himself as having been abandoned and, in the reenactment, not getting what he needed.

When the pattern was identified and examined in an empathic therapeutic environment, the mother was able to recognize the internal experience that motivated her response to the child's rejection. She was also able to appreciate how the pattern was a co-construction of the two of them; mother and son both set up a situation in which the mother would feel like a failure and the boy would feel abandoned. The therapist explained that "getting to know" this unhappy dance between mother and son—both intellectually and also through the vivid visual and affective experience of the video—could alert the mother to its emergence in the early moments and allow her to interrupt it, freeing herself and her child from its destructive effects.

Parent Consultation Model of Child Evaluation

The Parent Consultation Model (PCM), which I developed, derives from clinical experience with young children and from infant research (Downing 2005; Harrison 2005; Tronick 2001, 2005). In the PCM, the child psychiatrist takes the role of a consultant to the parents. The goal of the PCM is to explore the concerns and questions that parents have about their child's behavior and help them find answers as they figure out how best to help their child.

The PCM consists of five steps (Table 7–1). It begins with a telephone call in which the consultant listens to the parent's concerns, explains the model ("Let me tell you how I work, and you can see if it suits you"), and invites the parent to discuss the model with the child's second parent (if there is one) and call the consultant back if they wish to move forward. This is an important step, because it supports the collaborative process between the two parents. If the parent who calls expresses certainty that the other parent will agree, it is important to politely insist that the parents talk it over first and get back to the consultant.

In Step 2, the first of the three face-to-face sessions, the consultant meets with the parents alone to hear their concerns about their child, to get a history of the child and the family, and to generate consultation questions for the psychiatrist as the parents' consultant. During Step 3, the second face-to-face meeting, the consultant meets with the whole family for a play session (or talk session with older children, or a combination of the two) that is designed to gather data to answer the parents' questions. In the play session, the identified patient child plays first with the mother, then with the father, and then they play all together. If there is more than one child in the family, the second child or children play with the alternate parent. These are almost always pleasant meetings, which the consultant directs and in which the consultant does not let anyone feel put on the spot. The consultant video records these family sessions, to gain the maximum benefit from the observational data. The videotape is strictly confidential. During Step 4, the last of the three face-to-face consultation meetings, the consultant analyzes the recording and generates impressions that specifically address the parents' questions.

In Step 5, a final face-to-face meeting, the consultant meets again with the parents alone to review the list of consultation questions from the first meeting and address them one by one, using video clips to illustrate suggestions, recommendations, or points of deeper understanding.

TABLE 7–1.   Parent Consultation Model

Step 1	In telephone call, explain to parent the five steps of consultation and evaluation.
Step 2	Meet with parents alone. Discuss concerns and developmental and family history. Develop and clarify consultation questions.
Step 3	Meet with entire family. Videotape family play session as child plays with one parent, then the other (if two present), then all together. Play with child while parents converse together. In the case of older children, the family talks as well as plays.
Step 4	Analyze videotape and generate impressions that address parents' questions, in preparation for final meeting.
Step 5	Meet with parents only. Answer questions and brainstorm what parents want to do.

The family meeting (Step 3) is designed to obtain data to answer the parents' questions and draws from the Lausanne triadic play model (Fivaz-Depeursinge 1999). The consultant welcomes the family into the office and explains that they will begin by "playing in partners," so that the father and the identified patient-child play together, while the mother and the other child or children play in the same room. If there is only one child, the mother observes. After about 10–15 minutes, the consultant asks the family to "change partners." Although it is not an accurate Strange Situation test (Main and Solomon 1990; see also Chapter 6, "Attachment Theory"), the "mini-reunion" of the child with the mother often results in interesting observations. Next, the consultant asks the family to "all play together." After a period of time, the consultant asks the parents to sit in two chairs in the office and have a conversation with each other while the children continue to play. Finally, the consultant gets down on the floor and plays with the children in a way that contributes to his or her assessment of the patient-child's competence in pretend play and the identification of some central symbolic play themes.

One advantage of using this model is that it is rarely necessary to see the identified problem child alone to answer the parents' questions, and in those cases in which it is important, a subsequent visit can follow naturally from new questions that arise in the third parent meeting (Step 4). This means that the consultant does not immediately begin to make an individual connection with a child who may not become a patient, and the consultant remains focused on parental concerns. Another advantage is that the consultant is free to make important observations of the child in the context in which he or she lives—how the child and family express affect, how they communicate verbally and nonverbally, and how the family manages transitions and sets and maintains boundaries. These observations are in addition to the usual ones a child psychiatrist or analyst makes about the content of the child's speech or symbolic play.

Example 1: Aggressive Behavior

Two-year-old Joseph was brought for consultation because of aggressive behavior in pre-school. On the day of the family meeting, Joseph was pestering his parents and his two older sisters in the waiting room before the family meeting. He greeted the consultant at the door with a friendly smile and showed her his new dinosaur toy. When the meeting started, the consultant made the request for Joseph to play with his father while his sisters played with his mother, but Joseph refused. After a lot of cajoling, he began to play with his father, but he kept straying back to join his mother and sisters. In the meeting, Joseph demonstrated himself to be a well-developed boy with good language and motor skills. The symbolic content of his play was about his dinosaur eating all the other figures, and he made fierce munching noises while doing so. After viewing the video, the consultant was most struck by the visual image of the father, with his body stretched out on the floor and his arms reaching out to Joseph, who had gone to join his mother. As this was taking place, the mother was laughing, but doing nothing to redirect Joseph.

The parents' first question had been how to help Joseph stop his aggressive attacks on his sisters and his peers at school. The consultant saw many complex patterns in the family interaction and in Joseph's play, but she restricted herself to one of them as she focused on answering their question. She said that she thought the family had many positive qualities, and showed them some examples on the tape, but she explained that the parents were having trouble establishing and maintaining clear boundaries. She showed the parents the video of the father reaching out for Joseph, with a pleading look on his face. The father was struck by the image and exclaimed, "It looks as if I am begging him to listen to me!" The parents and the consultant then talked about how the parents could establish clearer and firmer boundaries and how the mother could support the father's position of shared authority in the family.

Example 2: Temper Tantrums

Older parents with a 3-year-old daughter, adopted at age 22 months, consulted the child psychiatrist because of the child's temper tantrums. They asked what caused the tantrums and what to do to stop them. Sophisticated professionals, they knew all the ins and outs of the adoption process and had attended multiple adoption seminars. In the family meeting, the child chose the puppet of a turtle to play with, the father chose a black-and-white dog puppet, and the mother chose a brown puppy puppet. In the play, the two dog puppets kept tapping on the turtle's shell, asking it to "come out and play." The girl anxiously kept poking the turtle's head and legs back into the shell when one or the other popped out. Finally, she had a full-fledged tantrum, screaming and kicking, until her parents carried her out to the car.

When the parents were viewing the video recording with the consultant, the father said, "When I was a boy, we had a dog, and when my family moved, the dog kept running away back to the old neighborhood; we had to give him to a neighbor in that neighborhood, because he could never get used to his new home." The mother looked at her husband in astonishment. "When I was a girl," she said, "we had a dog, and when we moved, my parents thought we couldn't keep the dog in the new home, so we gave him to a neighbor in the old neighborhood, but he kept running away from that family to our new home in the next city and barking at the door to be let in. My parents finally agreed to keep him in our new house." Neither parent had been aware of the other parent's story about the family dog that could not adjust to his new home. Although the parents had become familiar with the multiple reactions common to adoptive parents through their seminars and readings, the visual image of them with their child suddenly confronted them—they had a shared unconscious fear that their little daughter would not "bond" to them and become "adjusted to her new home." The consultant pointed out the turtle's self-protective response to the tapping on her shell, and the parents appreciated the turtle's need for a more graded and respectful approach to making a connection. They understood that it was their insecurity about their bond with their daughter that led them to behave in an intrusive way. The answer to their question was that the child was having tantrums partly in response to their overcontrol and that she needed them to become more respectful of her sensitivity to intrusion.

Example 3: Trouble Hearing Each Other

A grandfather was given temporary custody of his 4-year-old grandson because the boy's parents were unable to take care of him. The little boy had a speech articulation disorder as well as some behavioral problems. The grandfather's question was what to do about the fact that his grandson would "not listen," by which he meant not only "not listen" but also "not comply." The grandfather was hard of hearing. In the play session, as they were making individual LEGO constructions side by side, the grandfather asked the boy, "How do you like my house?" holding his construction up for the boy to see. At first the boy did not answer. The grandfather asked again, "How do you like my house?" The boy mumbled, "Bootiful." The grandfather turned back to his building. In the parent feedback part of the consultation, the grandfather was shown this sequence of video. "What did you hear him say when you asked him if he liked your house?" the consultant asked the grandfather. "Nothing," the grandfather responded. "He said it's 'bootiful,'" the consultant corrected. "Oh," the grandfather responded, "I have a hearing problem." The consultant continued, "You know, you were asking him an important question. I think you were asking him how he liked your home, living with you." The grandfather became tearful and answered, "I think that is right. I am insecure about whether he likes living with me." The answer to the grandfather's questions were that the two of them loved each other but one had a hard time speaking and the other a hard time hearing; together they had a hard time talking to each other. The grandfather was offered psychotherapy for his grandson and ongoing parent consultation for himself, both of which he accepted.

Sandwich Model of Therapeutic Action

The Sandwich Model of Therapeutic Action (SMTA) derives from my clinical experience and my study of infant research, and it aims to supplement my psychodynamic model with developmental theory in clinically useful ways (Tronick 2009) (Figure 7–1). The developmental model that I have chosen to integrate with psychodynamic theory is Tronick's Dyadic Expansion of Consciousness Model (Tronick 2009). This model is particularly effective for this purpose because it emphasizes the multiple simultaneous meaning-making processes that constitute developmental growth. I am proposing that we include a symbolic psychodynamic way of making meaning as one of these many ways. The SMTA deals with different temporal levels and conceptualizes therapeutic activity as simultaneously taking place in these different levels, much like taking a bite of a sandwich with two slices of bread and filling (meat or veggies). The top slice of bread represents the broader temporal perspective that explains that all open systems behave according to certain general principles governing change in nonlinear systems. The filling is the level of psychodynamic theory that deals with time over minutes, hours, and years, in which meaning is made using language and other symbols, and change is traced along a largely linear path. The bottom slice of bread is the level of the microprocess, of seconds and split-second time intervals shorter than the time required to create language, and where change is governed again by nonlinear rules. This level of therapeutic action requires the analysis of videotape. The importance of the top level is the least intuitively obvious to the clinician: its importance derives from its emphasis on multiple simultaneous actions that are occurring not only in centuries but in all time frames big and small, because the principles that guide change in these broad sweeps of time are also operative in changes such as traffic and weather and also in very short events. The key hypothesis of the sandwich model is that insight into therapeutic action is enhanced by studying this three-level simultaneous interactive process that includes different time scales and different modes of communication or interaction.

The benefit of the SMTA is that it allows the clinician to formulate a case and follow the progress of the case using his or her favorite psychodynamic theory, while also feeling confident in judging whether the case is moving forward according to the principle of growth in nonlinear systems—that is, whether it is increasing in complexity and coherence. In addition, the sandwich model allows the child clinician to take into account the microprocess—that is, "the music and the dance" of therapeutic action. Another advantage of this model is that it allows the child psychiatrist to make use of nonsymbolic meanings in domains that are typically the focus of other child clinicians, including pediatricians and pediatric subspecialists, psychotherapists, physical therapists, educators, nurses, occupational therapists, and so on, in a way that fosters collaboration.

For example, 3-year-old Chloe, who had severe temper tantrums, a sleep disorder, and tactile hypersensitivity demonstrated by chronic scratching of the bridge of her nose and a highly restricted wardrobe (i.e., old sweat pants and other worn, loose clothing), was brought to me for a second opinion after she was diagnosed in a major teaching hospital with a mood disorder for which risperidone was recommended. The most troubling symp-

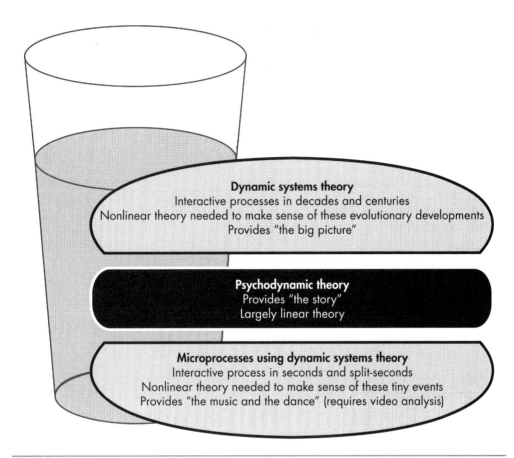

FIGURE 7–1. The Sandwich Model of Therapeutic Action: three temporal levels.

tom was her tantrums, in which she would scream for hours, calling out to her mother, "Mommy, come!" but when her mother appeared, she would cry, "Mommy, go!" This excruciating cycle continued until she and her mother were exhausted.

The medical history included a hospitalization of Chloe 3 days after birth for a urinary tract infection, involving multiple painful medical procedures. During the procedures, her parents were often asked to leave the room and could only listen through the door to their baby screaming while the technicians tried to get a vein. One might imagine that both child and parents were traumatized by this experience. I conducted the evaluation according to the PCM. In the family meeting, Chloe's demands dominated the activity, and the transition out of the playroom was so difficult that Chloe and her parents and younger brother could not leave the building for 20 minutes after the meeting ended. Video illustration to her parents demonstrated positive parenting in protecting the younger sibling and good scaffolding of pretend play, as well as significant mutual overcontrol and expressed helplessness. The answers to the parents' questions focused on Chloe's diagnosis (including that a diagnosis of mood disorder was premature) and the desirability of play therapy that included child and family.

My treatment began with Chloe and her mother in the playroom. The most frequently repeated play theme was that of a sick baby. Chloe would get the doctor kit and ask for her mother's help in examining the baby doll. She would tell her mother that the baby was sick and ask her mother to cry for the baby. She and her mother tried all sorts of things to comfort the baby, but no matter what they did, they could not make the baby better. I thought of Chloe's rocky neonatal period and her mother's inability to protect her from the painful medical procedures. My intervention did not complete this interpretation, but in a slow, repetitive way corresponding to the repetition of the play theme, I would point out how sad it was that no matter what this mommy tried to do, she could not help her baby feel better. This intervention, of course, also addressed the mother, who was present in the room.

During this treatment, I had frequent contact with Chloe's parents through meetings, telephone calls, and e-mail. The aim of our work was to help them break some of the painful patterns of struggle and overcontrol with Chloe so that the family could stop "walking on eggshells" and find more comfortable ways of being together. To do this, I used a combination of practical strategies and helping Chloe's parents "imagine Chloe's mind." In this kind of urgent situation, it is easy to feel the pull to find "silver bullets" to help a desperate family. Sometimes, parents will be seduced by the promise of a quick or certain cure through concrete methods. By contrast, the sustained presence of an empathic therapist who is willing to consider alternative treatments and to work with other professionals but who always keeps *the relationship with the family* at the center point of the treatment is the best approach, in my experience. I have found that there are no "unknown strategies" or "magic fixes" for parenting a child. Instead, the goal is to help the parents feel secure enough that they can reflect on what they are doing that is not working and let go enough to try something new, all in the context of the holding relationship with the therapist.

Because of Chloe's sensory hypersensitivity, throughout her treatment I collaborated with an occupational therapist by telephone, e-mail, and meetings to share our clinical experiences. In addition, I contributed to a school plan designed to make Chloe feel comfortable in the classroom with regulatory breaks and to support her play with her peers. Finally, I prescribed a low dose of sertraline for Chloe due to the exacerbation of her irritability after beginning the school year in a regular classroom. All these interventions were important in Chloe's treatment.

Later, in individual sessions with Chloe, I allowed her to come and go in the office and the playroom so that she would feel in control of the distance between us. In spite of this she would sometimes have tantrums with me and would scream at me to go away. I spoke to Chloe about how awful it must feel when no one could comfort her, when no one made her feel better. In one session, I began to construct a simple block construction on the floor next to the couch under which she was hiding, intending to give her an object on which to focus her aggression. In this way, I was using the symbolism of her behavior in the play to create what I hoped would be a shared symbolic meaning of her polarized internal images of her mother (and of herself) as "nice" when she could comfort her and "mean" when she could not, and how these images related to her anger and panic. I said that when she kicked over my block structure, it reminded me of when she said, "Mommy, go!" only this time she was saying, "Dr. H, go!" I told her that at that moment I must be the "mean Dr. H" to her and that must make her feel so much worse. Slowly, Chloe began to creep out from under the couch and at first angrily, then playfully, knock down the blocks of my building. In the play that followed, Chloe called attention to old and broken toys and told me a story of falling off her bicycle. She also told me with fascination about her daddy's iPhone and mused about the difference between boys and girls. Later, her mother told me that she spent a peaceful evening at home.

I thought that if Chloe could begin to appreciate how her own projected anger frightened her, she and I could start to explore her fearful anger and aggression and their effect on her behavior. I thought that Chloe had been born with a high-arousal temperament. I also had in mind research showing infants' sensitivity to mothers' angry facial expressions and how infants reacted with either withdrawal or distress to this emotional display (Malatesta and Wilson 1988). I thought that the mother's trauma related to Chloe's newborn illness might have interfered with the mother's capacity to tolerate Chloe's distress states, and I imagined that her mother might have responded to Chloe's distress by not being able to "follow" or empathically join her distress (Beebe et al. 2012).

Observations About the Microprocess

In the microprocess of the video, in which second-by-second vocalizations and actions are measured, there are characteristic patterns of Chloe interrupting me and taking repetitive brief turns, both associated with disjointed attention. At one point, Chloe stamps her foot repetitively when declaring that she likes the color pink, apparently emphasizing the meaning of the word *pink,* but the quality of repetitive bursts suggested to me an attempt to regulate a high-arousal state. Interestingly, Chloe does not interrupt me in the middle of my vocal turn. Almost always, she interrupts me just at the end of my vocalization. In some ways, that has a greater subjective disruptive effect on me than if she interrupted me at the beginning or in the middle. That is because in my efforts to join her, I attempt to match my vocal turns to hers; for example, I try to match the duration of her previous vocalization. If she cuts me off just before the end of my turn, I cannot match her previous turn; mine is shorter. Had she cut me off in the middle or the beginning of my turn, I might have implicitly adjusted my expectation and even my behavior to accommodate to a different rhythm instead of expecting a matched duration. Instead, in this pattern in the microprocess, Chloe and I seem to repeat the painful "Mommy, come! Mommy, go!" pattern.

Top Slice of Bread: Dynamic Systems Theory

Chloe's attempts to make meaning of her life experiences in helping relationships have been disrupted by frightening and painful bouts of distress. My intention is to offer her the scaffolding of my regulatory capacities and my analytic competency to identify her intention in the play and help her accomplish it. In that sense, I am the adult working in her zone of proximal development (Vygotsky 1967, 1978). I am hoping that the interaction between Chloe and me will increasingly create new, more flexible and adaptive organizations and, in the process, take apart Chloe's rigid patterns ("mean" and "nice") of making sense of herself in relationships.

Filling (Meat/Veggies): Psychodynamic Theory

Psychodynamic theory helps me make sense of Chloe's fear of aggression in intimate relationships. Her ambivalence toward her mother is revealed in the "transference" responses to me in the playroom. Her sense of herself as defective and bad is revealed in her interest in the old and broken toys and her story of falling off her bicycle, and her fascination with her daddy's equipment indicates a new (one might say "oedipal") interest in her daddy. These behaviors suggest intense conflicts about dependent longings, emerging romantic love, and frightening aggressive wishes in her primary relationships. The "Mommy, come! Mommy, go!" pattern characterizing the exclusive connection she had with her mother at the beginning of the treatment has developed into a more complex set of feelings and fantasies including her daddy as well as her mother.

Bottom Slice of Bread: Microprocesses

The disjointed rhythms of the microprocess, the fragmented attention, and the repetitive bursts of mild aggression Chloe presents me with are dysregulating and confusing to me (Jaffe et al. 2001). My experience is that of being pulled toward her by my straining for a connection, and then being cut off by her interruptions or shifting attention. The effect of her repetitive bursts of vocal and action turns is to commandeer my attention, in that it is difficult to organize my own thoughts in the presence of this kind of insistent unpredictable behavior in my partner. My subjective experience is at times one of fatigue, confusion, and sometimes helplessness, but at other times one of respect and tenderness.

Looking Toward the Future

Professionals in many disciplines care for children with emotional problems. Each discipline includes a repertoire of techniques and rests on a conceptual framework that attempts to explain these techniques. Whereas some disciplines offer unique therapeutic approaches that have proven helpful to many children and families over the years, few have provided empirical evidence to support their efficacy. The behavioral methods, chief among them cognitive-behavioral therapy, claim the greatest validation in research, including randomized controlled studies. However, even the best studies have to contend with problems of single versus multiple diagnoses (few real people actually have a single diagnosis), short durations of follow-up, and an enormous problem of confounding of variables. In addition to the problems attending the evaluation of efficacy in these studies, there is the problem of "rebranding," in which a "new" method is proclaimed when various concepts and techniques are drawn from previously existing methods and grouped together with a new name. Almost always the new method is simpler to articulate and to understand than the old methods from which it has been derived and gives the appearance of greater coherence, though usually at the expense of complexity. Unfortunately, many of these methods claim a unique legitimacy and seek to distinguish themselves from alternative methods rather than looking for common ground.

In my opinion, it is the task of the child psychiatrist to study the available information and do what the proponents of the individual methods rarely do: create syntheses of techniques that have a coherent conceptual base and seem to be helpful to children and their families. This task not only requires continuing efforts to keep up with new knowledge. It also requires the capacity to discriminate and to eschew the temptation of the silver bullet. Examples of such an integrative approach include the use of cognitive-behavioral therapy techniques in a psychodynamic therapy, the introduction of occupational therapy techniques aimed at regulation in a play therapy, and the use of medication in a psychodynamic therapy. Most of these syntheses represent efforts to put together multiple levels of meaning in the therapeutic endeavor—regulatory motor, cognitive, sensory, and symbolic meaning. An integrative approach can include the use of medication to regulate attention or arousal state. It requires putting together the body with the mind and also with the environment—the home and school. In many cases the child psychiatrist will choose to collaborate with other professionals, but in some cases—whether due to scarce resources in terms of time and money, or just because the addition of alternative techniques seems necessary in a dynamic therapy—the child therapist will adopt these techniques himself or herself.

Conclusion

In this chapter, I have attempted to set forth the basic foundation of psychodynamic play therapy for young children, beginning with Freud's psychoanalytic theory and the work of the early child analysts, and up through the present, when child psychiatrists frequently work as part of a team that includes not only the parents but also other professionals treating children. I have introduced two new models—the PCM and the SMTA—that integrate current developmental models and techniques with psychodynamic theory.

The case of Chloe illustrates this integration. At the end of 2 years of (mostly) weekly sessions, her tantrums were better, she had friends, and she had made gains in school. What was the source of this positive outcome? Was it the occupational therapy that eased her bodily experience of the world? Was it the sertraline that helped calm her irritability? Was it her parents' increasing ability to disengage from the patterns of struggle and overcontrol? Was it my work with the dyad in which I helped her mother "imagine Chloe's mind," while at the same time better understand her own? Was it the increasing maturation gained by academic and social learning at school in a supportive atmosphere? Or was it the individual therapy in which Chloe began to make sense of the terrifying threat of being left alone to suffer unbearable pain—even when the current unbearable experience was in her own mind and generated by her own rage? We cannot know the answer to this question, not because the answer is unknown, but because in the growth process, multiple interacting elements work together to make change happen, and we cannot predict which elements, at which time and to which degree, will have an effect. To understand therapeutic change in children, we must use a nonlinear model both to formulate a problem and to plan an intervention. To do that well, we must reach beyond our individual practices to collaborate with colleagues who can offer their experience and knowledge to an integrative approach that enriches what we have to offer our patients.

KEY POINTS

- Sigmund Freud introduced the idea that the unconscious mind has a powerful influence on our behavior and on the meanings we make of our experience. The unconscious reveals itself in symbols—in language and in the play of children.
- All human beings are unique, but as a group they can have corresponding experiences and common developmental outcomes. When research studies involving large populations with similar observable characteristics are brought together with clinical studies involving in-depth knowledge of one person at a time, they can together correct the tendency of either to suggest reductive solutions.
- The Sandwich Model of Therapeutic Action incorporates three different temporal and organizational levels of meaning making, and conceptualizes therapeutic activity as occurring simultaneously in all three levels in a constantly evolving process comparable in many ways to natural development. The model can be summarized as including 1) the broad perspective, including temporal periods of decades and centuries, wherein all open systems behave according to general principles governing change in nonlinear systems (example is evolution); 2) the psychodynamic theory level dealing with minutes, hours, and years, in which change is traced along a largely linear path and meaning is made using language and other symbols; and 3) the level of the microprocess, of seconds and split-second intervals shorter than the time to create language, where change again is governed by nonlinear rules (this level of therapeutic action requires videotape analysis).
- The growth and change process occurs in the context of multiple interacting elements that work together to make change happen. We cannot predict which elements, at which time and to what degree, will have an effect. To understand therapeutic change in children, we must use a nonlinear model both to formulate a problem and to plan an intervention.

References

Ablon SL: The therapeutic action of play. J Am Acad Child Adolesc Psychiatry 35:545–547, 1996
Beebe B, Lachmann F, Markese S, et al: On the origins of disorganized attachment and internal working models: paper I. A dyadic systems approach. Psychoanal Dialogues 22:253–272, 2012

Bion WR: Learning From Experience. London, Heinemann, 1962

Bion WR: Attention and Interpretation. New York, Basic Books, 1972

Downing G: Emotion, body, and parent-infant interaction, in Emotional Development: Recent Research Advances. Edited by Nadel J, Muir D. New York, Oxford University Press, 2005, pp 229–249

Erikson E: Childhood and Society. New York, WW Norton, 1950

Erikson E: Toys and Reasons. New York, WW Norton, 1977

Ferro A: The Bi-Personal Field: Experiences in Child Analysis. London, Routledge, 1999

Fivaz-Depeursinge E: The Primary Triangle: A Developmental Systems View of Mothers, Fathers, and Infants. New York, Basic Books, 1999

Fonagy P, Gergely G, Jurist E, et al: Affect Regulation, Mentalization, and the Development of the Self. New York, Other Press, 2002

Fraiberg S: Clinical notes on the nature of transference in child analysis. Psychoanal Study Child 6:286–306, 1951

Fraiberg S: Further considerations of the role of transference in the child. Psychoanal Study Child 21:213–236, 1966

Fraiberg S, Adelson E, Shapiro V: Ghosts in the nursery: a psychoanalytic approach to the problems of impaired infant-parent relationships. J Am Acad Child Adolesc Psychiatry 14:387–421, 1975

Freud A: The ego and the mechanisms of defense (1936), in The Writings of Anna Freud, Vol 2. New York, International Universities Press, 1966

Freud A: Normality and pathology in childhood, in The Writings of Anna Freud, Vol 6. New York, International Universities Press, 1965, pp 25–63

Freud A: A psychoanalytic view of developmental psychopathology, in The Writings of Anna Freud, Vol 7. New York, International Universities Press, 1974, pp 181–198

Freud S: The interpretation of dreams (1900), in The Standard Edition of the Complete Psychological Works of Sigmund Freud, Vols 4 and 5. Translated and edited by Strachey J. London, Hogarth Press, 1953, pp 1–715

Freud S: Jokes and their relation to the unconscious (1905a), in The Standard Edition of the Complete Psychological Works of Sigmund Freud, Vol 7. Translated and edited by Strachey J. London, Hogarth Press, 1953, pp 135–172

Freud S: Three essays on the theory of sexuality, I: the sexual aberrations (1905b), in The Standard Edition of the Complete Psychological Works of Sigmund Freud, Vol 7. Translated and edited by Strachey J. London, Hogarth Press, 1953, pp 135–172

Freud S: Creative writers and day-dreaming (1908), in The Standard Edition of the Complete Psychological Works of Sigmund Freud, Vol 9. Translated and edited by Strachey J. London, Hogarth Press, 1959, pp 143–153

Freud S: Analysis of a phobia in a five-year-old boy (1909), in Standard Edition of the Complete Psychological Works of Sigmund Freud, Vol 10. Translated and edited by Strachey J. London, Hogarth Press, 1955, pp 1–149

Freud S: Beyond the pleasure principle (1920), in Standard Edition of the Complete Psychological Works of Sigmund Freud, Vol 18. Translated and edited by Strachey J. London, Hogarth Press, 1955, pp 1–64

Greenspan S: The Challenging Child. New York, Addison-Wesley, 1995

Greenspan S, Shaker S: The First Idea. Cambridge, MA, Da Capo Press, 2006

Harrison AM: Herding the animals into the barn: a parent consultation model of child evaluation. Psychoanal Study Child 60:128–157, 2005

Jaffe J, Beebe B, Feldstein S, et al: Rhythms of dialogue in infancy: coordinated timing and infant development. Monogr Soc Res Child Dev 66:i–viii, 1–132, 2001

Klein M: The psychoanalytic play technique. Am J Orthopsychiatry 25:223–237, 1955

Klein M, Heimann P, Isaacs S, et al (eds): Developments in Psycho-Analysis. London, Hogarth Press, 1952

Lieberman A: Child-parent psychotherapy: a relationship based approach to the treatment of mental health disorders in infancy and early childhood, in Treating Parent-Infant Relationship Problems. Edited by Sameroff AJ. New York, Guilford, 2004, pp 97–122

Lieberman A: Still searching for the best interests of the child. Psychoanal Study Child 62:211–238, 2007

Mahler M: The Psychological Birth of the Human Infant. New York, Basic Books, 1975

Main M, Solomon J: Procedures for identifying infants as disorganized/disoriented during the Ainsworth Strange Situation, in Attachment in the Preschool Years: Theory, Research, and Intervention. Edited by Greenberg MT, Cicchetti, Cummings EM. Chicago, IL, University of Chicago Press, 1990, pp. 121–160

Malatesta CZ, Wilson A: Emotion cognition interaction in personality development: a discrete emotions, functionalist analysis. Br J Soc Psychol 27 (Pt 1):91–112, 1988

Modell A: "The holding environment" and the therapeutic action of psychoanalysis. J Am Psychoanal Assoc 24:285–307, 1976

Osofsky J: The effects of the exposure to violence on young children. Am Psychol 50:782–788, 1995

Slade A, Wolf DP: Children at Play. New York, Oxford University Press, 1994

Tronick E: Emotional connections and dyadic consciousness in infant-mother and patient-therapist interactions. Psychoanal Dialogues 11:187–194, 2001

Tronick E: Why is connection with others so important? The formation of dyadic states of consciousness: coherence governed selection and the co-creation of meaning out of messy meaning making, in Emotional Development. Edited by Nadel J, Muir D. New York, Oxford University Press, 2005, pp 293–315

Tronick E: The Neurobehavioral and Social-Emotional Development of Infants and Children. New York, WW Norton, 2009

Vygotsky L: Play and its role in the mental development of the child. Soviet Psychology 5:6–18, 1967

Vygotsky L: Mind in Society: The Development of Higher Psychological Processes. Edited by Cole M, John-Steiner V, Scribner S, et al. Cambridge, MA, Harvard University Press, 1978

Winnicott DW: The parent-infant relationship (1960), in The Maturational Process and the Facilitating Environment, New York, International Universities Press, 1982, pp 140–152

Winnicott DW: The Piggle: An Account of the Psychoanalysis of a Little Girl (1971), Madison, CT, International Universities Press, 1977

Yanof J, Harrison A: Technique in child analysis, in Textbook of Psychoanalysis, 2nd Edition. Edited by Gabbard GO, Litowitz BE, Williams P. Washington, DC, American Psychiatric Publishing, 2012, pp 361–376

CHAPTER 8

Interpersonal Neurobiology, Mindsight, and Integration

The Mind, Relationships, and the Brain

Benjamin W. Nelson, B.A.

Suzanne C. Parker, B.A.

Daniel J. Siegel, M.D.

Interpersonal neurobiology is an interdisciplinary field that uses a consilient approach in finding the common principles that arise through diverse fields in examining development, experience, and, ultimately, what it means to be human. This synthesizing approach provides a perspective from the neuronal and physiological to the relational and societal factors that shape the functioning of the mind. Interpersonal neurobiology is a home to both the objective lens of science and the subjective world of the human mind. One central feature of interpersonal neurobiology is the offering of a definition of the mind. In this chapter, we use the perspective of interpersonal neurobiology to explore the nature of how the mind develops in the setting of attachment relationships between a child and caregiving figures, and how this lens can inform both the parent's and the therapist's approach to cultivating the growth of a healthy and resilient mind.

Mind, Brain, and Relationships

Through an extensive synthesis of a range of sciences, interpersonal neurobiology suggests that an important aspect of the mind is *an embodied and relational process that regulates the flow of energy and information*. In addition to the fundamental properties of consciousness and subjective experience, this regulatory aspect of the mind can be defined as being an emergent property that arises as energy and information flow through the neurophysiological processes of the body and the relational experiences that occur, especially between people.

Individuals are both embodied in their neural systems and embedded in their social networks of interpersonal connections.

The embodied brain, or nervous system embedded within the body as a whole, is a complex system composed of interconnected parts that are integrated in a hierarchical organization. The brain is composed of various levels of complexity, including over 100 billion neurons, each with an average of 10,000 connections to each other; trillions of glia cells that serve a supporting function; and circuits of neurons, regions, and hemispheres that are linked together to create a functional whole system. Furthermore, the brain is dynamic (in a continual state of change), open (influenced by its environment), and nonlinear (small inputs can have large, unpredictable effects on the functioning of the system). Because this system is open and capable of chaotic functioning, it meets the criteria of a complex system. The architectural and functional complexity of the brain is furthered by its direct connections to the body through the central and peripheral nervous systems and the endocrine, vascular, immune, gastrointestinal, and hormonal systems, among others. In this way, the "embodied brain" can be viewed as the mechanism through which energy and information flow within the body. We refer to this embodied mechanism of energy and information flow simply as "the brain," but keep in mind that this term, as we are using it here, refers to the whole system of the body that permits electrochemical energy transformations to occur within a person. Relationships are how energy and information flow and are shared between people. As interpersonal neurobiologists, we see the mind as not simply the output of the brain, but rather as an emergent process that arises as energy and information flow in the complex system that comprises the embodied brain and the relationships between an individual and others. To conceptualize this process, you can picture a triangle of well-being in which energy flows bidirectionally between the mind, relationships, and the brain.

Complex systems have an innate or "emergent" property that arises from the interaction of fundamental elements, which constitute the "self-organization" system. Our suggestion is that the system from which the self-organizing aspect of mind arises is the energy and information flow of the embodied brain and a person's relationships. The self-organizing facet of mind is both within a person and between people.

Interpersonal neurobiology provides a definition of relationships as the sharing of energy and information. This exchange of energy and information across time arises through diverse modalities incorporating verbal communication and nonverbal exchanges, including facial expression, tone of voice, gestures, timing and intensity of response, touch, and posture. In this chapter, we offer a perspective on how the mind emerges both from neural developmental processes and from interpersonal communication patterns. With this definition of one aspect of mind being the embodied and relational self-organizing process that both emerges from and regulates energy and information flow within these internal and interpersonal systems, we can examine the interplay of physiological and interpersonal processes in the unfolding of the developing mind. The ability to sense and ultimately intentionally shape this energy and information flow in both body and relationships is called

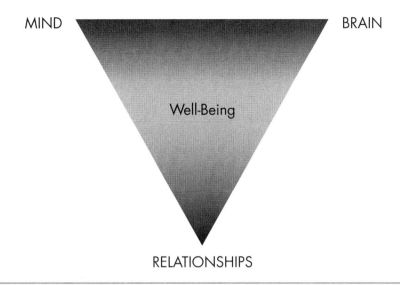

FIGURE 8–1.   The Triangle of Well-Being.
The harmony of integration is revealed as empathic relationships, coherent mind, and integrated brain. Brain is the mechanism of energy and information flow throughout the extended nervous system distributed throughout the entire body; relationships are the sharing of this flow; mind is the embodied and relational process that regulates the flow of energy and information.
Source.   Copyright © 2010 by Mind Your Brain, Inc. Used with permission by Daniel J. Siegel, M.D., from *Mindsight: The New Science of Personal Transformation.*

mindsight. By conceptualizing and understanding the mind in this way, parents and therapists can increase their effectiveness in helping shape the healthy growth of a child's brain.

Interpersonal Neurobiology and Early Development

Interpersonal relationships are crucial to neurodevelopment, providing the stimulus to either facilitate or inhibit the experience-expectant and experience-dependent maturation of brain structure and function. Genetic information inherited through evolution provides for the growth of synaptic connections that "expect" certain experiences to unfold. The brain responds in an experience-dependent way by activating certain neural pathways that then grow with a specific stimulus. Experience stimulates the activation of neurons. This activation can lead, in some circumstances, to the turning on of specific genes that lead to the transcription of DNA into RNA, and the translation of RNA into proteins by the ribosomes. This protein production, stimulated by gene activation in response to neural firing, is how the brain changes in response to experience—a process called *neuroplasticity.* This is the process for learning and development.

Particularly important to the investigation of infant and child mental health are the fields of developmental neurobiology and attachment research, which elucidate how early relationships influence the regulation of the nervous system's development and how communication inherent to this relationship organizes representations, thought patterns, emotional regulation, narratives, and memory development. Studies now demonstrate, too, how early relationships shape the molecular mechanisms that regulate gene expression in a process called *epigenetics* (Roth and Sweatt 2011; see also Chapter 10, "Behavioral Epigenetics and the Developmental Origins of Child Mental Health Disorders"). Experience, therefore, has both direct effects by creating neural activations that impact neuroplastic changes in synaptic connections and indirect effects by impacting the alteration in the regulation of gene expression, with subsequent modifications in synaptic growth. These effects of experience are how relationships shape the neural architecture of the developing brain.

In a general statement that emerges from a long line of reasoning (Siegel 2012a, 2012b), we can state that *relationships that are integrative*—that is, ones that honor differences and promote linkages—*stimulate the activation and growth of integrative fibers in the brain*. It is these integrative fibers, those that link differentiated areas to one another, that can be seen as the fundamental mechanism underlying regulation. Integration enables the coordination and balance of different regions within a system. In other words, the patterns of communication between caregiver and infant are a major source of the experience that shapes brain development in the early years of life. Naturally, genetics plays an important role in shaping a child's temperament. Other factors, such as in utero exposure to toxins, stress, and teratogens, also influence the innate propensities of the child's nervous system at birth. However, experience also plays a crucial role in influencing how neural development unfolds and interacts with these innate neural proclivities. Understanding these early experiential influences on brain development, a study in its infancy itself, is a focus of this chapter.

Our proposal is that the pattern of communication between caregiver and infant provides the primary experiential influence that shapes the unfolding of neural development. Healthy brain development relies on attuned, integrative interpersonal relationships in which differences are honored and compassionate linkages cultivated. One way that a parent promotes the healthy neuronal development of an infant is through the process of attunement, which is fundamental to secure infant-parent attachment; this process is facilitated by the parent's ability to reflect on mental life and to "see" the internal world of the child and of the parent beyond simply observing external behaviors.

Mindsight and Attunement

Attuned communication allows a parent to focus attention on the inner mental experience of a child and then to resonate with that internal state. Attunement incorporates alignment of psychobiological states of the child-parent dyad (Field 1985; Schore 1994) as well as resonance with the other person's state, even when it is very different from one's own. In fact, caregiver attunement to the internal state of the infant as his or her signals are perceived, made sense of, and responded to in a timely and effective manner—what is called "contingent communication"—is thought to be the basis of secure attachment. Such communication "sees" the mental life beneath external behaviors, and attunement involves the process of mindsight in which the mind is "seen" or perceived as a valued and tangible entity. The internal subjective mental world of the child's feelings, thoughts, memories, and states of mind are honored for what they are and linked through attuned communication. In this way, parents who use mindsight to communicate with their child are promoting integration in their relationships.

Integrative communication between infant and caregiver may be facilitated by a so-called resonance circuit that allows members of a dyad to attune to the intentions of the other. This resonance circuit involves mirror neurons in the cortex and other nonmirror neuron areas that create a functional linkage between the superior temporal cortex, insula, and middle prefrontal regions (Siegel 2007). These mirror neurons and the resonance circuits of which they are a part soak in the intentions of another, creating a cascade of neural firing downward through the insula to create shifts in the limbic system, brain stem, and body. Iacoboni and colleagues (Iacoboni 2009; Iacoboni et al. 2007) conducted studies on the mirror neuron system to demonstrate that it connects the occipital, temporal, and parietal cortices (perception of the outer world) to motor areas (mediating behavioral action) in the frontal lobe. This system enables a representation of the intention of another and then creates the response of mimicking behavior (imitation) and simulating the internal state of another (interpersonal resonance).

The process of resonance occurs when changes in the body are relayed back up through spinal lamina I and the vagus (tenth cranial) nerve upward to the brain stem and limbic regions before terminating in the posterior insula—especially on the right side of the brain—to create a primary representation of the physiological condition of the body (Craig 2004). Carr et al. (2003) suggest that the mirror neuron system is intimately involved with emotional processes mediated through the insula, which serves as a circuit transferring information between the cortex and the lower subcortical regions, including the limbic areas, brain stem, and body proper. The insula can carry information from cortical mirror neurons downward to alter subcortical states, and other parts of the insula can carry subcortical information about somatic, brain stem, and limbic states upward to the prefrontal regions of the cortex. Prefrontal input about the interior subcortical state then directly influences how an individual comes to feel another's feelings and it serves as the gateway to empathic understanding. This flow is ultimately mediated through several resonance circuit components—the insula, the anterior cingulate, and the medial prefrontal cortex—and allows a person to appraise the physiological condition of the body and the subsequent emotional processes as a part of interoception, the perception of the interior.

When one person attunes to another in this way, he or she internally approximates the psychobiological processes occurring in the other person. As Iacoboni (2009) explains, "Neural mirroring solves the 'problem of other minds' (how we can access and understand the minds of others) and makes intersubjectivity possible, thus facilitating social behavior" (p. 653). In this way, the "resonance circuitry" provides the foundation on which to view the attunement between parent and child. One cognitive neuroscience perspective providing a window into the mechanisms that may allow one mind to directly affect the neuronal firing of another brain is offered by Hasson et al. (2012) in a process of "brain-to-brain coupling": "Seeing or hearing the actions, sensations or emotions of an agent trigger [*sic*] cortical representations in the perceiver (so-called vicarious activations). If the agent has a similar brain and body, vicarious activations in the perceiver will approximate those of the agent, and the neural responses will become coupled" (p. 115). Affect regulation is a learned skill that relies on healthy parent attunement to the internal world of the infant (Feldman 2007). This regulation is based on the integration of various regions of the brain—the coordination and balance of the nervous system that permits differentiated regions to be linked to one another. As we stated in the section "Interpersonal Neurobiology and Early Development," integrative relationships—those that honor differences and promote compassionate linkages—can be proposed to stimulate the activation and growth of the integrative regions of the brain. When one uses mindsight to focus attention on the internal state of another, the individual's own state is changed and the person becomes linked to the other in a noncognitive manner. Through this process, a child can "feel felt" by the parent, and a state of "being with" is created, which we propose is at the heart of attachment security. These integrative experiences with the engagement of the resonance circuit between infant and caregiver allow for flexible and adaptive self-regulation to develop within the child because they permit coordination and balance the internal and interpersonal systems of the developing mind. Integration—within and between individuals—is the central mechanism underlying healthy regulation.

Affect Regulation

Affect regulation is the ability to modulate psychobiological states of activation and involves the capacity of the mind to monitor and modify the flow of energy and information both *intra*personally (self-regulation) and *inter*personally (dyadic regulation). Dyadic regulation depends on the attachment figure's capacity to attune and resonate with the child's internal state. Facilitated by the parent's own mindsight abilities, repeated patterns of dyadic states of regulation shape the architecture of the child's developing brain, serving as a fundamental way in which attachment relationships sculpt the development of self-regulatory capacities in infants and children. The earliest dyadic interactions during the first year of life have significant influences; research has shown that mother-infant interaction patterns when the infant is age 4 months correlate with attachment classification at age 12 months (Beebe et al. 2010).

During the first year of life, genetic overproduction of synaptic connections in cortical and subcortical regions occurs, causing the brain to more than double in size (Knickmeyer et al. 2008). The relationship between infant and parent is a dominant "environmental influence" that contributes to the stimulation and strengthening of specific neural networks. Such neuroplastic effects of caregiving are mediated by the activation of epigenetic mechanisms controlling gene expression. Synaptic connections least vital to environmental information may become obsolete, and the ensuing parcellation or pruning of synaptic connections allows organization of brain structure to take place. Schore (2001) posits, "From late pregnancy through the second year the brain is in a critical period of accelerated growth, a process that consumes higher amounts of energy than any other stage in the lifespan, and so it requires sufficient amounts of not only nutrients…but also regulated interpersonal experiences for optimal maturation" (p. 11). In more recent work, Schore (2012) cites Leckman and March (2011), who stated,

> Over the past decade it has also become abundantly clear that in addition to the remarkable cascade of genetic, molecular and cellular events that ultimately lead to the formation of the billions of neurons that inhabit the human neocortex, the in utero and immediate postnatal environments and the dyadic relations between child and caregivers within the first years of life can have direct and enduring effects on the child's brain development and behavior.…[T]he enduring impact of early maternal care and the role of epigenetic modifications of the genome during critical periods in early brain development in health and disease is likely to be one of the most important discoveries in all of science that have major implications for our field. (p. 334)

The emotional communication inherent to the dyadic relationship between infant and parent during this critical period of brain development supports the growth of brain systems involved in affect regulation (Tronick 2005). It is in this way that the parent's mature brain structure and function influence the organization of the infant's brain structure. As Siegel (2012a) explains, "After birth our social experiences will directly shape the intricate connections established within our growing cortical structures. Because the regulation of the subcortical areas appears to depend on the coupling of prefrontal areas to them, it is natural, then, to see how interpersonal interactions shape both the growth of connections and the epigenetic regulation of brain regions responsible for control of these emotional systems" (p. 316). Therefore, the energy and information flow that occurs in attuned psychobiological states between parent and infant allows for the infant's brain organization to unfold during the first few years. At the heart of such attachment experiences is mindsight—that is, the way the parent senses the internal subjective world of the infant and honors that mental sea inside.

Neural Systems Theory and Early Development: Mindsight in Parenting

The development of the neural systems underlying affect regulation may be directly influenced by the caregiver's capacity to make sense of the internal mental state of the child. The general process of representing the mind within perception has various names, including *theory of mind, mind-mindedness, psychological mindedness, reflective function, mentalization,* and *mindsight.* Peter Fonagy and colleagues' empirical work on mentalization and reflective functioning explores the ability of a parent to understand the mental and affective state of the child through reflection (Allen et al. 2008; Fonagy et al. 2007). As discussed in the earlier section "Mindsight and Attunement," the term *mindsight* refers not only to the ability to perceive the mental state of self and of other, but also to the capacity to move those states toward integration. Mindsight involves the sensing of the internal world of another and of the self, and then incorporating the interoceptive and emotional correlates of "feeling felt" through resonating cognitively, emotionally, and physically.

Early experiences with warmth and sensitivity—ones that are integrated and in which differences are honored and compassionate communication is enacted—foster this ability to perceive the inner state of another. At the heart of this process of attunement is the open, receptive state of the parent, or "parental presence." Presence involves being open to another's signals rather than distorting them through the lens of expectation and judgment. In this way, presence is a fundamental part of what is termed "mindful awareness" or simply being mindful (Siegel 2007, 2010b). With presence, relationships are enhanced and even one's own physiological mechanisms are moved toward health (Parker et al., in press). Parental presence facilitates early attunement between caregiver and child and lays the groundwork for the child to develop presence, to be able to reflect with mindsight on his or her own internal world and sense, and to honor the mental lives of others. Later, this mindsight ability allows resonance both with other people and with oneself without the scaffolding a parent initially provides. These interpersonal interactions and subsequent intrapersonal neural structural changes reveal the fundamentally social nature of the brain and indicate how different attachment patterns may influence the development of the mind (Siegel 2012a).

Research on the Adult Attachment Interview (AAI; George et al. 1996) suggests that parents' own capacity to reflect on how their childhoods shaped their development is in fact the best predictor of how a child will become attached to them. In essence, a "coherent narrative" of a parent is how he or she has used mindsight to make sense of his or her life, reflecting on the past, aware of the present, and imagining a desired future. Mindsight permits this "mental time travel" (Tulving 2002) that allows integration of past, present, and future. The ability to be present for the experience of reflecting on the past and being curious, open, and accepting of whatever arises in memory suggests that making sense of one's life requires elements of mindful awareness, and adult security of attachment has been found in a preliminary study to overlap with mindfulness traits (DiNoble 2009). In these ways, parental mindsight abilities would correlate with parental presence, adult security, and a child's secure attachment. Fortunately, mindsight is a teachable skill, one that may be at the heart of how clinicians can support parents in making sense of their lives and being fully present for their own children.

Attachment, Integration, and Mindsight

An understanding of attachment theory is crucial to comprehending the interplay between mindsight—the capacity that enables presence, attunement, and resonance with the state of the infant—and the child's intrapersonal and interpersonal patterns later in life. Because attachment theory is the topic of Chapter 6 of this volume, we present only a brief overview here from the interpersonal neurobiology view of integration and mindsight. Ultimately, attachment is the way a child is seen, feels safe, is soothed, and comes to feel secure. The four attachment patterns distinguished by researchers including Mary Ainsworth, John Bowlby, Mary Main, and Alan Sroufe (see Cassidy and Shaver 2008) are characterized as secure, avoidant, ambivalent, and disorganized. These terms describe the relationship between a child and a particular caregiver and are not used to describe a child. Research across more than three decades (Sroufe et al. 2005) reveals that attachment is based on the patterns of communication between attachment figure and child during early childhood development. By the time an individual reaches adolescence, the set of mental models based on early caregiver interactions is thought to begin to coalesce in yet-to-be-understood ways into a single state of mind with respect to attachment. As the adolescent moves into adulthood, this state of mind can be examined using the AAI and a single category of attachment can be assigned. As mentioned in the previous paragraph, it is this AAI attachment status of the parent that is the best predictor of the child's attachment to that parent.

A secure attachment relationship involves a caregiver who attunes to the internal state of the infant. From an interpersonal neurobiology view, secure attachment results from interpersonal integration, which stimulates the growth of neural integration within the child. The proposal is that the child's integrative prefrontal cortex develops the ability to independently modulate inner states and respond flexibly to a variety of situations given this set of secure attachment experiences. The infant feels seen by the parent; is safe with the parent; is soothed when distressed; and comes to feel secure in exploring the external world as well as a wide range of internal states that will be perceived by the parent, understood, and responded to appropriately (Siegel 2012a). These functions emerge directly from the parent's own mindsight abilities. A convergence occurs between a child's ability to attune to and modulate his or her own internal state and the ability to later discern and respond to the internal state of another. A secure pattern often later results in children who are socially aware and adept at both interpersonal and intrapersonal attunement (Sroufe and Siegel 2011). Being taught mindsight during childhood offers children a skill that supports integrative, mindsight-dependent relationships later in life.

An avoidant attachment pattern involves a parent whose response to the child may be uninvolved or misattuned (Sroufe et al. 2005). In this relationship, parental mindsight is at a minimum and there is a diminished amount of shared emotion about the internal state between parent and child, which may result in a lack of development of circuits that facilitate excitement, joy, and active, shared interest. In many ways, these low-affect states can be seen as diminished neural integration (Siegel 2012a). For a child who has been repeatedly disconnected from the parent's emotional life, this pattern can generalize to a distance from the affective states of others, which may persist later in life. A sense of self may be disconnected as well. People can be seen as sources of behavior rather than as centers of inner subjective mental life. This avoidant pattern can influence the expression of emotion and the awareness of the internal states of both oneself and others unless the neural areas responsible for these functions are nurtured, such as in therapy or other secure attachment relationships that may unfold in the future. Avoidance as a family pattern can be considered a state of minimal application of mindsight within or between family members.

An ambivalent pattern of attachment between parent and child is characterized by an inconsistency in attunement and at times an intrusiveness of the parent's own state into that of the child. The mindsight lens in this situation can be seen as distorted, such that what is seen of the inner mental world is not seen clearly. The child may have his or her emotions responded to, but not in an attuned way in which "feeling felt" is experienced with a sense of authenticity and accuracy. This pattern can lead to a confused sense of self and the child's inability to rely on self for emotional regulation, which is especially detrimental to a sense of security because he or she is likely experiencing large swings in his or her own affect due to the inability to be reliably seen and soothed by the parent. Such challenges to affect regulation can be viewed as emerging from restricted growth of the integrative fibers of the brain. Such "synaptic shadows" of the developmental past persist, and this form of insecurity later in a child's life is coupled with a sense of insecurity in social situations, and the child may become increasingly sensitive to emotional experiences without having fully developed the brain regions responsible for regulating these strong affective responses.

Lastly, a disorganized pattern occurs when parents are a source of fear—directly terrifying the child or exhibiting fear themselves—such that their responses are disorganizing for the child. There is contradictory activation of both the attachment circuit dominant in the limbic region that drives the child toward the parent to be soothed on the one hand, and the survival fight/flight/freeze brain stem–mediated circuit that moves the child away from that same figure on the other hand. This simultaneous activation of two incompatible motivations—to move toward and to move away—makes such disorganizing attachment experiences a "biological paradox." Often, the result is that the child cannot learn to appropriately modulate his or her own states of arousal because he or she does not have a secure model for affect regulation and emotional resolution, but rather has a cause of reactivity. Not only is the integration in such attachment patterns impaired, as in the avoidant and ambivalent patterns, but it is "disintegrated," as revealed in the association of this pattern with clinical forms of dissociation. A frequent outcome of this attachment pattern for the child is fragmentation of a sense of self and a lack of internal stability, sometimes revealing dissolution of the continuity of consciousness, especially under stressful conditions, and the psychiatric findings of dissociation (Dutra et al. 2009). During moments of frightening ruptures in the relationship, mindsight has become terrifyingly absent and the break in interpersonal connection creates a break in the child's continuity of connection to the internal self. Such frightening ruptures characterize the disorganized attachment relationship, and these children have the most significant negative developmental outcomes (Cassidy and Shaver 2008).

Mindsight and Infant Development: The Therapist's Experience

The various attachment patterns are important for the therapist to understand because therapy harnesses the power of neuroplasticity to create change. One goal of clinical intervention with an individual with a history of insecure attachment is to identify the form of attachment relationship pattern that has shaped that individual's developing nervous system. The framework of mindsight and integration can provide one way of understanding the role of clinical intervention. Interpersonal neurobiology suggests that integration is the basis of health. Integrated states move with flexibility and coherence across time, while nonintegrated states are prone to moving away from this "river of harmony" and toward either pole of chaos or rigidity. Secure attachment involves interpersonal integration and the cultivation of the child's own neural integration that permits mindsight to flourish in the child's inner and interpersonal life.

Insecurity (avoidance, ambivalence, and disorganization) involves various forms of impaired integration. Rigidity is found, for example, in the internal and interpersonal life of those with avoidant patterns with emotional numbing and lack of self-awareness. Chaos is present in the lives of those with ambivalent patterns, as noted in their intrusive emotional arousals and tendencies toward anxiety (Sroufe and Siegel 2011). Individuals with disorganized patterns have elements of both chaos and rigidity, with abrupt shifts in internal states (chaos) and emotional numbing (rigidity) experienced during affective dysregulation and dissociation. These variations of chaos and rigidity reveal how the brain is not well integrated as a result of such early impediments to affect regulation and attunement in these patterns of insecure attachment.

Within the experience of a clinician with a patient, whether in psychotherapy, a medical setting, or another context, elements of a person's attachment history may shape how the clinical relationship unfolds over time. Some individuals with avoidant attachment histories may not be readily connected to their own internal states or attuned to those of others, including the clinician. Those individuals exhibiting patterns of ambivalent attachment may be exquisitely sensitive to the clinician's state of mind and at times respond with intense reactions that may either amplify the emotional significance of an interaction or distort its meaning. For those with disorganized attachment histories, the presence of dissociation may be revealed when stressful information leads to a fragmentation of the client's experience and impairments to remembering conversations clearly and recalling information. Developmental studies reveal that children can successfully elicit from their teachers patterns of interaction and treatment similar to how they are treated at home by their parents—even though the teacher has no knowledge of the interactional patterns of treatment between the child and parent at home (Sroufe and Siegel 2011; Sroufe et al. 2005). Knowing this, a clinician can work from a "prepared mind" in using these interpersonal experiences and his or her own clinical internal response to get a sense of how attachment patterns have shaped the individual's mind. Offering the AAI may be useful for adolescents and adults in treatment. In therapy, individuals with insecure attachment histories can change across the life span (Siegel 2010a, 2010b). The therapist serves as a mindsightful stable figure who, although he or she may have been lacking early in life, can now serve as a "neuro-architect" who provides a way to rewire the brain toward integration. Schore (2012) cites Glass (2008): "Recent research in brain imaging, molecular biology, and neurogenetics has shown that psychotherapy changes brain function and structure. Such studies have shown that psychotherapy affects regional cerebral blood flow, neurotransmitter metabolism, gene expression, and persistent modifications in synaptic plasticity" (Glass 2008, p. 1589). The patient can actively grow and develop within the attuned, stable system of therapeutic relationships that allows him or her to "feel felt" and to be understood. The therapist offers mindsight at the heart of the therapeutic relationship such that the clinician's *presence*, *attunement*, and *resonance* create a foundation of *trust* (Table 8–1). This is the PART we play as therapists in the growth toward integration (Siegel 2010a).

Given that the prefrontal cortex remains plastic throughout life (Davidson and Begley 2012), the fundamental element in therapeutic efficacy is that therapist and patient successfully work together to create an integrated form of communication, which we propose is the essential experience that stimulates neuronal activation and growth of integrative regions of the brain. It is these regions that are the underlying mechanism of healthy regulation in the brain that allows the patient to fully develop adaptive self-regulation and engage in mutually rewarding social relationships. It is these prefrontal integrative circuits that enable mindsight to develop as well. The potential for the prefrontal cortex to develop throughout life creates the possibility of neurally shaping the way this region mediates neurophysiological mechanisms involved in various domains that are responsible for social attunement, response flexibility, and emotion regulation (Siegel 2012a). The ability to perceive and make sense of nonverbal signals is also important for the ability to perceive the internal states of others, and developing this integrative prefrontal area holds a great deal of potential for a therapist. We as therapists are not really "shrinks"; we are "integrators."

We are suggesting that clinical intervention harnesses the early developmental pathways in which mindsight-based relationships shaped the regulatory integrative circuits of the brain. Contingent communication early in life—the integrative experience of energy and information exchange with an attachment figure—leads to stimulation and growth of the nervous system that facilitates social resonance and self-regulation early on and then later in life. The absence of reliable, early, integrative communication, and its repair when ruptured temporarily, may be the developmental foundation of insecure attachment. For the one-third of the general population with insecure attachment, a result may be the underdevelopment of the integrative fibers that possibly lead to ingrained maladaptive states of the mind and integration of the nervous system (Siegel 2012a). For these reasons, clinicians in all branches of health care may benefit from knowledge about attachment and the development of self-regulation. Furthermore, the presence that is at the heart of these integrative relationships is something that can be taught to clinicians (Siegel 2010a) in order to provide the mindful awareness and receptivity to connect with the patient's experience as it unfolds in the moment. Such presence and the mindsight it entails enable the clinical relationship itself to become integrative. It is these experiences within psychotherapy that harness the power of the brain to change across the life span. Research has shown that therapists trained in mindfulness have better patient outcomes (Grepmair et al. 2007), and even a patient's visit to a physician for a common cold can be made more effective when the clinician is open and empathic (Rakel et al. 2009). When a physician has empathic presence, the patient's immune system is improved and patients recover from the

---

TABLE 8–1.   The PART therapists play

Presence
Attunement
Resonance, which collectively create a foundation of
Trust

Source.   Siegel 2010a.

---

common cold a day sooner. Mindfulness training for primary care physicians has been associated with decreased burnout and increased empathy (Krasner et al. 2009). Therapeutic presence, like parental presence, and the mindsight it permits should be the core stance clinicians take to support development of the mind, whether in the psychotherapy suite, examination room, home, or other settings where therapeutic contact occurs.

Conclusion

Interpersonal neurobiology provides a conceptual framework, drawn from the synthesis of scientific disciplines, to offer a definition of the mind and of mental health. In addition, the mind is a self-organizing, emergent property that both arises from and regulates energy and information as they flow within the embodied brain and between people in relationships. Helping parents and others to regulate this flow is facilitated by the central concept of mindsight, the ability to perceive energy and information flow within and between the self and others. Mindsight entails the capacity not only to perceive mental life, but also to move that flow of energy and information toward integration—the linkage of differentiated parts of a system—within one's body and in relationships.

Mindsight is a teachable skill wherein one learns a stability of presence so that what is perceived is "seen" with more detail, depth, and clarity. With such increased focus, it becomes possible to move that flow toward integration. Interpersonal neurobiology permits individuals to embrace a range of domains of integration (Siegel 2010b, 2012a) that can become the focus of clinical intervention and parental strategies (Siegel and Bryson 2011). By teaching parents mindsight skills to perceive and honor the mental lives of self and other and to move that life toward integration, clinicians empower parents to teach their children those same skills. Science has demonstrated that how parents make sense of their lives is the best predictor of how their children will become attached to them, and approaching parenting "from the inside out" (Siegel and Hartzell 2003) is a scientifically grounded way of facilitating secure attachment and the interpersonal and internal integration it entails. It is never too late to make sense of one's life, and never too late to develop mindsight skills and move one's life toward integration.

Clinicians and parents who know this approach can make sense of their lives as they cultivate their presence to help the development of others, and of themselves. Presence is the gateway toward integration, and integration made visible is kindness and compassion.

Our challenging work as parents and clinicians—to cultivate the healthy development of children—offers us a way to give a gift that keeps on giving across the generations. Along the way, we can join with each other as we take on the exciting challenge of learning new skills that empower us to help one another and to deepen how we both enjoy and care for our precious relationships with each other, with the planet, and with ourselves.

KEY POINTS

- Interpersonal neurobiology is an interdisciplinary field that uses a consilient approach in examining development, experience, and, ultimately, what it means to be human. The domain of interpersonal neurobiology combines many fields of science into one perspective.

- Three aspects of one human reality are represented in the Triangle of Well-Being (Figure 8–1): 1) mind—a self-organizing, emergent process that is both embodied and relational and that regulates the flow of energy and information; 2) relationships—the sharing of energy and information; and 3) brain—the mechanism through which energy and information flow.

- Early relationships shape the regulatory integrative circuits of the brain. This shaping occurs through neuroplasticity and the epigenetic regulation of gene-environment interactions and gene expression to create a degree of resilience or risk for the developing child.

- Mindsight is a term referring to one's ability to monitor and modify the energy and information flow both within and between oneself and others toward integration. In the therapeutic context, mindsight employs insight and empathy to harness the ability of neuroplasticity to move neural networks toward integration.

- Integration is the linkage of differentiated parts. Integration is proposed to be the foundational mechanism of health. Integrative relationships involve the respecting of differences and the compassionate communication between people. This type of communication stimulates the growth of integrative fibers in the brain. These are the neural circuits that facilitate the coordination and balance of disparate regions, creating the capacity for harmony with flexible and adaptive functioning.

References

Allen JG, Fonagy P, Bateman A: Mentalizing in Clinical Practice. Washington, DC, American Psychiatric Publishing, 2008

Beebe B, Jaffe J, Markese S, et al: The origins of 12-month attachment: a microanalysis of 4-month mother-infant interaction. Attach Hum Dev 12: 3–141, 2010

Carr L, Iacoboni M, Dubeau MC, et al: Neural mechanisms of empathy in humans: a relay from neural systems for imitation to limbic areas. Proc Natl Acad Sci 100:5497–5502, 2003

Cassidy J, Shaver PR (eds): Handbook of Attachment: Theory, Research, and Clinical Applications, 2nd Edition. New York, Guilford, 2008

Craig AD: Human feelings: why are some more aware than others? Trends Cogn Sci 8:239–241, 2004

Davidson RJ, Begley S: The Emotional Life of Your Brain: How Its Unique Patterns Affect the Way You Think, Feel, and Live—and How You Can Change Them. New York, Penguin Group/Hudson Street Press, 2012

DiNoble A: Examining the relationship between adult attachment style and mindfulness traits. Unpublished doctoral dissertation, California Graduate Institute of the Chicago School of Professional Psychology, 2009

Dutra L, Bureau J-F, Holmes B, et al: Quality of early care and childhood trauma: a prospective study of developmental pathways to dissociation. J Nerv Ment Dis 197:383–390, 2009

Feldman R: Parent-infant synchrony: biological foundations and developmental outcomes. Curr Dir Psychol Sci 16:340–345, 2007

Field T: Attachment as psychobiological attunement: being on the same wavelength, in Psychobiology of Attachment and Separation. Edited by Reite M, Field T. New York, Academic Press, 1985, pp 415–454

Fonagy P, Gergely G, Target M: The parent-infant dyad and the construction of the subjective self. J Child Psychol Psychiatry 48:288–328, 2007

George C, Kaplan N, Main M: The Adult Attachment Interview. Unpublished manuscript, University of California, Berkeley, 1996

Glass RM: Psychodynamic psychotherapy and research evidence: Bambi survives Godzilla? JAMA 300:1587–1589, 2008

Grepmair L, Mitterlehner F, Loew T, et al: Promoting mindfulness in psychotherapists in training influences the treatment results of their patients: a randomized, double-blind, controlled study. Psychother Psychosom 76:332–338, 2007

Hasson U, Ghazanfar AA, Galantucci B, et al: Brain-to-brain coupling: a mechanism for creating and sharing a social world. Trends Cogn Sci 16:114–121, 2012

Iacoboni M: Imitation, empathy, and mirror neurons. Annu Rev Psychol 60:653–670, 2009

Iacoboni M, Kaplan J, Wilson S: A neural architecture for imitation and intentional relations, in Imitation and Social Learning in Robots, Humans, and Animals: Behavioural, Social, and Communicative Dimensions. Edited by Nehaniv CL, Dautenhahn K. New York, Cambridge University Press, 2007, pp 71–87

Knickmeyer RC, Gouttard S, Kang C, et al: A structural MRI study of human brain development from birth to 2 years. J Neurosci 28:12176–12182, 2008

Krasner MS, Epstein RM, Beckman H, et al: Association of an educational program in mindful communication with burnout, empathy, and attitudes among primary care physicians. JAMA 302:1284–1293, 2009

Leckman JF, March JS: Editorial: developmental neuroscience comes of age. J Child Psychol Psychiatry 52:333–338, 2011

Parker SC, Nelson BW, Epel ES, et al: The science of presence: a central mediator of the interpersonal benefits of mindfulness, in Handbook of Mindfulness: Theory and Research. Edited by Brown KW, Creswell JD, Ryan RM. New York, Guilford (in press)

Rakel DP, Hoeft TJ, Barrett BP, et al: Practitioner empathy and the duration of the common cold. Fam Med 41:494–501, 2009

Roth TL, Sweatt JD: Annual Research Review: epigenetic mechanisms and environmental shaping of the brain during sensitive periods of development. J Child Psychol Psychiatry 52:398–408, 2011

Schore A: Affect Regulation and the Origin of the Self: The Neurobiology of Emotional Development. Mahwah, NJ, Erlbaum, 1994

Schore A: Effects of a secure attachment relationship on right brain development, affect regulation, and infant mental health. Infant Ment Health J 22:7–66, 2001

Schore A: The Science of the Art of Psychotherapy. New York, WW Norton, 2012

Siegel DJ: The Mindful Brain: Reflection and Attunement in the Cultivation of Well-Being. New York, WW Norton, 2007

Siegel DJ: The Mindful Therapist: A Clinician's Guide to Mindsight and Neural Integration. New York, WW Norton, 2010a

Siegel DJ: Mindsight: The New Science of Personal Transformation. New York, Bantam, 2010b

Siegel DJ: The Developing Mind: How Relationships and the Brain Interact to Shape Who We Are, 2nd Edition. New York, Guilford, 2012a

Siegel DJ: Pocket Guide to Interpersonal Neurobiology: An Integrative Handbook of the Mind. New York, WW Norton, 2012b

Siegel DJ, Bryson TP: The Whole-Brain Child: 12 Revolutionary Strategies to Nurture Your Child's Developing Mind, Survive Everyday Parenting Struggles, and Help Your Family Thrive. New York, Delacorte Press, 2011

Siegel DJ, Hartzell M: Parenting From the Inside Out: How a Deeper Self-Understanding Can Help You Raise Children Who Thrive. New York, Penguin Putnam, 2003

Sroufe LA, Siegel DJ: The verdict is in: the case for attachment theory. Psychotherapy Networker, March–April 2011

Sroufe LA, Egeland B, Carlson EA, et al: The Development of the Person: The Minnesota Study of Risk and Adaptation From Birth to Adulthood. New York, Guilford, 2005

Tronick EZ: Why is connection with others so critical? The formation of dyadic states of consciousness and the expansion of individuals' states of consciousness: coherence governed selection and the co-creation of meaning out of messy meaning making, in Emotional Development: Recent Research Advances. Edited by Nadel J, Muir D. Oxford, UK, Oxford University Press, 2005, pp 293–315

Tulving E: Episodic memory: from mind to brain [in French]. Annu Rev Psychol 53:1–25, 2002

Additional Resources

Mindsight Institute: www.mindsightinstitute.com. This is an educational center dedicated to providing a scientific understanding of the mind and well-being in order to cultivate a more compassionate society. Numerous live and recorded classes and workshops are available.

Norton Series on Interpersonal Neurobiology: http://books.wwnorton.com/books/index.aspx. The series includes books on interpersonal neurobiology.

CHAPTER 9

Basics of Counseling in Infant-Parent and Early Childhood Mental Health

Barbara Stroud, Ph.D.
Michael M. Morgan, Ph.D., L.M.F.T.

Professionals in the infant-parent and early childhood mental health field are charged with the task of supporting optimal developmental outcomes by promoting attentive and responsive relationships between caregivers and young children. To facilitate quality interpersonal interactions within family systems, providers need to employ strong relationship skills, including the foundational core counseling skills of active listening, empathic responding, validating observed strengths, and honoring differences (Cochran and Cochran 2006; Duffey and Somody 2011). As professionals use such relational counseling skills in supporting parents, a parallel process invites sensitive and responsive caregiving by these parents.

These counseling skills support interpersonal development and positive social-emotional outcomes (California Department of Education, WestEd Center for Child and Family Studies 2009), and healthy interpersonal interactions are essential in supporting development across domains, including early neurodevelopment (Shonkoff and Phillips 2000). In infant mental health practice, counseling interventions target social-emotional competence, early brain development, and emerging interpersonal skills. Every professional engaging a caregiver-infant dyad has the potential to model a relationship of support that encourages positive developmental outcomes.

In this chapter we outline some of the basic interdisciplinary counseling skills necessary to support positive child development outcomes, highlight the importance of a dyadic focus, and suggest specific ways that practitioners can evaluate the dyadic relationship. Although basic counseling interventions can be practiced and are encouraged within the broad scope of the infant-parent and early childhood mental health field, some caregiver-child dyads may benefit from more targeted psychotherapeutic interventions that are specific to a trained and duly authorized psychotherapist. An appropriate referral can be critical in such cases, and we describe important considerations for making good referrals.

Counseling and Psychotherapy

Among the range of services offered by practitioners to young children and their families, counseling and psychotherapy need to be distinguished. Although many professionals increasingly use the terms interchangeably (Day 2008), doing so blurs some important distinctions that can guide professional practice. Practitioners who understand the relationship between the two are better able to maximize their own role in helping clients within their expertise and scope of practice, and to make referrals to allied professions.

Crago (2000) captures some of the discussion about how counseling and psychotherapy are related. Counseling is often framed as a relatively short-term, less intensive service focused on helping clients resolve important but relatively transient and conscious concerns of living. Psychotherapy, on the other hand, has been described as a longer-term, more intensive form of treatment that often seeks to help clients make deeper personality changes through work with unconscious material. Crago rejects these simple categorical distinctions and suggests that counseling and psychotherapy can best be understood to fall along a more fluid continuum of helping, and notes that practitioners are likely to shift along the continuum depending on the circumstances of their work with a particular client. Although Crago's description improves on the idea that counseling and psychotherapy are distinct (but allied) approaches to creating change, it still suggests that at any given moment a practitioner will be at some specific point between the two, either closer to counseling or closer to psychotherapy.

We believe that this view misses the most significant and powerful relationship between the two approaches—namely, that basic counseling skills form the foundation for all successful helping. According to our view, effective practitioners will use core counseling skills no matter where their services might fall on the continuum suggested by Crago (2000). Psychotherapy (as a more intensive, long-term helping approach) builds on core counseling skills, rather than moving away from them toward a different skill set. Professionals offering psychotherapy add specific theory and interventions to the fundamental counseling skills, based on the unique needs of individual clients and the practitioner's conceptualization of those needs. It is important to note that we are not trying to define the relationship between professional fields or to enter into the debate about the qualifications, helpfulness, or prestige of those who define themselves as counselors or psychotherapists. Rather, we are trying to articulate a pragmatic relationship between salient skill sets that can ultimately improve the work of practitioners.

Within certain jurisdictions (e.g., countries or states), professional licensing boards and legally defined scopes of practice may authorize, certify, or endorse individuals as psychotherapists or counselors. This practice can be confusing not only to the public at large but also within professional circles when practitioners are engaging in referral or consulting activities. Some titles, such as psychologist, may imply that one is a psychotherapist, yet many psychologists are not psychotherapists. Likewise, many psychotherapists are not psychologists, but instead are marriage-family therapists, social workers, nurse practitioners, and so on. The professional activity of "counseling" becomes even more confusing because counseling skills are shared across multiple disciplines such that professional licenses and scopes of practice can have substantial overlap. To add to this confusion, some therapies limit training to licensed psychotherapists but not all psychotherapists are trained in these treatment modalities, whereas other treatment approaches that rely heavily on counseling skills are used in the training of both psychotherapists and nonpsychotherapists.

Recent trends suggest that fewer and fewer psychiatrists spend time providing psychotherapy to their clients. Mojtabai and Olfson (2008) found that the percentage of outpatient psychiatric visits including psychotherapy declined from 44% in 1996–1997 to only 29% in 2004–2005. This ongoing trend is likely due, they assert, to the combined effects of third-party reimbursement policies and the ongoing shift in psychiatry toward psychopharmacology or pharmacotherapy. However, in discussing this decline, the authors suggest that even when psychiatrists are not providing psychotherapy per se, they can learn and use some key psychotherapeutic techniques in their practice. Therefore, familiarity with and proficiency in basic counseling skills will benefit all practitioners working in infant and early childhood mental health, even though only some will have the disposition, additional skills, and legal authority to provide more extensive and/or specific types of psychotherapy.

Basic Counseling Skills

The counseling skills that we suggest can be helpful to all infant-parent and early childhood mental health practitioners focus largely on the establishment and maintenance of an effective working relationship with clients. The cumulative research on what leads to a positive outcome in effective mental health services has identified the relationship between practitioner and client as an important component in successful treatment (Lambert and Barley 2002; Norcross 2010). The most studied aspect of the relationship is the working alliance (Norcross 2010). The working alliance typically involves agreement between professional and client on treatment goals and tasks, coupled with a relationship bond that includes trust and attachment (Bordin 1979; Hatcher and Barends 2006). An impressive review of the research supporting the contribution of the working alliance to outcome, across multiple professions and modalities of treatment (including even outcomes in pharmacotherapy), is presented by Norcross (2010). The working alliance is not unlike the shared meaning making created within the context of the infant-parent dyad as discussed in Chapter 3, "Typical and Atypical Development." Additionally, the need for an emotional bond within the professional relationship clearly parallels the need for strong elements of trust, attunement, and attachments for all successful relationships.

One key dimension of the working alliance is the quality and strength of the bond between practitioner and client (Bordin 1979). Carl Rogers (1957) is credited with some of the earliest and most enduring contributions to the understanding of the therapeutic relationship. His ideas and subsequent research have demonstrated that three key conditions form the core of a helpful relationship: accurate empathic understanding, warmth and positive regard, and congruence. At the same time, effective professionals refrain from blaming, criticizing, or in any way rejecting clients (Binder and Strupp 1997; Lambert and Barley 2002). The fact that these qualities of the relationship are important to outcome should not be surprising given how they parallel what is known about the importance of relationships for healthy child development. As practitioners seek to build an attuned, supportive relationship with parents, they are providing the same kind of attachment experience and coregulatory scaffolding for parents that we hope parents will later be able to provide for their children (see Chapter 3 and Chapter 6, "Attachment Theory"). Birch (2008) asserts that a primary way practitioners help caregivers improve their parenting is through the type of relationship practitioners build with caregivers, perhaps most poignantly stated as "do unto others as we would have others do unto others" (Pawl and St. John 1998, p. 7).

Practitioners can use several skills to help create a strong working alliance with clients. However, the skills are in some ways secondary to a broader philosophy or way of being in the world. The point here is that the development of a successful helping relationship is contingent first on a certain way of being in the world. This reflects Rogers's (1957) concepts of congruence and positive regard. A practitioner is not being congruent if he or she is experiencing negative thoughts and feelings about a client's choices while attempting to use warm and respectful language of support. The ideals suggested in Brazelton's (1995, 1999) Touchpoints model articulate the kind of philosophical foundation needed for effective helping relationships. In addition to providing an outline of developmental challenges, Brazelton suggests that practitioners shift from the predominant deficit model to a more positive view of clients. Brazelton specifies several guiding principles and assumptions about parents that, when fully adopted by practitioners, form a foundation for both congruence in the relationship and the type of supportive experience that research has associated with positive outcome (see Chapter 4, "Brazelton's Neurodevelopmental and Relational Touchpoints and Infant Mental Health," for additional details about the approach).

Practitioners who approach their professional relationships with this kind of supportive philosophy can use some specific counseling skills to communicate warmth and empathy and to help establish a solid working alliance. The skills are not technically difficult; however, at initial use they can feel awkward, and some practice and perhaps reflective mentoring are required before professionals can integrate counseling skills into a way of being with clients. The first task of any helping professional is to comprehend the client's experience—both the content of the person's story and the emotional experience—and to communicate that understanding so that the client perceives the professional as genuinely attuned to his or her experience. There are several skills that can help a practitioner develop a deeper level of empathy with clients and better communicate this level of understanding. The process, however, is not quite as linear as suggested here. Emotional understanding and then communicating this level of personal knowledge is often a process of approximations, with the professional tentatively inquiring about how well he or she is interpreting the content of a client's dialogue, the emotional experience of the client, and the personal meaning the experience has for the client.

Empathic understanding, within the process of a relationship based on mutual positive regard, comes first. To empathically understand another is to enter into the other's subjective world and to in some small way share the experience (Cochran and Cochran 2006). Fonagy's (1998) concept of mentalizing (similar to reflective functioning) provides a useful template to encourage empathic understanding. Mentalizing is the process whereby a professional (or parent) learns about the mental state (thoughts, intentions, feelings) of self and others (see Chapter 20, "Attachment, Intersubjectivity, and Mentalization Within the Experience of the Child, the Parent, and the Provider"). Practitioners become aware of the mind of others and their affects, intentions, and meanings through two separate but related channels (Shai and Belsky 2011). First, practitioners can intuitively perceive others' intentions and mental states through an *implicit or embodied* process. Pragmatically, this requires practitioners to tune into their gut as a source of data in the relationship. As they actively listen to the client, practitioners consider how they themselves feel. One must take care to ensure that they are not superimposing their own emotions onto the client, but with a careful, reflective attention, this intuitive approach can help practitioners perceive things that the client may not have clearly articulated. The more *explicit* process for understanding a client's mental state requires practitioners to consciously listen and look for the emotional clues a client will give (e.g., tone of voice, facial expression, body posture), as well as to mentally put themselves into the place of the client and reflect on what the clients' experience would be like. Practitioners might ask themselves how they would feel, and how they would make sense of the world if they were in the client's place.

When the practitioner has a sense that he or she understands something about the client or the client's situation, the practitioner can communicate that understanding to the client. The skills of paraphrasing and reflecting are used to accomplish this goal. Interested readers are encouraged to see the lengthier descriptions of these skills provided by Chen and Giblin (2002) and Cochran and Cochran (2006). To paraphrase, the practitioner re-states *in his or her own words* the content of what the client has shared. Reflecting focuses on the emotional experience of the client, as well as the personal meaning the client makes of the experience. To reflect, the counselor states as clearly as possible, again in his or her own words, the emotion the client is experiencing, along with any thoughts, values, or aspirations that might be behind the client's experience. The practitioner need not wait to be absolutely sure about what he or she is going to reflect. Even when the practitioner's understanding is not entirely correct, the attempt to paraphrase and reflect communicates to the client a desire to deeply and empathically understand, strengthens the therapeutic relationship, and invites the client to provide additional information. The practitioner will have additional opportunities to adjust and attune his or her response until the client acknowledges feeling understood.

For example, suppose that a father, with weariness in his eyes and voice, describes his experience over the past several nights of trying to get his colicky daughter to sleep at night. He mentions rocking, walking, trying to feed her, driving her around, and ultimately giving up while she cried in his arms. While he speaks, the practitioner tunes into her own body's internal sensations, and notes a sense of desperation and frustration. As she listens, she notes his eyes and voice, and reflects on how she would feel if she had tried so hard, with great patience and care, to help a distressed child settle and sleep. When the father finishes, she paraphrases the content and reflects both feeling and meaning. "You worked so hard and tried so many things to help your daughter. You wanted her to be able to settle, and you need your rest too. When she continues to cry despite all your efforts, it sounds like you feel frustrated and helpless, and might even wonder if you can be a good father." The practitioner not only paraphrases and reflects the father's feeling, but also acknowledges his desire to be a good father (validating this strength). The client in this case might nod his head and affirm the response, and may feel both understood and validated. He may begin to see the practitioner as an ally in his efforts to be a good parent.

In paraphrasing and reflecting, it is important that the practitioner attend to the client's response, both nonverbal and verbal, and adjust what he or she says and how he or she communicates it to fit with the client's particular needs. Teyber and McClure (2011) describe this as *client response specificity*, a process that parallels the type of attuned, contingent responding that parents must learn in order to be able to forge a healthy attachment relationship with their child. Some clients will need more emphasis on the emotional aspect of their experience, whereas others may pull back from overt emotional expression. In the first case, the practitioner may need to emphasize the emotion more, going into more detail and validating more overtly the client's experience. In the latter case, a brief naming of emotion may suffice. By adjusting their responses in this way, practitioners reinforce for the client that they understand and can be trusted.

Effective practitioners also work to imbue their interactions with clients with attempts both to identify and validate any observed strengths and competencies and to recognize and honor differences. These counseling skills (Duffey and Somody 2011) parallel many of Brazelton's (1999) Touchpoints principles. Practitioners are encouraged to look for opportunities to support mastery, while assuming that caregivers want to be good parents and want the best for their children, even when the caregivers' behaviors may not currently reflect these aspirations. Because society is increasingly diverse, practitioners must recognize that there are likely differences between themselves and each of their clients, even when there are no obvious differences in language or ethnicity (Cochran and Cochran 2006). A practitioner honors those differences by inviting and initiating conversations about caregivers' perceptions, goals, and ways of understanding concerns and solutions, and by behaving with clients in ways that recognize the caregivers as the experts on their particular children.

One final counseling skill is critical in forging a strong working relationship. Inevitably, as in all human relationships, there will be difficulties in the developing relationship between practitioners and clients. There will be misunderstandings, missteps, and transference-countertransference reactions. More important than any misstep, however, is how the practitioner responds to it (Teyber and McClure 2011). When a professional can recognize and overtly address these difficulties, the relationship is strengthened, and the clients come to see that the practitioner is invested in having a healthy, respectful relationship with them.

Discussing with clients what is happening in the relationship as it occurs is referred to as the skill of immediacy (Chen and Giblin 2002) and is a key way for practitioners to be genuine in how they relate to clients. The recognition of a mismatch, followed by explicit efforts by the practitioner to repair the relationship, also parallels the kinds of interactions that are necessary for healthy attachment between parents and children, as articulated by Tronick in his work (see Chapter 3). Practitioners who employ this sort of relational immediacy and repair demonstrate for caregivers a way to strengthen their relationships with their children.

Working With Child-Caregiver Dyads

The field of infant and early childhood mental health is unique among helping professions in that its focus is not on an individual (either the parent or the child) but rather on the dyadic relationship between the child and the caregiver (Birch 2008; see also Chapter 20). The emotional health and overall physical wellness of infants and young children are embedded in relationships or dyadic interactions. Therefore, it is through strengthening these relationships that practitioners can best support healthy long-term development for the child and parent. Once a practitioner (of any discipline) decides to work in a dyadic fashion, the standard clinical rules are shifted. Whether providing psychotherapy, counseling, speech and language services, occupational therapy, or developmental guidance, the therapist using a dyadic approach must be mindful of the various internal processes of each member of the dyad as these processes affect the relationship. Imagine the often simple and effortless act of breast-feeding, which for some infant-parent dyads can be very challenging and create distress in both mother and infant, as well as in their relationship. In an optimal situation, the mother is attuned to the infant, by sharing glances and perhaps speaking, singing, or gently humming to the baby. The infant in this moment of emotional and physical connection experiences not only nutritional sustenance but emotional nourishment and the experience of joyful engagement. The infant learns that "I can bring pleasure to my mother, and she can offer joy and emotional support to me." However, how does this interaction change if one or both members of the dyad are stressed or emotionally unavailable? Consider a mother experiencing mild baby blues or postpartum depression. How does this relationship change if the mother is unable to meet the infant's gaze, offer calming verbal support, or participate in reciprocal smiles? Such an interaction may lead to an infant who experiences his or her mother as emotionally unavailable or a mother who begins to view herself as ineffective because she gets little joy in response from her baby. Now consider an infant with severe gastrointestinal issues as expressed in poor feeding, excessive crying, and frequent reflux responses to breast-feeding. Even a very attentive and emotionally available mother may withdraw from such a challenging infant. The infant may experience his or her world as increasingly painful with little emotional or physical relief.

It is important to remember that each member of the dyad brings to the relationship his or her internal experience. At the same time, the shared actual experience of the relationship becomes blended with each member's perceived understanding, and this creates the internal meaning of the relationship (Tronick and Beeghly 2011). Each dyad member internalizes an answer to the question "What does this relationship interaction mean to me and how does it shape my understanding of other relationships?" When working from a dyadic perspective, the practitioner is considering not only the outward experience of each member of the dyad, but the way in which that experience is understood and internalized by each individual. Each experience of the dyad is shaped by the mind and held as a mental representation or internalized idea of the infant's or parent's place in the relationship. In other words, the child's and caregiver's perceptions of themselves, as well as their internal understanding of other relationships, will be shaped by the meaning each of them makes about their relationship together.

Whether providing counseling or psychotherapy interventions with a dyad, the practitioner must regularly attend to how moment-to-moment interactions are shaping and shaped by the ongoing meaning-making process of both child and caregiver. Sroufe (2000) discusses the balanced and artful interactions of support that caregivers provide their infants to fine-tune emerging regulation skills. The quality, timing, and tone of the caregiver's response to the various needs of the infant help to shape internal regulation skills. This capacity for self-regulation is just one of the multiple factors that support the success or failure of the dyad. Regulation, or the ability to return to calm in the face of new experiences or stressful events (Greenspan et al. 1998), is another indicator of successful interpersonal development. Practitioners will also observe in a successful dyad evidence of back-and-forth nonverbal and verbal communication flow, elements of shared joyful interacting, and the ability to work together to recover from distress or miscues in the relationship (Greenspan et al. 1998). This same activity of recovery or relationship repair is evident in the basic counseling skills of immediacy, discussed in the previous section, "Basic Counseling Skills." Adequate regulation skills within the dyad assist in encouraging positive relationship interactions across the life span.

Dunn (2004) speaks about the ways that a child's response to sensory information can impact regulation and the working relationship of the dyad. Young children are regularly adapting to their sensory environment, and how they manage this process should be supported by a nurturing caregiver. The dyad's success is therefore also influenced by how each member individually responds to or organizes sensory information, in addition to how the dyad in unison interprets new sensory experiences in order to reach or maintain a state of calm. Consider, for example, the sensory information present in a pediatrician's office: bright lights, hard examining table, a sometimes-cold stethoscope, and so on. How does the young child respond or adapt to this new sensory information, and perhaps more importantly, how does the parent support the child's integration of this information such that the child can return to a state of calm?

An individual's response to stress and the skills of stress recovery as mediated by the developing autonomic nervous system are embedded in relationships (Lillas and Turnbull 2009). This concept is discussed in greater detail in Chapter 5, "The Neurorelational Framework in Infant and Early Childhood Mental Health." Stress results in dysregulation (or disequilibrium) of the dyad's ability to interact in a mutually supportive style. Dyads struggle with universal stressors (e.g., childhood illness, caregiver separation, sleep management) as well as family-specific stressors (e.g., poverty, mental illness, community violence). Stress recovery methods are individualized and influenced by constitutional issues, family practices, and cultural expectations (Axia and Weisner 2002). The dyad's observed capacity to respond to and recover from stress provides the practitioner with more insight into the relational success of the dyad.

Emotional experiences shape the workings of a relationship and also influence the parent-child dyad. Interpersonal relationships can be experienced as joyful, distressing, or at times fearful. More successful dyads demonstrate a range of affective responses and may be experienced by an observer as joyful and active (Thompson 2012). The caregiver will demonstrate the ability to expand on the young child's joyful participation in the relationship as well as effectively calm the child when distressed. Additionally, an attuned caregiver will be able to predict when the interaction, environment, or emotional experience of the child is overwhelming, too arousing, or creating stress. In an effective dyadic interaction, the caregiver offers a measured balance of responses and engagement that meets the emotional needs of the infant or young child. This process is often referred to as coregulation (Fogel 1993), or the adequate reading of and appropriate responding to the cues of the infant or young child. The parent's capacity to coregulate the child not only supports self-regulation skills, but this back-and-forth interaction of supportive cueing and measured responsiveness serves the attachment system as well.

To build a deeper understanding of the quality of the dyadic relationship as well as the emotional meaning-making taking place within the dyad, a practitioner may want to consider the following questions: What am I observing in the dyad that provides an understanding of the emotional experiences of each member of the dyad? (What is the meaning making developed by both parties?) How does each member of the dyad influence the affective tone of the relationship? (How does the behavior of the child affect the feelings of the caregiver, and vice versa?) Does this dyad struggle to recover from distressing emotions? Is this caregiver able to support the developing emotional understanding of this young child? (Can the caregiver name the feelings the child is experiencing, thus helping to bridge from raw sensation to cognitive awareness?) How does the family's internalized and expressed demonstration of cultural practices influence the parent-child relationship? Are the observed interactions appropriate within the cultural context of this family? What are the specific strengths and capacities that each member of the relationship can bring to influence the quality of the dyadic experience? These are the questions that will provide the practitioner with a better understanding of how the dyad supports regulation in the face of intense emotions and whether a psychotherapy referral may be appropriate.

In thinking about the psychological needs of a parent-child dyad and the supports to achieve optimal developmental outcomes, practitioners should use skilled observation techniques to assess the quality of the dyadic interactions and to determine the capacity of the relationship to promote healthy child development. A dyad that demonstrates relationship challenges may benefit from a psychotherapy intervention. Table 9–1 has been designed to

TABLE 9–1. Assessment and planning in dyadic intervention	
Practitioner's question	Observed relationship concern
Assessment of dyadic interaction	
1. How does this dyad recover or respond to dysregulation in their relationship rhythms?	Regulation issues—establishing and maintaining a state of calm
2. How does this dyad manage and make use of sensory information?	Sensory regulation—caregiver recovery and support to infant
3. How does the caregiver in this dyad manage personal stress and, furthermore, support the stress recovery systems of the child?	Managing stress responses—dyad's established methods of stress recovery
4. What is the capacity of the dyad to maintain a regulated emotional state?	Affective tone of the relationship—how feelings are expressed and experienced in the dyad
Planning: is referral necessary?	
5. Do the observed concerns within the dyad negatively impact the child's developmental success?	Whether the concern(s) of this dyad will be best addressed by a counseling intervention or a psychotherapy referral

assist practitioners as they observe the infant-parent interaction in an effort to assess relationship successes and challenges.

Making an Appropriate Referral

When the practitioner observes over time that the infant-parent dyad has significant difficulty in maintaining regulation, recovering from distress, or managing intense affect, and furthermore that these observed difficulties are hampering developmental success, a psychotherapy referral may be appropriate. In the same way that issues of "goodness of fit" between parent and child will promote healthy development (Thomas and Chess 1977), an effective referral will match the needs and abilities of the dyad with a specific psychotherapy approach that can likewise best meet their needs and promote healthy development. The referring practitioner should consider the following attributes: the developmental level of the child, any atypical sensory needs of the child or parent, the child's and parent's ability to tolerate stress, the parent's capacity for self-reflection and ability to gain insight from examining his or her own behavior, and the caregiver's ability to tolerate intense affect.

In considering a therapy referral, the practitioner should examine theory as it impacts practice. Infant mental health practices follow theory. When considering an appropriate referral, a practitioner should also consider the best theoretical match for the dyad. Models of infant-parent psychotherapy as envisioned by Selma Fraiberg (1980) have stimulated multiple therapeutic frameworks and evidence-based practices within the field. These more psychodynamically influenced practices often focus on the reflective functioning or internal narrative of the parent (e.g., Infant-Parent Psychotherapy; Child-Parent Psychotherapy; Mindful Parenting; Watch, Wait, and Wonder) as well as on how the caregiver's implicit memory of being parented influences his or her current parenting activities. From this perspective, not only are the events of the parent's past significant to current parenting, but the parent's internal understanding of those historical events also guides caregiving activities. When making a referral to a more psychodynamically oriented intervention approach, the referring practitioner should consider whether the parent has the skills and competencies needed to fully benefit from such an intervention.

Some infant mental health practices take a more directive or coaching approach. Models that offer directed behavioral training, parental skill building, or coaching in the moment of dyadic engagement often have their roots in a cognitive-behavioral perspective or in social learning theory (e.g., Parent-Child Interaction Therapy, Video Intervention Therapy, Floortime, Filial Play Therapy, Theraplay, Circle of Security). These intervention models may be a good fit for families that can incorporate new learning quickly and are eager to gain new skills and are highly motivated to participate. With cooperative families, many of these models can produce timely improvement when implemented with fidelity and when there is an absence of chronic pathology in the family system. More systematic and structured parenting support and teaching interventions may also prove valuable to parents who lack strong internal regulation skills, benefit from external structures, and find success in more directive approaches to change.

Elements often associated with a humanistic theoretical framework are embedded in many infant and child mental health practices. Infant and child mental health practitioners seek to use strength-based approaches with families and to implement clinical interventions that empower and engage caregivers as the agents of systems change while seeking to maximize the developmental potential of all children. Optimal social-emotional success or emotional wellness is the desired outcome (Center on the Social and Emotional Foundations for Early Learning 2013). All practitioners across disciplines can and should be using excellent counseling skills as a strategy for supporting positive change in the sphere of relevant relationships (e.g., the parent-child dyad, the parent-therapist dyad, the parent-parent dyad). Through the parallel process, "the way the staff person interacts with a child, parent, or colleague can then positively spill over and influence the parent's relationship with her child" (Heffron and Murch 2010, p. 9). When applied to the use of basic counseling skills, this parallel process becomes a key way that practitioners can positively influence the parent-child relationship.

Each of the basic counseling practices we have discussed (empathic understanding, immediacy, paraphrasing, reflecting, and so on) serves as a parallel to the type of relationship practitioners should aim to support between infants and caregivers. The working alliance is a parallel to the attachment bond. Within the concept of empathic understanding, practitioners can see the building blocks of emotional attunement as practiced by a caregiver toward a child. The counseling skill of immediacy parallels the parental need to consistently attend to the parent-child relationship and work to repair it as ruptures occur. In the counseling skill of paraphrasing, the counselor is in fact accurately reading and responding to the cues of the client. As practitioners model these skills to parents, they provide a new potential for the quality of the relationships. Through this experience, parents can create a change in their relationship experience with their child. The type of intrapersonal change necessary to create this level of relationship change may stem from an intervention based on parental insight or direct coaching and practice. The lived and felt experience of "being different" in an intentional manner can create the small shift for parents and children, and may create new potentials for how to be in relationships. Some dyads may need to feel the change first before they can embrace and live the change. The way practitioners interact with families can be the beginning of that felt, purposeful, and relational change.

When seeking an infant mental health therapy referral, what should the referring practitioner be looking for in the therapist? If the practitioner's state offers some form of infant mental health endorsement, designed to identify practitioners with the knowledge and expertise to work within this specialized field, he or she should seek out these professionals and learn more about the services they provide.

Clinical interventions designed for children from birth to age 5 years follow a developmental perspective, and support a healthy parent-child relationship as outlined in this chapter. Highly qualified infant mental health practitioners not only will include the parent in the clinical work but will adapt the clinical intervention to the developmental needs and emotional availability of the parent as well as the child. For example, preverbal children are offered more sensory- or relationship-based therapies, as opposed to more narrative approaches.

In the dyadic or family-focused lens of the infant mental health field, and from a deeper understanding of the family as the primary change agent for the child, understanding and honoring family strengths, vulnerabilities, and adaptations become integral to the clinical work. Existing family strengths can serve as a learning tool for the family and the practitioner, as a means to combat vulnerabilities, while the family's adaptations to stress or change provide a window into current coping skills within the family system. Best practice demands that therapists provide services in line with the family's cultural expectations and linguistic preference. In the earliest of relationships, culture is embedded in every caregiving activity (Rogoff 2003). Cultural practices shape the very expression of emotion and define socially appropriate behaviors (California Department of Education, WestEd Center for Child and Family Studies 2009). Infant mental health practitioners of high quality have a strong understanding of and respect for individual differences and family cultural variance, and adapt their interventions to meet the specific needs of various cultural groups. All of these treatment values should be evident in practitioner referrals for relationship-based infant mental health services.

The shared understanding of the parent's role in treatment may also shape referral decisions. It is the role of the referring practitioner to offer the caregivers direction and guidance as to the reason for the referral. Furthermore, caregivers need to be empowered to offer their voice in the defined activities of treatment and the outcomes that indicate success for their child. Thus, the concept of "parents as partners" in the treatment process should be understood from the point of referral. The better the referring practitioner can prepare and explain the reasons behind the therapy referral, the greater the likelihood of treatment participation and success.

Conclusion

Although many practitioners may not do the specific work of psychotherapy with parent-child dyads, all have opportunities to promote positive change and healthy development by cultivating and using basic counseling skills, such as empathy, reflecting feelings, paraphrasing, and others discussed in this chapter, in their work with clients. Use of these basic counseling skills creates a strong therapeutic alliance to support change, while also modeling a nurturing dyadic relationship that best supports healthy child development. Relationships underlie healthy child development and serve as the vehicle for assessment and intervention within the infant and early childhood mental health field. Therefore, practitioners must also become sensitive to the nuanced manner in which each member of the dyad is influencing the quality of the dyadic experience, and look for opportunities to support an optimal dyadic relationship. When a referral is appropriate, practitioners can ensure a good fit between the dyad and the service referral by assessing the contribution of each member of the dyad, as well as strengths, needs, cultural considerations, and so forth. Some dyads may benefit from a more psychodynamic approach, whereas others may benefit from a more concrete coaching intervention. In all referrals, practitioners should ensure that the other provider is knowledgeable and sensitive to developmental and cultural issues. All professionals within the infant mental health field, whether providing counseling or psychotherapy, need to remain ever mindful of the impact of their interventions on the overall development, social-emotional health, and future functioning of the child.

KEY POINTS

- Professionals of every discipline working with young children and their families should use basic counseling skills to build an effective working alliance with caregiver-child dyads and to support their healthy development.
- Professionals can develop and enhance a beneficial working alliance by cultivating and communicating empathic understanding with clients, identifying and validating client competencies, and showing a willingness to openly and nonreactively work through with clients any challenges or difficulties that emerge within the professional relationship.
- Through the parallel process, the way in which practitioners interact with parents, particularly when showing respect, presence, and empathy, can support positive change in the sphere of relevant relationships (e.g., parent-child dyad, parent-therapist dyad, parent-parent dyad).

- Psychotherapists come from many different disciplines with a range of training, specialization, and experience. Before making a psychotherapy referral for a client or dyad, the referring professional should determine the background, focus, training, approaches, and other capacities of the intended referral provider to determine whether he or she can best meet the client's needs.
- Professionals should consider a psychotherapy referral for clients when they observe any of the following in the parent or within the child-caregiver relationship:
  1. Difficulties with regulation, affect, and mood
  2. Challenges with stress recovery
  3. Histories of trauma, maltreatment, relationship difficulties, or attachment problems
  4. Other signs of mental health conditions, including risk to self or others, substance use or other addictions, self-harming behaviors, prolonged grief, problematic mood changes, extreme phobias, debilitating interactional patterns, anxiety disorders, and eating disorders
  5. Other conditions or situations in which psychotherapy could be a primary or adjunctive therapy

References

Axia VD, Weisner TS: Infant stress reactivity and home cultural ecology of Italian infants and families. Infant Behav Dev 25:255–268, 2002

Binder JL, Strupp HH: "Negative process": recurrently discovered and underestimated facet of therapeutic process and outcome in the individual psychotherapy of adults. Clinical Psychology: Science and Practice 4:121–139, 1997

Birch M: The reason for such a book, in Finding Hope in Despair: Clinical Studies in Infant Mental Health. Edited by Birch M. Washington, DC, Zero to Three, 2008, pp 1–28

Bordin ES: The generalizability of the psychoanalytic concepts of the working alliance. Psychotherapy: Theory, Research, and Practice 16:252–260, 1979

Brazelton TB: Working with families: opportunities for early intervention. Pediatr Clin North Am 42:1–9, 1995

Brazelton TB: How to help parents of young children: the Touchpoints model. J Perinatol 19:S6–S7, 1999

California Department of Education, WestEd Center for Child and Family Studies: California Infant/Toddler Learning and Development Foundations. Sacramento, California Department of Education, 2009

Center on the Social and Emotional Foundations for Early Learning: Research synthesis: infant mental health and early care and education providers. 2013. Available at: http://csefel.vanderbilt.edu/documents/rs_infant_mental_health.pdf. Accessed March 28, 2013.

Chen M, Giblin NJ: Individual Counseling: Skills and Techniques. Denver, CO, Love Publishing, 2002

Cochran JL, Cochran NH: The Heart of Counseling: A Guide to Developing Therapeutic Relationships. Belmont, CA, Brooks/Cole, 2006

Crago H: Counselling and psychotherapy: is there a difference? Does it matter? Australian and New Zealand Journal of Family Therapy 21:73–80, 2000

Day S: Theory and Design in Counseling and Psychotherapy, 2nd Edition. Boston, MA, Lahaska, 2008

Duffey T, Somody C: The role of relational-cultural theory in mental health counseling. Journal of Mental Health Counseling 33:223–242, 2011

Dunn W: A sensory processing approach to supporting infant-caregiver relationships, in Treating Parent-Infant Relationship Problems: Strategies for Intervention. Edited by Sameroff AJ, McDonough SC, Rosenblum KL. New York, Guilford, 2004, pp 152–187

Fogel A: Developing Through Relationships: Origins of Communication, Self, and Culture. Chicago, IL, University of Chicago Press, 1993

Fonagy P: Prevention: the appropriate target of infant psychotherapy. Infant Ment Health J 19:124–150, 1998

Fraiberg S (ed): Clinical Studies in Infant Mental Health: The First Year of Life. New York, Basic Books, 1980

Greenspan SI, Wieder S, Simons R: The Child With Special Needs: Encouraging Intellectual and Emotional Growth. Boston, MA, Perseus Books, 1998

Hatcher RL, Barends AW: How a return to theory could help alliance research. Psychotherapy (Chic) 43:292–299, 2006

Heffron MC, Murch T: Reflective Supervision and Leadership in Infant and Early Childhood Programs. Washington, DC, Zero to Three, 2010

Lambert MJ, Barley DE: Research summary on the therapeutic relationship and psychotherapy outcome, in Psychotherapy Relationships That Work: Therapist Contributions and Responsiveness to Patients. Edited by Norcross JC. New York, Oxford University Press, 2002, pp 17–32

Lillas C, Turnbull J: Infant/Child Mental Health, Early Intervention, and Relationship-Based Therapies: A Neurorelational Framework for Interdisciplinary Practice. New York, WW Norton, 2009

Mojtabai R, Olfson M: National trends in psychotherapy by office-based psychiatrists. Arch Gen Psychiatry 65:962–970, 2008

Norcross JC: The therapeutic relationship, in The Heart and Soul of Change: Delivering What Works in Therapy, 2nd Edition. Edited by Duncan B, Miller S, Wampold B, et al. Washington, DC, American Psychological Association, 2010, pp 113–141

Pawl JH, St. John M: How You Are Is as Important as What You Do in Making a Positive Difference for Infants, Toddlers, and Their Families. Washington, DC, Zero to Three, 1998

Rogers CR: The necessary and sufficient conditions of therapeutic personality change. J Consult Clin Psychol 21:95–103, 1957

Rogoff B: The Cultural Nature of Human Development. New York, Oxford University Press, 2003

Shai D, Belsky J: When words just won't do: introducing Parental Embodied Mentalizing. Child Dev Perspect 5:173–180, 2011

Shonkoff JP, Phillips DA (eds): From Neurons to Neighborhoods: The Science of Early Childhood Development. Washington, DC, National Academy Press, 2000

Sroufe LA: Early relationships and the development of children. Infant Ment Health J 21:67–74, 2000

Teyber E, McClure FH: Interpersonal Process in Therapy: An Integrative Model. Belmont, CA, Brooks/Cole, 2011

Thomas A, Chess S: Temperament and Development. New York, Brunner/Mazel, 1977

Thompson R: How emotional development unfolds starting at birth. Zero Three 3:6–11, 2012

Tronick E, Beeghly M: Infants' meaning making and the development of mental health problems. Am Psychol 66:107–119, 2011

CHAPTER 10

Behavioral Epigenetics and the Developmental Origins of Child Mental Health Disorders

Barry M. Lester, Ph.D.

Carmen J. Marsit, Ph.D.

Cailey Bromer, B.S.

Nature and nurture discussions have been rekindled with new dimensions as neuroscience and the field of epigenetics advance. The term *epigenetics* refers to "the interactions of genes with their environment, by which genotype gives rise to phenotype and brings the phenotype into being" (Waddington 1940), or to the ways in which the developmental environment influences the mature phenotype (Van Speybroeck 2002). This rapidly growing field focuses on heritable alterations in gene expression, resulting from changes in chromosomes without alteration of the DNA sequence.

Epigenetics research sheds light on the interplay of genetics, gene control, gene-environment interaction, fetal programming in utero, and the impact of infancy and early childhood experiences, including the caregiving environment, on human health, well-being, and disease. This rapidly advancing science has significant importance for infant mental health (IMH) clinicians, and this chapter is intended to offer a baseline understanding of epigenetics and explore a number of related concepts and theories.

There is clear evidence that epigenetic changes can 1) be transmitted vertically (transgenerationally), 2) result from influences in the prenatal environment, and 3) occur from postnatal influences. Waterland and Jirtle (2003) demonstrated in agouti mice that a spe-

This work was supported in part by NIH grants U10 DA24119 and COBRE P20RR018728. Thanks to the patients and families who stimulated these ideas.

cifically enriched maternal prenatal diet could silence a gene that influences coat color and the development of obesity, cancer, and diabetes before the mice are 100 days old—a lifelong impact from a prenatal environmental exposure. Champagne et al. (2003) demonstrated in rats that low maternal licking and grooming behaviors in the days after birth alter genes that inhibit stress responses, resulting in rats with lifelong difficulties regulating the stress arousal system. This maternal neglect inhibited growth hormones and created a stress response in the pup that in turn altered (i.e., methylated) part of the genome impacting the number of glucocorticoid receptors in the hippocampus. Methylation of genes in pups reared by low-licking dams could be blocked by transferring litters to known high-licking dams in the first week after birth, and was intergenerational. The experience of high- and low-licking traits passed from mother to females cared for in the first week of life, whether or not the female was a biological daughter. Findings also showed that even known high-licking dams became low lickers when they were stressed during pregnancy—a transfer of the mother's environmental experiences to the genome, neural anatomy, and neural functioning of offspring (Weaver et al. 2004).

Similarly, but in humans, Radtke et al. (2011) demonstrated that methylation of the glucocorticoid receptor gene occurs in fetuses in utero when mothers experience intimate partner violence during pregnancy. This methylation was not seen if the intimate partner violence occurred before or after the index pregnancy. The methylation of this gene persists at least to age 19 and likely beyond, and has lifelong consequences, including playing a key role in child, adolescent, and adult psychosocial behavior, and increasing the risk for mental health disorders.

Research on the developmental origins model of health and disease in adults suggests that in response to environmental signals, the fetus makes adaptations through programming to "prepare" for his or her unique postnatal environment. These adaptations are thought to be due, in part, to epigenetic mechanisms and raise questions, including 1) whether this process can explain some mental health disorders, 2) how the process is influenced by the postnatal environment, 3) whether mental health–based preventive interventions should begin prior to or in pregnancy, and 4) whether postnatal interventions can ameliorate epigenetic risks. This application of epigenetics to the study of behavior—the emerging field of behavioral epigenetics—will heavily influence IMH.

In this chapter, we summarize basic epigenetic principles, describe the new field of behavioral epigenetics, and provide a summary of the current related literature. We discuss the developmental origins model of health and disease in the context of mental health outcomes and the significance of prenatal stress on the intrauterine neuroendocrine environment. We then synthesize these concepts and present a developmental origins model of child mental health disorders in which prenatal environmental stressors impact placental gene expression, altering both the hippocampus and the hypothalamic-pituitary-adrenal (HPA) axis set points, as well as the infant's responsivity to postnatal environmental conditions, potentially affecting liability to child and adult mental health disorders. Epigenetic effects on key placental genes increase fetal exposure to cortisol, altering the infant's response to the postnatal environment. This biophysiology, coupled with the combination of "goodness of fit" (or relative match or mismatch of the infant's capacities with caregiver approaches and sensitivity) and the level of adversity in the postnatal environment, influences risk for mental health disorders.

Basics of Epigenetics

In the term *epigenetics,* as defined earlier in this chapter, the prefix *epi* implies that the epigenome is above, around, or in addition to the DNA-based genome. By understanding this process, IMH clinicians can appreciate the malleability of the genome as it is relevant to the periods in development addressed by the field.

Although debate about the definition of *epigenetics* continues (Bird 2007), it is probably safe to describe epigenetics as the inheritance of information based on gene expression control rather than gene sequence (Gallou-Kabani and Junien 2005); epigenetic modifications lead to heritable yet environmentally susceptible changes in gene expression without altering DNA sequences. DNA, like any molecule, is subject to alteration, and such acquired changes involve enzymes, primarily large protein molecules, that facilitate the change—the methylation—in DNA. Chromatin is a key player and one of five elements responsible for compressing DNA from a 6-foot strand to fit within a cell nucleus; for protecting DNA loss over time, including during cell division; and for controlling gene expression, the phenomenon with which we are concerned here. DNA methylation involves the addition of a methyl group to cytosine, one of the four bases that define the code of DNA. Methyl groups are the "change agents" that enact a stable DNA change that alters or perpetuates gene expression but does not alter the DNA sequence. A methyl group makes certain segments of DNA unreadable, and when this DNA methylation is found in gene promoters, transcription proteins cannot activate the gene and it is silenced.

Behavioral Epigenetics

Thousands of epigenetics studies have been conducted over the last 40 years; however, the application of epigenetics to the study of behavior is just beginning. Behavioral epigenetics is described as the application of the principles of epigenetics to the study of physiological, genetic, environmental, and developmental mechanisms of behavior in human and nonhuman animals (Lester et al. 2011). It typically investigates, at the level of chemical changes, gene expression and biological processes that underlie normal and abnormal behavior, including how behavior affects and is affected by epigenetic processes. Behavioral epigenetics is interdisciplinary in its approach and draws on sciences such as neuroscience, psychology, psychiatry, genetics, biochemistry, sociology, and psychopharmacology.

In a 2011 PubMed search of published articles fitting the definition of behavioral epigenetics described above, 178 articles met these criteria, with the majority published in the preceding few years. Analyzing the articles by the major construct studied identified the most investigated categories to be psychiatric illness, substance abuse, learning and memory, neurodevelopment, parenting, and stress—all relevant to the IMH field. In this review, identifying genes that were studied in each of the behavioral categories provided insight into some of the mechanisms that are being investigated. For example, *NR3C1* is the glucocorticoid receptor gene that cortisol and other glucocorticoids bind to and is prominent in parenting studies. This gene impacts the HPA axis and is key to the developmental origins model of child mental health disorders presented later in this chapter.

Developmental Origins Model of Health and Disease

Evidence from preclinical, prospective clinical, and epidemiological studies suggests that early development has echoes across one's lifetime (Barker et al. 1995; Gluckman and Hanson 2004). Early work showed that measures of birth size are related to adult risk of coronary heart disease and other metabolic syndromes, including hypertension, stroke, insulin resistance, type 2 diabetes, and dyslipidemia (Barker 1998; Barker and Osmond 1988). The relationship between impaired fetal growth and an increased incidence of cardiovascular disease, hypertension, and type 2 diabetes was especially strong in individuals who became obese in adolescence or adulthood. Disease burden increases when there is a "mismatch" between limited prenatal nutrients/calories and postnatal nutrient/calorie-rich environments (Gluckman and Hanson 2004).

The literature on the influence of prenatal stress on offspring suggests that many biological factors acting during prenatal life are associated not only with the development of common adult cardiovascular and metabolic disorders, but also with neurobehavioral and behavioral disorders (Allin et al. 2006; Barker 2002; Hales et al. 1991; McMillen and Robinson 2005; Thompson et al. 2001). Low birth weight is related to mental illnesses, including schizophrenia, depression, and psychological distress (Alati et al. 2007; Cannon and Rosso 2002; Cheung et al. 2002). It is generally accepted that birth size is not at the heart of these disorders, but rather is a proxy for underlying mechanisms, and that there are common factors that influence intrauterine growth as well as adult physiological systems (Welberg and Seckl 2001). These observations on "developmental origins" are due, in part, to environmental factors acting early in fetal life with effects on developing systems that alter structure and function, and likely behavioral expression. It has been suggested that the biological purpose of this "programming" is to alter the set points or to "hardwire" physiological systems to prepare the fetus for optimal adaptation to the postnatal environment.

Role of the Neuroendocrine System

There are few settings in which gene-environment interactions are more profound, critical windows are of a more narrow duration, and the latency to onset of effect is shorter than the influence of an adverse intrauterine environment on neuroendocrine and neurobehavioral functioning in the newborn. Neuroendocrine physiology is unique during intrauterine life. Fetal neuroendocrine function is almost exclusively autonomous from that of the mother, and there are robust placental mechanisms that create a barrier to passage of maternal hormones and neurotransmitters across the placenta, including all of the peptide hormones and releasing factors, glucocorticoids, catecholamines, and all but a trace amount of thyroid hormones. A very high endogenous secretion rate of catecholamines by the fetus conditions the prenate's capacity for a huge increase in norepinephrine and epinephrine secretion at birth to facilitate postnatal adaptation (Padbury and Martinez 1988). The fetus is protected from a hyperadrenergic state in utero by placental mechanisms for the uptake and degradation of catecholamines. This situation, however, renders the fetus exquisitely vulnerable to the effects of catecholamine uptake inhibitors (e.g., cocaine and amphetamines) or drugs that increase catecholamine secretion (e.g., nicotine).

Developmental Origins Model of Child Mental Health Disorders

Lester and Padbury (2009) describe the effects of prenatal cocaine exposure as a stressor producing an adverse intrauterine environment with altered regulation of catecholamines and glucocorticoids. As a stressor, cocaine programs the HPA axis, which controls, among other functions, the release of cortisol within the neuroendocrine system to mediate the stress response. This action impacts behavior due, in part, to plasticity of brain neurotransmitter monoamine systems. The cocaine exposure model is but one example of whole classes of stressors that impact and modify these systems. We have integrated these concepts into a more generic model of the developmental origins of child mental health disorders (see Figure 10–1; Lester et al. 2012). The model is heuristic to illustrate how developmental origins could relate to child mental health disorders, and to describe one of many pathways that may be involved. The model shows the impact of an adverse intrauterine environment, encompassing maternal stress, environmental exposures, inadequate or poor nutrition, or other adverse conditions, on placental gene expression affecting cortisol and altering the infant's responsivity to environmental factors affecting liability to mental health disorders.

There are several candidate genes involved in responsivity and control of the HPA axis in the placenta during gestation. It is important for IMH practitioners to be aware of genes and pathways currently being investigated and to monitor theories and published findings, because these may present unique opportunities and/or specific targets for preventive and therapeutic interventions. Genes currently being researched include those for 1) the norepinephrine transporter (NET), 2) the steroid metabolic enzyme 11β-HSD2, and 3) the glucocorticoid receptor NR3C1. Placental NET and 11β-HSD2 genes are pivotal placental genes that program the intrauterine neuroendocrine environment, protecting the fetus from the harmful effects of excess catecholamines and glucocorticoids (Meyer 1985). From our preliminary findings, we hypothesize that the association of prenatal stress and altered fetal development is mediated by effects on the 11β-HSD2 gene. As a result, the altered HPA set points and neurobehavioral reactivity predispose the child to the devel-

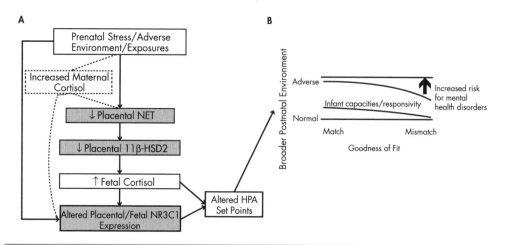

FIGURE 10–1. Developmental origins model of child mental health disorders.

The model illustrates one of many pathways in which prenatal environmental stressors could impact placental gene expression altering hypothalamic-pituitary-adrenal HPA set points and the infant's responsivity to postnatal environmental conditions affecting liability to mental health disorders. (A) Epigenetic effects on key placental genes *(shaded)* increase fetal exposure to cortisol, altering the abilities of the infant to respond to the postnatal environment, which includes both parenting and broader environmental conditions (e.g., poverty). (B) The "goodness of fit" or relative match or mismatch between the infant's capacities and the kind of parenting appropriate for the infant's capacities in the context of the degree of adversity of the broader postnatal environment will determine the probability of risk for mental health disorders. This risk is maximized when the infant has restricted behavioral capacities that clash (are a mismatch) with parenting styles in the context of environmental adversity.

11β-HSD2=corticosteroid 11β-dehydrogenase isozyme; NET=norepinephrine transporter; NR3C1=glucocorticoid receptor gene.

Source. Developed by Lester, Marsit, Conradt, Bromer, and Padbury and partially adapted from Gluckman and Hanson 2004. First published in: Lester BM, Marsit CJ, Conradt E, et al.: "Behavioral Epigenetics and the Developmental Origins of Child Mental Health Disorders." *Journal of Developmental Origins of Health and Disease* 3:395–408, 2012. Permission for use granted from JDOHD by RightsLink Copyright Clearing House.

opment of mental health disorders. In the model, an adverse intrauterine environment and/or prenatal stress alters expression of key placental genes increasing fetal exposure to cortisol and altering HPA set points, which, in turn, alter the capacity for neuroendocrine and neurobehavioral responses to the postnatal environment. These "acquired" effects could be exacerbated in situations where there is already a genetic predisposition for a mental health disorder such that the added epigenetic effects increase the likelihood that the disorder will reach threshold and be expressed. A more sensitive genotype in the presence of epigenetically induced altered gene expression from prenatal stress puts the infant at greater risk for mental health disorders than a more resistant genotype with the same prenatal stress.

In the model, the larger (distal) postnatal environment in which these altered HPA set points are now expressed can range from "typical," even enriched, to adverse, including the "usual suspects" of poverty, low socioeconomic status, low level of education, poor quality of the home and neighborhood, race and ethnicity, community violence, and others. The more immediate (proximal) postnatal environment involves parenting or "relationship" factors, most notably the goodness of fit of the child with the parenting or caregiving environment.

The goodness of fit concept has its origin in the field of infant temperament (Chess and Thomas 1991) but has broader applicability as a framework to understand developmental processes involving both infant and parent as they dynamically modify each other's behavior through continual positive or negative feedback. A good fit occurs when there is a match between the caregiving environment and the child's capacities (including behavior) that promotes the child's optimal developmental outcome. A poor fit involves a mismatch between child characteristics and the caregiving environment, leading to poorer developmental outcome. For example, infants' cognitive and language development were enhanced when mothers were better able to read their babies' cry signals (Lester et al. 1995). Goodness of fit may explain findings relating HPA reactivity in infants to the quality of the attachment relationship (Gunnar 1994; Spangler and Grossmann 1993) and to face-to-face interaction (Haley and Stansbury 2003). In the model, the goodness of fit between the caregiving environment and the infant's neurobehavior, in the context of the broader distal environment, determines the infant's relative risk for developing mental health disorders. A good match is when the type of parenting provided is compatible with the child's fetally programmed neurobehavior, thus fostering optimal development. In a mismatch, parenting is not suitable for the infant's neurobehavior. The probability of developing mental disorders is increased when an infant's capacities (altered by HPA set points) and the parenting are a mismatch in the context of postnatal environmental adversity. In the context of an adverse distal environment, such as poverty, a good match between the caregiving environment and the infant's neurobehavior would serve as a protective factor.

Environmental-Developmental Perspective

So far in this chapter, we have described how an altered HPA axis and altered behavioral responsivity could lead to child mental health disorders depending on the fit with the postnatal caregiving environment. However, from an evolutionary perspective there may also be adaptive value to these fetally programmed neuroendocrine and behavioral modifications. This understanding comes from the field of evolutionary developmental biology ("evo-devo") and is based on the recognition that gene-environment interactions are ubiquitous and extend to the activation of genetic activity by nongenetic influences. In addition to being agents of heredity, genes are now seen as playing a key role in the organization and regulation of development (Carroll 2005; Hofer 2006). Developmental outcomes are epigenetic, not just genetic, and this is also true as part of the evolutionary process. The view of development within evolutionary biology recognizes that changes in evolution reflect changes in development. In addition to the "traditional" evolutionary processes of random genetic mutation, drift, and recombination that produce phenotypic variation and are acted upon by natural selection, epigenetic processes are now seen as contributing to individual ontogeny and adaptation to the more immediate environment.

One of the evolutionary functions of development is the production of variability in developmental patterns to adapt to environmental change. Developmental interactions play a role in evolution as a source of novel variation such that what becomes maladaptive may depend on the circumstances. For example, rats and monkeys raised in adversity show behavioral and physiological responses similar to those of children raised in poverty and social upheaval (Cameron et al. 2005). Under experimental adversity (frequent separations), mothers become less attentive. Their offspring show maternal behavioral differences, but they also grow up to be fearful with highly reactive adrenocortical responses, and to have increased appetite, depression, cognitive deficits, and rapid sexual maturation. In humans, these behaviors would typically be classified as psychopathological or maladaptive. Strikingly, the animal work shows that these traits are transmitted to the next generation even when the adverse conditions are no longer present. What these behaviors have in common is that they indicate increased behavioral and physiological variability that could increase the chances that a greater number of offspring will adapt and survive in chaotic and threatening situations in future generations. Offspring with "normal" behavior and physiology may be less successful in chaotic and threatening conditions.

Behavior belongs to the class of allostatic systems (McEwen 1998) in which the ability to achieve stability through change is vital for survival. In contrast to homeostatic systems that must be maintained within narrow boundaries, such as blood pH or body temperature, allostatic systems (including the HPA axis) have broader boundaries that enable humans to cope with internal (e.g., infection) and external (e.g., poverty) demands. A narrow behavioral repertoire, which could appear "economical" in the short term by being less negatively affected by postnatal environmental challenges, would, over time, be less adaptable to a wide range of environmental conditions. The sobering thought is that what is labeled as "dysregulated" behavior today could be beneficial in a different environment (Hofer 2006). The increased vigilance and fighting behavior related to cortisol in animal studies could have survival value in hostile environments.

Similarly, although we might be tempted to classify the altered neuroendocrine and behavioral responses in our model as maladaptive, we can also hypothesize that this increased variability could be beneficial for long-term adaptation in more unpredictable environments. Also, how the fetus is reprogrammed in response to an environmental signal obviously depends on the nature of the environmental signal. If the signal is poor nutrition, the reprogramming involves changing the set points of metabolic pathways. In this example, we have the case of a specific insult that triggers specific and directional effects. Our model is different because we are proposing a stress model and the stress signal is nonspecific. In the same way that it makes sense for poor nutrition to affect metabolic pathways, it makes sense for stress signals to affect the stress (HPA) system. However, unlike poor nutrition, in which case the fetus has a specific environment to prepare for, the nonspecific nature of stress may not enable the fetus to prepare for a specific environment. The reprogramming has to enable the fetus to adapt to a wide variety of postnatal environmental conditions—a more unpredictable environment. Thus, rather than altering HPA set points in a specific direction, the alterations would more likely be bidirectional, resulting in increased HPA variability, enabling the fetus to prepare for a more unpredictable postnatal environment and increasing the number of infants who match their postnatal environment.

The infant's responsivity is reprogrammed to allow for a range of predictable environments. The left side of Figure 10–1 shows that there is a very low probability for developing mental health disorders when the infant's responsivity is maximized and there are ample opportunities for matching with parenting behavior in the normal broader postnatal environment. However, as shown on the right side of the figure, the infant's capacities are diminished by a poor fit with the parenting environment and further diminished by environmental adversity, leading to high risk for developing mental health disorders. Epigenetic processes could operate both prenatally and postnatally, affecting behavioral phenotypic expression and the dynamics of this system at the molecular level. A "cost" to this HPA and neurobehavioral reprogramming might be effectiveness in the short term but more rapid wearing down of these systems than would have occurred if the reprogramming had not taken place, perhaps leading to an earlier and/or more pronounced manifestation of mental health disorders (e.g., early onset of substance use).

Of course, this explanation is oversimplified. Different stressors or combinations of stressors will have different effects and multiple effects. Poor nutrition can affect metabolic pathways and also be a stressor. Poor nutrition can affect glucocorticoid regulation of body weight, and stress can affect birth weight. A single insult such as prenatal cocaine exposure could affect the hippocampus directly as a teratogen and can also be a stressor. The total number of stressors may be important, and there may be a threshold for the number of stressors depending, in part, on what they are.

Risk and Protective Factors

Risk and protective factors can be identified at several levels in the model, and most can be acted on by IMH clinicians either individually or within larger systems of care. Prenatal stress factors include a wide array of risks, ranging from a poor reproductive and/or nutritional history to a more immediate event (e.g., maternal ingestion of a teratogen such as cocaine). Prenatal risk factors, alone and in combination, create an at-risk intrauterine environment, setting off the cascade of prenatal events described in the model. Genetic risk factors include more sensitive genotypes with, for example, the single nucleotide polymorphism (SNP) profile related to mental health disorders. Genetic protective factors include the resistant genotype, absent that SNP profile. Developmental timing could be a risk factor if an insult occurs during a critical period. Epigenetic modification of specific fetal tissues can confer both risk and protection.

Although epigenetic changes can be related to negative behavioral outcomes in animal and human models, epigenetics can also be protective through gene expression control. DNA methylation, for example, can offset the effects of a deleterious polymorphism. The fact that epigenetic changes can be reversible and transgenerational suggests not only that protective factors can be "programmed" but also that therapeutic interventions may support such positive changes.

Infant behavior (and later temperament and personality) can be a risk factor or a protective factor and in our model would relate to variability in behavioral responsivity. Although increased behavioral variability could be a risk factor, it may also be adaptive depending on environmental context. The match between infant and parent is a protective factor that is likely important for resilience. Thus, the model's locus of resilience is the upper left quadrant (Figure 10–1), where the child is reared in an adverse environment, but there is a good fit between child behavior and parenting quality and the resulting risk for developing mental health disorders is low.

Populations at Risk

The application of modern biology and the developmental origins perspective has led to the identification of new populations at risk for child mental health disorders, as well as a different understanding or redefinition of populations already known to be at risk. Populations impacted by famine, poor nutrition, poverty, war, sociopolitical policies, or dislocation may require several generations for progeny to recover and to reach their full potential (Harper 2005). Thus, some of the current impacts of risk may actually be fallout from a prior generation, exacerbated by new impacts within the generation and placing the next generation at increasing peril. Behaviors, phenotypes, illnesses, and other traits once thought to be intergenerational or familial nongenetic heritable traits—that is, learned through caregiving and socialization or resulting from lifestyle, exposures, or other experiences—may be epigenetically inheritable or the result of epigenetic modifications induced by nutrition, parenting practices, and other experiences of the fetus, infant, and young child (Belsky 2008; Wakshlak and Weinstock 1990; Whitelaw and Whitelaw 2006).

Conclusion

The potential for epigenetically inheritable or modifiable behavior seems reasonable and forces new consideration of both the origin of traits once thought to be influenced solely by the child's environment and the therapeutic approaches built on these prior understandings. This potential also suggests that new approaches to understanding these mechanisms, their inheritance, and their importance need to be developed and applied, including in the field of behavioral epigenetics. New approaches are of particular importance for IMH providers as therapies, therapeutic strategies, the timing and target of interventions, and the concepts of prevention, promotion, and early intervention are examined through an epigenetic lens. Primary interventions for families deemed to be at risk may need to commence in early pregnancy, perhaps even prior to conception, to promote understanding of the environmental milieu of the fetus related to such issues as maternal stress, intimate partner violence exposure, and maternal mental health, and to monitor other elements of the prenate's environment as judiciously as maternal blood pressure and fetal biophysical indices are followed. Rethinking the concept of traditional therapy is warranted to define and create environmental enrichment therapies that address potential and known epigenetic risks through the active safeguarding of favorable prenatal and postnatal environments, with rapid therapeutic intervention begun when these environments are problematic. Also, such surveillance and action are necessary for the immediate postpartum parent-child interactions, including tactile communications (Sharp et al. 2012), and the global developmental milieu for the child age 0 to 5 years relative to stability, safety, resource aggregates, and caregiver attunement, sensitivity, and interactional congruence as measures of the relative goodness of fit for the child.

KEY POINTS

- Epigenetics is a field of study exploring the ways in which the epigenome affects changes in gene expression by modifying chromosomes without altering DNA sequences. Behavioral epigenetics focuses on the application of epigenetic principles to the study of physiological, genetic, environmental, and developmental mechanisms of behavior.
- Neuroendocrine physiology is unique and vulnerable during intrauterine life, rendering the fetus highly susceptible when exposed to drugs of abuse, nicotine, and high levels of maternal stress hormones.
- Such exposures can alter the hypothalamic-pituitary-adrenal (HPA) axis and neurobehavioral reactivity, predisposing the child to the development of mental health disorders when the adverse intrauterine environment and/or prenatal stress alters expression of key placental genes increasing fetal exposure to cortisol and altering HPA set points. This cascade can negatively alter neuroendocrine and neurobehavioral responses to the postnatal environment. These "acquired" effects could be exacerbated in situations in which there is already a genetic predisposition for a mental health disorder such that the added epigenetic effects increase the likelihood that the disorder will reach threshold and be expressed.
- The fact that epigenetic changes can be reversible and transgenerational suggests not only that protective factors can be "programmed" but that therapeutic interventions may support such positive changes.
- Outcome is not driven by epigenetics alone. Epigenetic processes operate both prenatally and postnatally, affecting behavioral phenotypic expression. One of the greatest predictors of outcome is the goodness of fit between the child's prenatal influences and the broader postnatal environment, including the proximal influence of parenting and the distal influences and resource base within the family, community, and society in general.

References

Alati R, Lawlor DA, Mamun AA, et al: Is there a fetal origin of depression? Evidence from the Mater University Study of Pregnancy and its outcomes. Am J Epidemiol 165:575–582, 2007

Allin M, Rooney M, Cuddy M, et al: Personality in young adults who are born preterm. Pediatrics 117:309–316, 2006

Barker DJ: Mothers, Babies, and Health in Later Life. New York, Churchill Livingstone, 1998

Barker DJ: Fetal programming of coronary heart disease. Trends Endocrinol Metab 13:364–368, 2002

Barker DJ, Osmond C: Low birth weight and hypertension. BMJ 297:134–135, 1988

Barker DJ, Osmond C, Rodin I, et al: Low weight gain in infancy and suicide in adult life. BMJ 311:1203, 1995

Belsky J: War, trauma and children's development: observations from a modern evolutionary perspective. Int J Behav Dev 32:260–271, 2008

Bird A: Perceptions of epigenetics. Nature 447:396–398, 2007

Cameron NM, Champagne FA, Parent C, et al: The programming of individual differences in defensive responses and reproductive strategies in the rat through variations in maternal care. Neurosci Biobehav Rev 29:843–865, 2005

Cannon TD, Rosso IM: Levels of analysis in etiological research on schizophrenia. Dev Psychopathol 14:653–666, 2002

Carroll SB: Endless Forms Most Beautiful: The New Science of Evo-Devo. New York, WW Norton, 2005

Champagne FA, Francis DD, Mar A, et al: Variations in maternal care in the rat as a mediating influence for the effects of environment on development. Physiol Behav 79:359–371, 2003

Chess S, Thomas A: Temperament and the concept of goodness of fit, in Explorations in Temperament: International Perspectives on Theory and Measurement. Edited by Strelau J, Angleitner A. New York, Plenum, 1991, pp 15–28

Cheung YB, Khoo KS, Karlberg J, et al: Association between psychological symptoms in adults and growth in early life: longitudinal follow up study. BMJ 325:749, 2002

Gallou-Kabani C, Junien C: Nutritional epigenomics of metabolic syndrome: new perspective against the epidemic. Diabetes 54:1899–1906, 2005

Gluckman PD, Hanson MA: Developmental origins of disease paradigm: a mechanistic and evolutionary perspective. Pediatr Res 56:311–317, 2004

Gunnar M: Psychoendocrine studies of temperament and stress in early childhood: expanding current models, in Temperament: Individual Differences at the Interface of Biology and Behavior. Edited by Bates J, Wachs TD. Washington, DC, American Psychological Association, 1994, pp 175–198

Hales CN, Barker DJ, Clark PM, et al: Fetal and infant growth and impaired glucose tolerance at age 64. BMJ 303:1019–1022, 1991

Haley DW, Stansbury K: Infant stress and parent responsiveness: regulation of physiology and behavior during still-face and reunion. Child Dev 74:1534–1546, 2003

Harper LV: Epigenetic inheritance and the intergenerational transfer of experience. Psychol Bull 131:340–360, 2005

Hofer MA: Evolutionary basis of adaptation in resilience and vulnerability: response to Cicchetti and Blender. Ann NY Acad Sci 1094:259–262, 2006

Lester BM, Padbury JF: Third pathophysiology of prenatal cocaine exposure. Dev Neurosci 31:23–35, 2009

Lester BM, Boukydis CF, Garcia-Coll CT, et al: Developmental outcome as a function of the goodness of fit between the infant's cry characteristics and the mother's perception of her infant's cry. Pediatrics 4:516–521, 1995

Lester BM, Tronick E, Nestler E, et al: Behavioral epigenetics. Ann NY Acad Sci 1226:14–33, 2011

Lester BM, Marsit CJ, Conradt E, et al: Behavioral epigenetics and the developmental origins of child mental health disorders. J Dev Orig Health Dis 3:395–408, 2012

McEwen BS: Protective and damaging effects of stress mediators. N Engl J Med 3:171–179, 1998

McMillen IC, Robinson JS: Developmental origins of the metabolic syndrome: prediction, plasticity, and programming. Physiol Rev 85:571–633, 2005

Meyer JS: Biochemical effects of corticosteroids on neural tissues. Physiol Rev 65:946–1020, 1985

Padbury JF, Martinez AM: Sympathoadrenal system activity at birth: integration of postnatal adaptation. Semin Perinatol 12:163–172, 1988

Radtke KM, Ruf M, Gunter HM, et al: Transgenerational impact of intimate partner violence on methylation in the promoter of the glucocorticoid receptor. Transl Psychiatry 1:e21, 2011

Sharp H, Pickles A, Meaney M, et al: Frequency of infant stroking reported by mothers moderates the effect of prenatal depression on infant behavioural and physiological outcomes. PLoS One 7:e45446, 2012

Spangler G, Grossmann KE: Biobehavioral organization in securely and insecurely attached infants. Child Dev 64:1439–1450, 1993

Thompson C, Syddall H, Rodin I, et al: Birth weight and the risk of depressive disorder in late life. Br J Psychiatry 179:450–455, 2001

Van Speybroeck L: From epigenesis to epigenetics. The case of C.H. Waddington. Ann NY Acad Sci 981:61–81, 2002

Waddington CH: Organisers and Genes. Cambridge, UK, Cambridge University Press, 1940

Wakshlak A, Weinstock M: Neonatal handling reverses behavioral abnormalities induced in rats by prenatal stress. Physiol Behav 48:289–292, 1990

Waterland RA, Jirtle RL: Transposable elements: targets for early nutritional effects on epigenetic gene regulation. Mol Cell Biol 23:5293–5300, 2003

Weaver IC, Cervoni N, Champagne FA, et al: Epigenetic programming by maternal behavior. Nat Neurosci 7:847–854, 2004

Welberg LA, Seckl JR: Prenatal stress, glucocorticoids and the programming of the brain. J Neuroendocrinol 13:113–128, 2001

Whitelaw NC, Whitelaw E: How lifetimes shape epigenotype within and across generations. Hum Mol Genet 15:R131–R137, 2006

CHAPTER 11

DC:0-3R

A Diagnostic Schema for Infants and Young Children and Their Families

Cherise Northcutt, Ph.D.
Barbara McCarroll, Ph.D.

The Diagnostic Classification of Mental Health and Developmental Disorders of Infancy and Early Childhood: Revised Edition (DC:0-3R; Zero to Three 2005) provides a systematic, developmentally based approach to the classification of mental health and developmental difficulties in the first 4 years of life. It was developed in response to the shortcomings and relative inattention to infants and young children in DSM-IV-TR (American Psychiatric Association 2000) and should continue to fill similar gaps with DSM-5 (American Psychiatric Association 2013). DC:0-3R is a complex, multiaxial schema that integrates findings from different contexts and over time. In addition to focusing on the individual, DC:0-3R places an emphasis on the caregiving relationships. The resulting diagnosis provides a classification of a disorder, not an individual. Clear communication to the family and among service providers is prioritized, and a multimodal intervention is facilitated. Although DC:0-3R was designed to be used with children from birth through age 3 years, most clinicians find the diagnostic classification system useful well into preschool ages.

DC:0-3R addresses the unique challenges of diagnosing mental health conditions in infants and young children; these challenges include the complexity and rapid pace of early childhood development and the central role of the environment and relationships in developmental progress. Other nosological schemes fail to capture the complex interplay between these factors. According to Egger and Emde (2011),

> the goal of a mental health assessment is to make sense of a child's mental health symptoms and the associated factors that include the parent-child relationship, the environmental context, the child's physical and developmental status, acute and chronic stressors, and biolog-

ical features. Understanding the interplay among these factors may begin with a nosological framework, but the domain of classification must be integrated with within-person, relationship-based, and environmental (including family, neighborhood, culture) approaches to understanding the risk for, emergence of, and persistence of impairing emotional, behavioral, and developmental symptoms in disorders of early childhood. (p. 103)

History of DC:0-3

In 1987, Zero to Three: National Center for Infants, Toddlers, and Families established a multidisciplinary task force that was cochaired by Stanley Greenspan and Serena Wieder and included clinicians and researchers from infant mental health centers throughout North America and Europe. The task force, which met for 7 years, was charged with systematically analyzing case reports from participating centers, identifying recurring behavioral problems, and describing categories of disorders, using expert consensus to identify and generate developmentally based descriptive categories of mental health and developmental disorders in infancy and early childhood. The first edition of the classification system, DC:0-3 (Zero to Three 1994), was published in 1994. An update, DC:03R (Zero to Three 2005), was published in 2005 to clarify ambiguities and incorporate new clinical experience and clinical and developmental research.

The American Academy of Child and Adolescent Psychiatry has also recognized the specific challenges in diagnosis with very young children. In 2001–2002, it proposed an addition to DSM-IV-TR, called the Research Diagnostic Criteria—Preschool Age (RDC-PA) (Scheeringa et al. 2002). RDC-PA was developed as a complementary and developmentally sensitive diagnostic system, modifying Axis I of the DSM-IV-TR diagnostic criteria for use with preschool children, age 2 years and older. The age range therefore differs from that covered by DC:0-3 and DC:0-3R, which focus on the first 3 years of life. In addition, the RDC-PA goal—to clearly define criteria to facilitate research on the diagnostic validity of psychiatric disorders in preschool children—differs from the goals of DC:0-3R. Nonetheless, whenever possible, criteria from RDC-PA were incorporated into DC:0-3R. At the same time, an effort was made in DC:0-3R to overcome some of the limitations of other nosologies.

DC:0-3R encourages clinicians to refer to DSM-IV-TR and the International Classification of Diseases (ICD) of the World Health Organization (1977, 1992) when formulating a diagnosis. With the release of DSM-5 (American Psychiatric Association 2013), clinicians are now encouraged to refer to DSM-5 when formulating a diagnosis.

In DSM-5, several changes have been introduced to the diagnostic system. The new system has been changed to a nonaxial organization that is more consistent with other, international diagnostic classifications, such as the ICD system. Disorders in DSM-5 are now arranged in chapters organized by general categories, and the clinician can account for subtypes and symptom severity. In addition, dimensional approaches that cut across available categories support a comprehensive process that serves clinicians, patients, families, and researchers. Another modification provides two options—other specified and unspecified designations—that replace not otherwise specified (NOS) categories and allow flexibility for conditions that do not fulfill diagnostic criteria. Axes I, II, and III from earlier editions of DSM have been combined under clinical diagnostic categories. The earlier Axes IV and V have been included in and combined with DSM-5 clinical disorders, with special notation for psychosocial and contextual factors and for disability. The World Health Organization Disability Assessment Schedule 2.0 (WHODAS 2.0; Üstün et al. 2010) replaces the Global Assessment of Functioning.

Reimbursement and Public Policy Implications

Few states support the DC:0-3R diagnoses for reimbursement. Several of the states that do not reimburse for services on the basis of DC:0-3R diagnoses, including Oklahoma, Arizona, Indiana, and California, have developed "crosswalks" for translating DC:0-3 and DC:0-3R to DSM-IV-TR. These crosswalks were designed to enable reimbursement rather than for clinical purposes (Egger and Emde 2011); they are suggestive rather than prescriptive. Such crosswalks were not designed, however, to be used to go from DSM-IV-TR or ICD-9 (World Health Organization 1977) or ICD-10 (World Health Organization 1992) to DC:0-3R. With the release of DSM-5, these crosswalks will need to be revised. Table 11–1 is a proposed crosswalk to translate DC:0-3R to DSM-5 diagnoses. It provides corresponding DSM-5 diagnostic numeric codes for DC:0-3R clinical disorders and alphanumeric ICD V and Z codes for DC:0-3R Axis II, relationship classification. The latter codes correspond to conditions that may be a focus of attention and may affect diagnosis, course, prognosis, or treatment. The newer Z codes offer greater specificity. For example, a physically abusive relationship classification on DC:0-3 Axis II crosses to DSM-5 child physical abuse with a corresponding ICD-9 V code, as well as ICD-10 Z code options to specify whether the abuse is by a parent or by someone other than the parent (American Psychiatric Association 2013).

The proposed crosswalk not only suggests corresponding diagnoses and codes for reimbursement but also provides a way of describing a child's mental health presentation and the many factors that broaden the clinical picture. It is an application that will continue to adapt to current and available data.

Diagnostic Process

The mutiaxial diagnostic framework organizes information into a comprehensive format. This diagnostic process involves a multidimensional approach that takes into consideration current and historical functioning of the identified child and his or her family. An in-depth assessment follows expressed concerns regarding impairment or deviations from typical in a child's functioning. Although a sign or symptom in a child is often the presenting problem (Axis I), a parent's maladaptive interactions with the child (Axis II) are often viewed as cen-

TABLE 11–1. Crosswalk between DC:0-3R and DSM-5

DC:0-3R disorders: five axial classifications	DSM-5 disorders: nonaxial classifications
Axis I: Clinical disorders	
100 Posttraumatic stress disorder	309.81 Posttraumatic stress disorder
	309.89 Other specified trauma- and stressor-related disorder
	309.9 Unspecified trauma- and stressor-related disorder
150 Deprivation/maltreatment disorder	313.89 Reactive attachment disorder
	313.89 Disinhibited social engagement disorder
200 Disorders of affect	
210 Prolonged bereavement/ grief reaction	309.0 Adjustment disorders, with depressed mood
	309.24 Adjustment disorders, with anxiety
	309.28 Adjustment disorders, with mixed anxiety and depressed mood
	308.3 Acute stress disorder
	311 Unspecified depressive disorder
220 Anxiety disorders of infancy and early childhood	Anxiety disorders
221 Separation anxiety disorder	309.21 Separation anxiety disorder
222 Specific phobia	300.29 Specific phobia
223 Social anxiety disorder (social phobia)	300.23 Social anxiety disorder (social phobia)
224 Generalized anxiety disorder	300.02 Generalized anxiety disorder
225 Anxiety disorder not otherwise specified (NOS)	300.09 Other specified anxiety disorder
	300.00 Unspecified anxiety disorder
230 Depression of infancy and early childhood	Depressive disorders
231 Type I: major depression	296.20 Major depressive disorder, unspecified, single episode
	296.30 Major depressive disorder, unspecified, recurrent episode
232 Type II: depressive disorder NOS	300.4 Persistent depressive disorder (dysthymia)
	311 Other specified depressive disorder
	311 Unspecified depressive disorder

TABLE 11–1. Crosswalk between DC:0-3R and DSM-5 *(continued)*

DC:0-3R disorders: five axial classifications	DSM-5 disorders: nonaxial classifications
Axis I: Clinical disorders (*continued*)	
240　Mixed disorder of emotional expressiveness	296.99　Disruptive mood dysregulation disorder
	300.9　Other specified mental disorder
	300.9　Unspecified mental disorder
300　Adjustment disorder	309.9　Adjustment disorders, unspecified
400　Regulating disorders of sensory processing	
410　Hypersensitive	
411 Type A: Fearful/cautious	300.02　Generalized anxiety disorder
412 Type B: Negative/defiant	313.81　Oppositional defiant disorder
420　Hyposensitive/ underresponsive	314.00　Attention-deficit/hyperactivity disorder, predominantly inattentive presentation
430　Sensory stimulation–seeking/ impulsive	314.01　Attention-deficit/hyperactivity disorder, predominantly hyperactive/ impulsive presentation
	314.01　Attention-deficit/hyperactivity disorder, combined presentation
	313.81　Oppositional defiant disorder
	312.81　Conduct disorder, childhood-onset type
	312.89　Other specified disruptive, impulse-control, and conduct disorder
	312.9　Unspecified disruptive, impulse-control, and conduct disorder
500　Sleep behavior disorder	
510　Sleep-onset disorder (protodyssomnia)	307.42　Insomnia disorder
520　Night-waking disorder (protodyssomnia)	307.46　Non–rapid eye movement sleep arousal disorders, sleepwalking type
	307.47　Nightmare disorder
	307.46　Non–rapid eye movement sleep arousal disorders, sleep terror type
	327.42　Rapid eye movement sleep behavior disorder

TABLE 11–1. Crosswalk between DC:0-3R and DSM-5 *(continued)*

DC:0-3R disorders: five axial classifications	DSM-5 disorders: nonaxial classifications

Axis I: Clinical disorders (*continued*)

600 Feeding behavior disorder	Feeding and eating disorders
	307.52 Pica
	307.53 Rumination disorder
601 Feeding disorder of state regulation	307.59 Other specified feeding or eating disorder
	307.50 Unspecified feeding or eating disorder
602 Feeding disorder of caregiver-infant reciprocity	307.59 Other specified feeding or eating disorder
	307.50 Unspecified feeding or eating disorder
603 Infant anorexia	307.59 Avoidant/restrictive food intake disorder
604 Sensory food aversions	307.59 Avoidant/restrictive food intake disorder
605 Feeding disorder associated with concurrent medical condition	307.59 Other specified feeding or eating disorder
	307.50 Unspecified feeding or eating disorder
606 Feeding disorder associated with insults to the gastrointestinal tract	307.59 Other specified feeding or eating disorder
700 Disorders of relating and communicating	315.8 Other specified neurodevelopmental disorder
	315.9 Unspecified neurodevelopmental disorder
710 Multisystem developmental disorder	299.00 Autism spectrum disorder
	315.8 Other specified neurodevelopmental disorder
	315.9 Unspecified neurodevelopmental disorder
800 Other disorders	300.9 Other specified mental disorder
	300.9 Unspecified mental disorder
	DSM-5 and ICD-10 psychiatric diagnoses if criteria met

TABLE 11–1. **Crosswalk between DC:0-3R and DSM-5** *(continued)*

DC:0-3R disorders: five axial classifications	DSM-5 disorders: nonaxial classifications
Axis II: Relationship classification	V codes correspond to ICD-9
Overinvolved	V61.20 Parent–child relational problem
	V61.8 High expressed emotion level within family
Underinvolved	V61.20 Parent–child relational problem
	V61.21 Child neglect
	V61.22 Child neglect by parent
	V62.83 Nonparental child neglect
Anxious/tense	V61.20 Parent–child relational problem
	V61.21 Child psychological abuse
	V61.22 Child psychological abuse by parent
	V62.83 Nonparental child psychological abuse
	V61.29 Child affected by parental relationship distress
Angry/hostile	V61.20 Parent–child relational problem
	V61.21 Child psychological abuse
	V61.22 Child psychological abuse by parent
	V62.83 Nonparental child psychological abuse
	V61.8 High expressed emotional level within family
	V61.29 Child affected by parental relationship distress
Verbally abusive	V61.20 Parent–child relational problem
	V61.21 Child psychological abuse
	V61.22 Child psychological abuse by parent
	V62.83 Nonparental child psychological abuse

TABLE 11–1. Crosswalk between DC:0-3R and DSM-5 *(continued)*

DC:0-3R disorders: five axial classifications	DSM-5 disorders: nonaxial classifications
Axis II: Relationship classification *(continued)*	
Physically abusive	V61.20 Parent-child relational problem
	V61.21 Child physical abuse
	V61.22 Child physical abuse by parent
	V62.83 Nonparental child physical abuse
Sexually abusive	V61.20 Parent-child relational problem
	V61.21 Child sexual abuse
	V61.22 Child sexual abuse by parent
	V62.83 Nonparental child sexual abuse
Parent-Infant Relationship Global Assessment Scale (PIR-GAS) (1–100) Documented maltreatment (1–10) to well adapted (91–100)	
Axis III: Medical and developmental disorders and conditions	
DSM-5 and ICD-10 nonpsychiatric diagnoses	Included in and combined with DSM-5 clinical disorders
Classifications used by physical and occupational therapists, speech and language pathologists, special educators, and other primary health care providers	315.8 Global developmental delay
	Intellectual disability (intellectual developmental disorder)
	317 Mild
	318.0 Moderate
	318.1 Severe
	318.2 Profound
	319 Unspecified intellectual disability (intellectual developmental disorder)
	315.39 Language disorder
	315.39 Speech sound disorder
	315.35 Childhood-onset fluency disorder (stuttering)
	315.39 Social (pragmatic) communication disorder

TABLE 11–1. Crosswalk between DC:0-3R and DSM-5 *(continued)*

DC:0-3R disorders: five axial classifications	DSM-5 disorders: nonaxial classifications
Axis III: Medical and developmental disorders and conditions (*continued*)	
	307.9 Unspecified communication disorder
	315 Specific learning disorder
	315.4 Developmental coordination disorder
	307.3 Stereotypic movement disorder
	307.23 Tourette's disorder
	307.22 Persistent (chronic) motor or vocal tic disorder
	307.21 Provisional tic disorder
	307.20 Other specified tic disorder
	307.20 Unspecified tic disorder
Axis IV: Psychosocial stressors	
Psychosocial and Environmental Stressor Checklist with type, onset, and severity	Included in and combined with DSM-5 clinical disorders *with special notation for psychosocial and contextual factors*
Axis V: Emotional and social functioning	
Capacities for Emotional and Social Functioning Rating Scale	Included in and combined with DSM-5 clinical disorders *with special notation for disability*
• Attention and regulation	
• Forming relationships/mutual engagement	plus
• Intentional two-way communication	World Health Organization Disability Assessment Schedule 2.0 (WHODAS 2.0), *modified for children*
• Complex gestures and problem solving	
• Use of symbols to express thoughts/ feelings	
• Connecting symbols logically/ abstract thinking	

tral to such presenting problems. Presenting problems, temperament, developmental progression, family dynamics, community, and culture are all considered. The recommended process is to be ongoing, flexible, and dynamic, necessitating modification as new data are considered. Multiple observations in typical settings are conducted over time (Lieberman et al. 1997) to evaluate a child's relational capacities and those of significant caregivers. Information is gathered from family members, nonfamily care providers, medical records, community support agencies, educators, and other relevant individuals. Thus, clinical formulation and treatment planning rely on information from multiple sources. The overall goal of the diagnostic process is a thorough investigation that leads to interventions to facilitate adaptive functioning of the child and family; these interventions can be carried out by a single discipline, individual clinicians, or interdisciplinary teams.

There are two core aspects to the diagnostic process: the assessment of the child and family and the classification of the disorders. Although the classification of the disorders may facilitate clear communication among professionals about descriptive syndromes, treatment plans and interventions are based on as complete an understanding of the child and the child's relationships as possible. Even when pressed for time, clinicians need to take into account all relevant areas of the child's functioning while conducting a complete diagnostic assessment. DC:0-3R recommends a minimum of three to five sessions to complete a comprehensive assessment. Sessions should involve obtaining a developmental history; direct observations of family functioning, family and parent dynamics, caregiver-child relationships, and interaction patterns; direct observation of and reports about the child's individual characteristics, language, cognition, and affective expression; and assessment of sensory reactivity and processing, motor tone, and motor planning. These are integrated to develop an understanding of the child's strengths and challenges, level of overall adaptive patterns, and capacities and functioning in the major areas of development; an understanding of the relative contribution of the different areas assessed to the child's overall competencies and challenges; and a comprehensive treatment or preventive intervention plan. Findings are summarized on the five axes, with Axes I, II, and III dealing with the classification of disorders and Axes IV and V reflecting the assessment of individuals in context.

Overview of the DC:0-3R Axes

Multiaxial classification systems have gained wide acceptance and provide a common language for infant mental health practitioners in a variety of collaborating disciplines, such as medicine, psychology, social work, and education. Academicians, theorists, and researchers use data accumulated in these schemata for research and theory development. In addition, the developing brains, cognitive levels, and emotional and relational abilities of young children require a classification system that is sensitive to the wide variations of evolving abilities and needs. Therefore, these systems need to encompass complexity and are most useful when used flexibly and dynamically. Axes II and IV of both DC:0-3 (Zero to Three 1994) and DC:0-3R (Zero to Three 2005) demonstrate sensitivity to the specificity of this young population. The DC:0-3R axes are detailed below. A comprehensive account is available in the DC:0-3R manual (Zero to Three 2005).

Axis I: Clinical Disorders

Axis I provides a classification of the prominent features of children's impairments and functioning. Table 11–2 lists the categories of Axis I clinical disorders.

TABLE 11–2. DC:0-3R Axis I: clinical disorders

100	Posttraumatic stress disorder
150	Deprivation/maltreatment disorder
200	Disorders of affect
210	Prolonged bereavement/grief reaction
220	Anxiety disorders of infancy and early childhood
240	Mixed disorder of emotional expressiveness
300	Adjustment disorder
400	Regulatory disorders of sensory processing
410	Hypersensitive
420	Hyposensitive/underresponsive
430	Sensory stimulation–seeking/impulsive
500	Sleep behavior disorder
510	Sleep-onset disorder (protodyssomnia)
520	Night-waking disorder (protodyssomnia)
600	Feeding behavior disorder
700	Disorders of relating and communicating
710	Multisystem developmental disorder
800	Other disorders

Source.   Zero to Three 2005.

Axis II: Relationship Classification

The dependency of infants and young children on their caretakers is not restricted to the provision of basic physical or even emotional needs. Emotional functioning, regulatory capacities, and relational abilities are developed in the context of the relationship with the primary caretaker, who is usually the parent. Axis II describes the quality and patterns of child-parent/caregiver relationships and identifies the affective tone of the connection and psychological involvement of the identified caretaker. Classification is specific to a relationship and describes the interactions between the child and the parent/caregiver. Assessment considers the following aspects of the relationship dynamic: overall functional level of both the child and the parent/caregiver; level of distress in both the child and the parent/caregiver; level of conflict and resolution between the child and the parent/caregiver; and effect of the quality of the relationship on the child's developmental progress. Maladaptive qualities in this axis include overinvolved, underinvolved, anxious/tense, angry/hostile, verbally abusive, physically abusive, and sexually abusive patterns. Impairment in an important relationship can derail development in one or several domains. It is the relationship that deserves the first line of intervention and the relationship that can provide the most effective repair.

Axis III: Medical and Developmental Disorders and Conditions

Physical and developmental diagnoses using other diagnostic classification systems are noted on Axis III. This axis includes specific classifications used by speech/language pathologists, occupational therapists, physical therapists, special educators, health care providers, and other primary health care providers.

Axis IV: Psychosocial Stressors

Axis IV provides a framework for identifying and evaluating psychosocial and environmental stressors that may influence the presentation, course, treatment, and prevention of mental health difficulties in infants and young children. These stressors might include challenges to a child's primary support group, social environment, and educational and child care; the family's housing, economic and occupational situation, and health care access; legal or criminal justice challenges; and the health of the child. The severity and duration of the stressors are also noted.

Axis V: Emotional and Social Functioning

Observations of interactions between a child and significant caregivers yield information about the child's social and emotional functioning. The child's dynamic interaction patterns with important caregivers are influenced by the child's constitutional-maturational patterns, caregivers, family, community, and culture (Interdisciplinary Council on Developmental and Learning Disorders 2005). A developmentally based relational approach is essential to the classification of the mental health of infants and young children.

Listed below are the categories for emotional and social functioning that are rated on the DC:0–3R Capacities for Emotional and Social Functioning Rating Scale (Zero to Three 2005):

1. Attention and regulation (typically observable beginning between birth and age 3 months)
2. Forming relationships/mutual engagement (typically observable beginning between ages 3 and 6 months)
3. Intentional two-way communication (typically observable beginning between ages 4 and 10 months)
4. Complex gestures and problem solving (typically observable beginning between ages 10 and 18 months)
5. Use of symbols to express thoughts/feelings (typically observable beginning between ages 18 and 30 months)
6. Connecting symbols logically/abstract thinking (typically observable beginning between ages 30 and 48 months)

The instrument provides a summary of the child's highest level of functioning at home and in other settings, using the following 6-point scale:

1. Functions at an age-appropriate level under all conditions and with a full range of affect states
2. Functions at an age-appropriate level, but is vulnerable to stress or has a constricted range of affect or both
3. Functions immaturely (i.e., has the capacity, but not at an age-appropriate level)
4. Functions inconsistently or intermittently unless special structure or sensorimotor support is available
5. Barely evidences this capacity, even with support
6. Has not achieved this capacity

Diagnostic Guidelines and Diagnostic Tools

DC:0-3R recognizes that for some infants and young children, more than one diagnostic classification may be appropriate. To assist with the diagnostic process, DC:0-3R provides guidelines for prioritizing and identifying Axis I diagnoses. Eleven guidelines are delineated and need to be reviewed prior to completing the diagnostic process.

Several tools have been developed to assist in the diagnostic process and for recording diagnostic information. Wright and Northcutt (2004), in consultation with Zero to Three and the DC:0-3R Training Task Force, mapped out the DC:0-3R diagnostic guidelines for Axes I, II, and V on flowcharts. The Relationship Problems Checklist (RPCL) and the Parent-Infant Relationship Global Assessment Scale (PIR-GAS) are used to assist with Axis II. PIR-GAS allows for a judgment about the relationship classification under consideration, whereas RPCL can assist clinicians in documenting problems or lack of problems in a relationship. The Psychosocial and Environmental Stressor Checklist is used to assist with Axis IV; this checklist provides a framework for identifying sources of stress experienced by the young child and noting the duration and severity. The Capacities for Emotional and Social Functioning Rating Scale is used to assist with Axis V; a child's overall pattern of emotional and social functioning can be summarized using this scale. All of these instruments are available on the Zero to Three Web site (www.zerotothree.org).

Case Example

The following case demonstrates the use of DC:0-3R diagnostic guidelines and tools to develop goals and interventions for a child.

> Poppy, an 18-month-old female Hispanic toddler, had been enrolled at a therapeutic child care center for a year when the staff expressed concern about her flat affect, narrow range of emotional expression, and sense of despair observed during encounters with her 27-year-old mother, Jen. Poppy and Jen lived in a homeless shelter, and Jen was attending a drug and alcohol recovery program. Poppy's father was serving a 6-month sentence for domestic violence and drug offenses. Poppy was born at 40 weeks' gestation with no complications. Med-

ical records reported asthma from age 1 month, and center staff noted recent frequent wheezing episodes. The toddler had experienced a significant period of developmental gain following enrollment and regular attendance at the therapeutic center, her mother's participation in recovery, and relational repair efforts. Ongoing multidisciplinary support of Poppy and her mother continued to scaffold the family through successes and failures.

Observations of the child and her relationships with her mother, her peers, and her teachers had been ongoing during her enrollment at the center. Poppy had been screened every 6 months using the Ages and Stages Questionnaire, 3rd Edition (ASQ-3; Squires and Bricker 2009), which can be used to monitor children from ages 2 to 60 months; five domains of functioning—communication, gross motor, fine motor, problem solving, and personal social—are screened to help identify children who are at risk for developmental delays. The enrollment ASQ-3, conducted in collaboration with Jen, had yielded weak communication scores, consistent with the mother's reports. However, between ages 8 and 17 months, Poppy's receptive and expressive skills had strengthened. All other developmental scores were consistently within normal limits. Poppy's mother had been attending her treatment program, and parent-child exchanges appeared mutually satisfying. Although Jen had lost custody of three older children, Jen was determined to be a good mother to her youngest daughter. Overall, Poppy had developed social and emotional competence appropriate for her age, and teachers described the toddler as being skillful at making her needs and intentions known. In the classroom, Poppy engaged in age-appropriate parallel and reciprocal play among peers, and mutual enjoyment was observed.

By age 12 months, the toddler was using vocalizations and nonverbal cues such as eye contact to ask for help to reach toys, request more food, and settle peer disputes. As her language skills grew, Poppy used two- and three-word sentences to ask for individual time with the psychologist. She said "Go walk" when she wanted to carry out the ritual of settling a baby doll in a stroller, walking the stroller outdoors, and periodically stopping to tend to the imagined needs of the doll. Each stop included nonverbal bids for mutual engagement. The outings, with the psychologist, routinely ended with Poppy laughing and squealing back to the center. Jen was able to join the walks at times, and on those occasions Poppy coached her mother on the routine activities that she had cocreated. Mother and child eventually began their own walks and developed new rituals together.

However, some difficulties emerged. Teachers described concerns about changes in Poppy's emotional life when she was age 17 months. Sad facial expressions were seen, smiles seemed effortful, and little joy was expressed during play. At mealtime, she seemed disconnected from the group and often stared outside. She seemed to find no enjoyment in food, and teachers noted an automatic quality to her playing and eating behaviors. Poppy's preferred teacher reported a regression in the toddler's language skills and changes in parent-child interactions. During separation and reunion with her mother, Poppy displayed a flat weary expression and ignored her mother's presence. Her mother often appeared preoccupied and disconnected from her child. Jen reported that Poppy would bang her head when angry, and Jen asked staff for help with discipline. She also said that she had relapsed and had not been attending her recovery program regularly. She acknowledged that she gave Poppy a bottle and put her in front of the television when she arrived home. Jen was being medicated for depression and felt overwhelmed by her recovery efforts, homelessness, and financial concerns.

In addition to having substance abuse histories, both of Poppy's parents reported being physically and emotionally abused as children. Jen was raised by a single mother who abused cocaine and lived with a variety of men during Jen's childhood. Poppy's parents frequently engaged in domestic violence, to which Poppy was exposed for the brief time the parents were together. Both parents were incarcerated during Poppy's early months, and she spent her first 2 months in foster care. Her father was in custody and unavailable for much of Poppy's life. This amalgam of these severe chronic stressors impinged on her social and emotional developmental progression.

Although other clinical disorders were considered during the assessment process, the DC:0-3R classification Type II: depressive disorder NOS was determined to be the best fit at the time of the assessment. Both posttraumatic stress disorder and deprivation/maltreatment disorder were discussed, but not enough supporting data were found.

From the diagnostic impressions of Poppy's case, summarized in Table 11–3, the staff developed a treatment plan for Poppy. The treatment plan was created with the intention of maintaining flexibility and making modifications when appropriate. The goals and interventions are listed below.

Goals

1. **Target clinical disorder (Axis I):** Reduce Poppy's depressed mood symptoms and her disengagement from and lack of interest in playing and eating.
2. **Target relationship disorder (Axis II):** Poppy avoided engagement with her mother and was minimally interactive with secondary caretakers. The relationships with caretakers were a focus. a) Maintain positive attachments to primary caregivers. Increase connectedness and engagement with Poppy through increasing the mother's responsiveness to Poppy's cues. b) Support the mother's relational capacities and increase her ability to take pleasure in interactions with Poppy.
3. **Target psychosocial and environmental stressors (Axis IV):** Jen reported a relapse in her recovery, which jeopardized her bids for housing and financial support. In addition, she had neglected her weekly sessions with her psychotherapist. Support the mother's recovery and make referrals for assistance with housing, financial, and mental health needs.
4. **Target emotional and social functioning (Axis V):** Poppy's previously gained social-emotional competence and her communication gains in particular had regressed. Coach the mother on ways to play with Poppy to support her skills and increase her social-emotional capacities.

Interventions

1. Staff psychologist provided daily infant psychotherapy.
2. Center staff provided parent-child psychotherapy at the center and in the home to enhance Poppy and her mother's relationship and interactions.
3. Early care educators ensured that stable, predictable routines were maintained in the child care center to reduce Poppy's distressful symptomatology. They also worked with the mother to assist her in developing stable, predictable routines at home to reduce Poppy's distress.

TABLE 11–3. Poppy's case: summary of history and observations

Axis	DC:0-3R diagnosis	Criteria indicators
I Clinical disorders	232. Type II: depressive disorder not otherwise specified	Depressed mood most of the day more days than not Diminished pleasure in play Difficulty responding to caregivers
II Relationship classification	Disordered: underinvolved, substantial evidence; Parent–Infant Relationship Global Assessment Scale score of 39	Maladaptive stressful parent-child interactions with dissociative features in child Mother disconnected from child Developmental regression in child's language
III Medical and developmental disorders and conditions	Asthma	Medical diagnosis
IV Psychosocial stressors	Multiple psychosocial stressors	Foster care, domestic violence, neglect, parental separation, parental mental illness and substance abuse, single parenting, multiple moves, economic challenges, unemployment, Child protective services involvement, parental incarceration
V Emotional and social functioning	Complex gestures and problem solving and emergent use of symbols to express thoughts and feelings	Functions with age-level capacities that are vulnerable to stress and with constricted affect

4. All center staff provided support for the mother and her recovery.
5. Center staff, community health assistants, social workers, and public health nurses linked the mother to appropriate resources and agencies to address psychosocial needs.

DC:0-3R: Considerations for the Future

The DC:0–3R task force recommends continued study and refinement of the classification system. Three proposed revisions are currently being considered for possible inclusion: a new axis focusing on the family and two new diagnoses for Axis I, disruptive behavior disorder and excessive crying disorder. The proposed new Axis VI, the family axis, would require information gathering and documentation of three areas: family history of mental illness, family structure and available supports, and family culture. With regard to disruptive behavior disorder, the problem for the task force is to distinguish developmentally appropriate, relatively normative, and transient levels of disruptive behaviors from early emerging symptoms of what may become differentiated patterns of disruptive behavior disorders later in childhood. For excessive crying disorder, the task force recommends a longitudinal, developmentally informed study.

Overall, there is an interest in understanding the general conditions under which the early, undifferentiated forms of distress seen in infancy and early childhood develop. Currently, knowledge of the specifics of symptomatology that emerges from birth to 24 months is limited. Clinically focused longitudinal studies of infants are needed that utilize more refined measures in order to understand this symptomatology. Such data would further understanding of infants and young children and help refine this classification system.

Another future consideration is a chronic stress disorder classification diagnosis that reflects the impact of chronic stress on infants and young children. A child living in chronically unsettled conditions experiences recurring stress that interferes with the ability to develop an organized strategy to cope with stress and regulate emotion. The stress would be viewed in the context of the child's individual characteristics and the parents' ability to provide a sense of safety in the relationship and help the child regulate emotion. In conjunction with unpredictable, inconsistent, and disorganized conditions, a chronic stress diagnosis would require signs and symptoms such as disturbances of mood, arousal, attention, regulation, biological rhythms, developmental progression, and relational capacities. Examples of chronically stressful conditions include parental substance abuse, mental health conditions, and protective services involvement, among others. The parent is likely to be impaired when overwhelmed or in distress and be unavailable to help the child regulate emotions and even to witness the child's everyday achievements. The experience of enduring chaos and stress may be one that the child cannot resolve, because paradoxically the parent is a source of fear and anxiety as well as the only haven of safety.

An additional consideration for the future is a provision for quantification of Axis IV items. A list of items relevant to the population of a therapeutic center has been selected from the DC:0–3R Psychosocial and Environmental Stressor Checklist as part of biannual assessments of infants and young children. For each item, there is a rating that corresponds to the severity of the stressor. The ratings are totaled and a score is assigned.

Conclusion

DC:0–3R offers a systematic, developmentally based approach to the classification of mental health and developmental difficulties during a child's first 4 years of life. The goal of the assessment and diagnostic process is to obtain a thorough understanding of the child in the context of the family and use a common language to summarize information. Findings from a comprehensive assessment are summarized in DC:0–3R on five axes, with Axes I, II, and III dealing with the classification of disorders, and Axes IV and V reflecting the assessment of individuals in context. This combination is intended to provide an integrative assessment and generate a well-informed, comprehensive treatment or preventive intervention plan.

KEY POINTS

- The Diagnostic Classification of Mental Health and Developmental Disorders of Infancy and Early Childhood: Revised Edition (DC:0-3R), provides a systematic, developmentally based approach to the classification of mental health and developmental difficulties in the first 4 years of life.
- DC:0-3R addresses the unique challenges of diagnosing mental health conditions in infants and young children, including the complexity and rapid pace of early childhood development and the central role of the environment and relationships in developmental progress.
- The multiaxial diagnostic framework organizes the findings from a comprehensive assessment on five axes: Axis I, clinical diagnosis; Axis II, relationship classification; Axis III, medical and developmental disorders and conditions; Axis IV, psychosocial (and environmental) stressors; and Axis V, emotional and social functioning.
- The clinician should review codes to assist in assigning appropriate codes required for reimbursement, thereby enhancing the availability of treatment for infants and young children.

References

American Psychiatric Association: Diagnostic and Statistical Manual of Mental Disorders, 4th Edition, Text Revision. Washington, DC, American Psychiatric Association, 2000

American Psychiatric Association: Diagnostic and Statistical Manual of Mental Disorders, 5th Edition. Washington, DC, American Psychiatric Association, 2013

Egger HL, Emde RN: Developmentally sensitive diagnostic criteria for mental health disorders in early childhood: the Diagnostic and Statistical Manual of Mental Disorders–IV, the Research Diagnostic Criteria—Preschool Age, and the Diagnostic Classification of Mental Health and Developmental Disorders of Infancy and Early Childhood—Revised. Am Psychol 66:95–106, 2011

Interdisciplinary Council on Developmental and Learning Disorders: Diagnostic Manual for Infancy and Early Childhood. Bethesda, MD, Interdisciplinary Council on Developmental and Learning Disorders, 2005

Lieberman AF, Wieder S, Fenichel E (eds): The DC:0-3 Casebook: A Guide to the Use of Zero to Three's Diagnostic Classification of Mental Health and Developmental Disorders of Infancy and Early Childhood in Assessment and Treatment Planning. Washington, DC, Zero to Three, 1997

Scheeringa M, Anders T, Boris N, et al: Research Diagnostic Criteria—Preschool Age (RDC-PA). August 17, 2002. Available at: http://www.infantinstitute.com/WebRDC-PA.pdf. Accessed March 29, 2013.

Squires J, Bricker D: Ages and Stages Questionnaires: A Parent-Completed Child-Monitoring System, 3rd Edition (ASQ-3). Baltimore, MD, Paul H Brookes 2009

Ustün TB, Chatterji S, Kostanjsek N, et al: Developing the World Health Organization Disability Assessment Schedule 2.0. Bull World Health Organ 88:815–823, 2010

World Health Organization: International Classification of Diseases, 9th Revision. Geneva, World Health Organization, 1977

World Health Organization: International Statistical Classification of Diseases and Related Health Problems, 10th Revision. Geneva, World Health Organization, 1992

Wright C, Northcutt C: Schematic decision trees for DC:0-3. Infant Ment Health J 25:171–174, 2004

Zero to Three: Diagnostic Classification of Mental Health and Developmental Disorders of Infancy and Early Childhood (DC:0-3). Washington, DC, Zero to Three, 1994

Zero to Three: Diagnostic Classification of Mental Health and Developmental Disorders of Infancy and Early Childhood: Revised Edition (DC:0-3R). Washington, DC, Zero to Three, 2005

CHAPTER 12

Fussy Babies

Early Challenges in Regulation, Impact on the Dyad and Family, and Longer-Term Implications

Larry Gray, M.D.

All babies cry; however, some cry more than others. Excessive crying can frustrate parents and pediatric caregivers. Parents often worry about the reasons for this crying and about their ability to console their crying child. In fact, excessive crying is one of the most common presenting complaints for which pediatric medical care is sought (Wade and Kilgour 2001). The purpose of this chapter is to focus on the challenge of excessive infant crying, review prevailing theories and current treatments, and highlight a recent approach that embraces the complexity of excessive and persistent infant crying.

The infant's first cry, a sign of physical robustness and health, is universally welcomed in the birthing environment. After the initial cry, which has immediate physiological benefits, crying primarily communicates to the mother or primary caregiver(s) the infant's basic survival needs. A hunger cry signals the need for nutrition and can even stimulate breast milk letdown before feeding ensues. A pain cry signals the need for immediate external intervention and has the distinct qualities of higher pitch, increased tenseness, and longer duration (Craig et al. 2000). Perhaps relating to survival fitness, most mothers reliably identify their own infant's hunger or pain cries (Abraham 1981). Attachment theorists have emphasized that in addition to signaling basic physical needs, infant crying results in caregiving routines that privilege close physical contact to the mother and form relationship patterns that are believed to lead to later secure attachment relationships (Bowlby 1958).

Normal and Excessive Crying

Although the amount of early infant crying individually varies, a consistent pattern of early infant crying has been identified. Called the "normal crying curve" (Barr 1990), the time infants spend crying progressively increases until it peaks at age 6–8 weeks, then gradually decreases until about age 4 months. This pattern includes a clustering of crying in the evening hours, most notably at the peak weeks of crying, and has been demonstrated despite different cultural caregiving practices (Barr et al. 1991). The mean duration for crying during this peak period is around 2 hours per day. The conventional standard for excessive infant crying has traditionally been the parent's report of total crying that surpasses 3 hours per day for more than 3 days in any 1 week (Wessel et al. 1954). In Western cultures, the prevalence of parents reporting early crying at this level ranges from 8% to 40%, depending largely on the definition used (Reijneveld et al. 2001), but 20% seems to be the most consistently reported prevalence rate (Wurmser et al. 2001).

Excessive crying is not the same thing as colic, but both share the core symptom of high levels of crying. Colic, by definition, is excessive crying plus additional features in a baby who is otherwise "healthy and well fed" (Wessel et al. 1954). The defining behavioral features of colic are 1) inconsolability (despite adequate parenting); 2) crying that begins and ends without warning; 3) a high-pitched quality to the cry; and 4) clenched fists, flexed legs, grimacing, or distended abdomen. The presence or absence of these cardinal features helps the clinician distinguish colic from excessive crying (Lester et al. 1990). These features may also cause concerned parents and medical providers to worry that the infant is in pain (Gudmundsson 2010) or has a serious medical condition (Poole 1991).

Causes of Excessive Crying

An interesting paradox exists regarding the origin and mechanisms of excessive crying in infants. Because an infant's cry typically precipitates an immediate response from the environment, the origin of this excessive crying has been viewed as "external" to the infant and as generated by nutritional inadequacy or physical separation from caregiving (Bowlby 1958). However, because excessive crying is also "paroxysmal" and persists despite increased caregiving, it also has been assumed to be caused by "internal" or "organic" causes.

Parents are concerned by the excessive and paradoxical nature of crying and accordingly use increased multiple health care services (McCallum et al. 2011). When excessive crying is not accompanied by additional features of high-pitched crying, arching of the back, regurgitation, vomiting, or diarrhea, the crying is unlikely to be caused by organic pathology (Lehtonen et al. 2000). Using these criteria, Gormally and Barr (1997) estimate that only 5%–10% of all excessively crying babies have a treatable medical or organic problem. Despite this low percentage, all infants require a thorough pediatric physical examination to rule out any painful cause for their crying. The differential diagnosis for colic is extensive (Reust and Blake 2000); however, the majority of causes of extensive crying are identified by a thorough history and physical examination, not laboratory testing (Freedman et al. 2009). Repeated examinations are often required to increase the sensitivity of the diagnostic process and can provide additional reassurance to parents that an identifiable and hence treatable cause for the crying does or does not exist.

When excessive crying is identified, the most common treatable causes include a cow's milk protein allergy, gastroesophageal reflux, and, in rare cases, a serious infection. Because the cause of excessive crying is seldom clear, families often try multiple treatments simultaneously to increase the odds of finding an effective treatment. Double-blind randomized controlled trials (RCTs) and meta-analytic systematic reviews have been advocated as the best indicators of effective treatments for excessive crying. In a recent systematic review, Hall et al. (2012) report that replacement of cow's milk protein with a hypoallergenic formula, maternal dietary restriction of milk products if breast-feeding, and reducing behavioral stimulation of the infant are effective in decreasing crying, with small to moderate effect sizes. These authors also reported that the anticholinergic pharmacological agent dicyclomine hydrochloride has been found effective, but its side effects (including death) clearly contraindicate its use.

Over the past two decades, gastroesophageal reflux and gastroesophageal reflux disease have been increasingly implicated as causes of excessive crying. The clinical diagnosis of reflux is complicated because a majority of babies "spit up" on a daily basis, and this may overlap with the natural increase in age-related crying or be a symptom of reflux. For most infants, however, this spitting up is "physiological" reflux and resolves on its own by age 1 year (Nelson et al. 1997). The increased number of infants diagnosed on clinical grounds with "reflux" may be related to hesitancy on the clinician's or parents' part to subject the infant to the invasive nature of the diagnostic testing for gastroesophageal reflux disease (pH monitoring or endoscopy) and to the ease of prescribing the now widely available acid-suppressing agents for infants and young children. This diagnostic trend parallels a 16-fold increase in use of antireflux medication for children between 1999 and 2006 and $13 billion in 2005 annual sales (Hassall 2012). To add to the clinician's dilemma, two expert pediatric gastroenterology consensus statements argue that gastroesophageal reflux disease is not a cause of excessive crying in the first months of life (Sherman et al. 2009; Vandenplas et al. 2009), and proton pump inhibitors are not indicated for treatment of excessive crying (van der Pol et al. 2011). Moreover, an RCT involving 103 infants age 9 months with persistent crying and mild reflux symptoms compared antireflux medication, placebo, and a maternal infant mental health consultation and found no differences among the three groups in crying reduction (Jordan et al. 2006).

This research represents the paradigm shift that is occurring in the theoretical and clinical treatment of the crying infant. The once-favored reductionistic and biomedical perspective is giving way to a systemic or family-centered approach (Douglas and Hiscock 2010). This new perspective counters the "shotgun" approach of covering all the known effective treatments in every case, and at the same time does not overlook common medical conditions. This family-centered perspective also embraces the complexity of excessive infant crying during the first 3 months and the potential for multiple presentations of persistent infant crying after the early months have passed. In the next section, we explore risks related to excessive and persistent crying. The recognition and severity of these risks have fueled the field to find a new perspective to address the adverse risks associated with early infant crying. These risks include shaken baby syndrome, also known as abusive head trauma; family stress; parental depression; parent-infant relationship distress; and behavioral and developmental problems.

Risks Associated With Excessive Crying
Abuse

A troubling association exists between excessive infant crying and shaken baby syndrome, now more commonly called abusive head trauma (AHT). Colic crying was first mentioned as a risk factor for shaken baby syndrome or child abuse in the classic 1987 article "Seven Deadly Sins of Childhood: Advising Parents About Difficult Developmental Phases" (Schmitt 1987). Using hospital discharge data from infants with AHT, Barr et al. (2006) demonstrated that the rate of AHT cases resembled the normal infant crying curve. The curves were similar in onset (at ages 2–3 weeks), had a clear peak (with AHT hospitalizations peaking 4–6 weeks after the typical crying curve peak), and declined by age 9 months. In addition, Barr and colleagues—using data from the National Center on Shaken Baby Syndrome—found that 28% of the AHT cases mentioned crying as the stimulus for the shaking episode (Lee et al. 2007). The recognition of crying as a trigger for abuse underscores the importance of preventive efforts to help families cope with the challenges of excessive crying.

Family Stress and Parental Depression

Parents report that having a baby who cries excessively disrupts almost all aspects of their lives and makes them feel that they are living "close to the edge" (Long and Johnson 2001). In focus groups conducted by Bayat et al. (cited in Gilkerson et al. 2005), parents shared that they were emotionally and physically exhausted ("No one said it would be this hard"); they felt isolated and criticized and often withdrew from their support systems ("When my mother-in-law said, 'I don't know what you're talking about, that baby is fine,' I thought I'm just going to stop talking [to her] about it"); they searched for the cause of crying and for what would help ("I tried everything. I'm still trying"); and they lost confidence in themselves ("I didn't want to be the parent I was turning into") and their baby ("It's supposed to be bliss. I'm just wishing [his] infancy away"). Given the frequency of uninvited advice and criticism, parents value nonjudgmental support ("Anyone who listened, helped") (Bayat et al., cited in Gilkerson et al. 2005, pp. 36–37) and want to have their experience validated by people who believe them and accept their reality ("I wanted someone to see what was going on and then recognize how awful it was for me") (Long and Johnson 2001, p. 159).

Mothers of excessively crying infants report higher parenting stress or stress around crying (Humphry and Hock 1989; Wake et al. 2006). In fact, from the prepartum to the postpartum period, distress levels increase for parents of excessively crying infants but decrease for parents of typically crying infants (Miller et al 1993). Families with excessively crying infants are at higher risk for parental anxiety, family conflict, and conflict between parenting partners (Papoušek and von Hofacker 1998; Räihä et al. 1995). Some evidence indicates that parenting stress may continue for years after the excessive crying has ended (DeGangi et al. 2000; Papoušek and von Hofacker 1998; Stifter 2001). Maxted et al. (2005) found that 45.2% of mothers who sought help for infant crying from an outpatient colic clinic reported moderate to severe symptoms of depression; however, the severity of depression was not related to the degree of colic symptoms. When there was co-occurrence of high maternal depression and intense crying symptoms, Maxted et al. found that all other areas of infant, parent, and family functioning were affected. There is increasing evidence that it is the parent's perception of the crying as problematic, rather than the actual amount of crying, that predicts maternal stress or maternal depression (Pauli-Pott et al. 2000), paternal depression (Katch 2012), or later behavioral problems (MacKenzie and McDonough 2009). In this broader view of excessive crying, it is important to consider the subjective meaning of the crying to the parent, rather than solely relying on the baby's behavior as a predictor of parental distress.

Parent-Infant Relationship Distress

Given the increased stress on the mother and overload on the family system, excessive infant crying can cause distress in the parent-infant relationship. Papoušek (2000) describes a cycle wherein the parent's psychobiologically attuned intuitive competence and coregulatory capacity can be thrown off by the persistent alarm state evoked by the infant's crying, and defines a clinical syndrome of excessive crying characterized by a triad of interacting parent-infant symptoms: 1) the infant's inconsolable crying with sleep-wake organization problems, 2) the parents' overload and psychosocial distress, and 3) frequent interactional failure that maintains or exacerbates the behavioral problems. Interestingly, Ziegler et al. (2004) found that the periods of parent-infant dysregulation, which they called "vicious cycles of negative reciprocity," occurred mainly when the parent was trying to help the infant with soothing or sleeping, not at other times. These authors emphasize the loss of pleasure in the relationship and the absence of "relaxed dialogue" between parent and infant: "The parents may do everything they can to soothe their infant, but are rendered silent in their attempts at dialogue and interaction with him" (Ziegler et al. 2004, p. 104). MacKenzie and McDonough (2009) question the concept of a fussy baby separate from the influence of the parent-infant relationship and highlight the importance of understanding the meaning of the infant's crying to the quality of the relationship.

Developmental and Behavioral Problems

Parents and professionals ask if excessive crying is predictive of later developmental or behavioral difficulties. The research is divided about this question, with some studies showing a relationship between persistent crying in early infancy and later behavior and development, and other studies showing no such relationship. Several studies tracked cognitive development in infants with excessive crying and found no differences between early cry and noncry groups at ages 12–18 months (Rautava et al. 1995; Stifter and Braungart 1992). Other research, however, suggests an association between persistent crying and long-term differences in later child behavior or development. Rao et al. (2004) reported that infants who showed prolonged average daily crying beyond age 12 weeks were at significant risk for cognitive problems at age 5 years. Wurmser et al. (2004/2008) found that in a clinical population of infants whose parents had sought help from the Munich Interdisciplinary Research and Intervention Program for Fussy Babies, the infants were still seen at 30 months as more difficult and stubborn and had more emotional and behavioral problems than a contrast group. Wolke et al. (2002) followed infants referred for crying problems at age 2 months until they were ages 8–10 years. Nearly half (48%) were still persistent criers at age 6 months and had significantly more externalizing problems in childhood; they had greater hyperactivity and conduct problems, had more negative emotionality, were more difficult and demanding, and were less adaptable than children who were not persistent criers in infancy (Wolke et al. 2002). DeSantis et al. (2004) found that a greater amount of time fussing at age 12 weeks was connected with a significantly higher incidence of sensory processing, coping, and behavioral/attention difficulties at ages 3–8 years. In a meta-analysis of 22 longitudinal studies involving children with crying, feeding, or sleeping problems (i.e., regulatory problems), Hemmi et al. (2011) found that children with previous crying problems have more later behavioral problems than do children with no similar history. A history of crying problems led to the highest effect sizes for general behavioral problems, externalizing behaviors, internalizing behaviors, and attention-deficit/hyperactivity disorder. Young children who had experienced excessive crying and who had numerous adverse risk factors—defined as social adversities, a depressed mother, or a negative family environment—showed more behavioral problems over time compared with children with excessive crying who did not have such experiences (Hemmi et al. 2011).

Although more research is needed on the long-term impact of excessive crying on a child's behavior and development, the current clinical understanding is that early infant crying may not be a time-limited factor confined to the early months, particularly when multiple family and environmental factors are present. Interventions to address the complexity of interacting infant, family, and contextual factors may be needed to prevent or ameliorate later behavioral or developmental problems.

Addressing the Complexity of Infant Crying

Given the multifaceted nature of early infant crying, a range of primary and secondary prevention and intervention services should be widely available to offer families support, address risk, and promote healthy infant and family development. In primary care, physicians and other health care providers can follow the Bright Futures recommendations from the American Academy of Pediatrics (http://brightfutures.aap.org) and ask parents about their infant's crying and how the parents are coping with the crying. The Touchpoints Model of Development offers pediatricians and other infant and family professionals guidance around partnering with families during stressful times when the child's development, such as infant crying, produces disruptions in the family system (Brazelton and Sparrow 2006; see www.brazeltontouchpoints.org/programs/professional-development). Also, delivery hospitals and primary care can incorporate primary prevention programs, such as Period of PURPLE Crying (Barr et al. 2009), to inform parents about normal infant crying, risks associated with crying, and strategies to use when they feel at the end of their rope. Models of collaborative care can be developed to address crying concerns. In an RCT, Salisbury et al. (2012) showed that faster improvement of excessive infant crying resulted from an outpatient family–based biopsychosocial treatment consisting of a developmental pediatrician combined with an early childhood mental health professional than from standard pediatric outpatient care. Primary care can be linked to infant mental health services for referrals for parent-infant psychotherapy to address relationship concerns as well as to early intervention for emerging developmental delays and/or disabilities.

Erikson Institute's Fussy Baby Network

Since 2003, we have offered a community-based, universally available, secondary prevention program, Fussy Baby Network (FBN), for any family in the Chicago area struggling with an infant's crying, sleeping, or feeding issues during the baby's first year of life (Gilkerson et al. 2005). Developed at Erikson Institute, FBN maintains a dual focus on helping parents in the "here and now" moment with their urgent concerns about their baby while building longer-term parenting capacities of confidence and competence in meeting their infant's needs. Now a national model, FBN has affiliate sites in 10 states and is funded to infuse its approach through FBN Advanced Trainings into two other evidence-based national home visiting models: Healthy Families America and Healthy Steps for Young Children.

FBN responds immediately to parents through Warmline telephone support and home visits within 24–48 hours of the first contact. Parents find out about the program from their pediatrician, the FBN Web site, or other parent-focused advertising. The length and intensity of service are decided with the parent, but assistance is typically short term (four to eight contacts). Infant mental health specialists with backgrounds in social work, counseling, and occupational therapy provide services. Developmental and behavioral pediatricians from the University of Chicago Comer Children's Hospital provide weekly team consultation and staff an FBN clinic as needed to offer infant assessment and parent consultation. Because of the complexity of concerns, FBN can serve as a portal of entry to longer-term services for the infant, parents, or family.

Core Intervention Processes

The FBN approach addresses the parents' urgent concerns using five core intervention processes, which were chosen to promote longer-term parenting capacities. The approach is referred to as FAN, because the visual representation of the core processes resembles a fan (Figure 12–1; Gilkerson 2010).

The outer rim of the FAN presents the essence of each core process in one word: feeling, calming, thinking, doing, and reflecting. *Empathic inquiry* is offered for support around parents' feelings about their baby and about themselves as parents; *mindful self-regulation* helps the visitor stay fully present and calm during engagement with the parent and baby; *collaborative exploration* involves joining with parents in developing a shared understanding of the baby, including the parents' perceptions of the baby; *capacity building* is used to help parents strengthen their confidence and competence in caring for their baby; and *integration* serves to help parents build reflective capacity and a coherent narrative around a stressful experience (for a more detailed description of the FAN approach, see Gilkerson 2009; Gilkerson et al. 2012). Using the FAN approach, the visitor reads parental cues and matches the core processes to what the parents are showing they most need and can make use of in the moment: If a parent is expressing feelings (verbally or nonverbally), then empathic inquiry is offered. If a parent's affect is more contained and he or she wants to understand the baby, then collaborative exploration is used. If the parent is focused on the baby and wants to try something, or if the baby begins to do what the parent is most concerned about, then capacity building is offered.

Arc of the Visit

To help bring a sense of coherence and containment, the visits typically follow an arc, beginning with empathic inquiry, an invitation for parents to share what it has been like *for them* to take care of their baby. In the middle, the visitor asks if the visit is getting to what the parents most hoped would be addressed. At the end, the visitor allows time for parents to reflect about their child (describe their baby in three words) and about what has been most meaningful to them (e.g., by asking, "We have talked about so many important things. I'm wondering if there is something you would like to remember or hold on to that would be helpful to you in the next week").

Matching Core Processes to Needs in the Moment

Outside of the arc questions, there is no specific order for the processes. The visits flow based on what the parents are showing they can use in the moment. A visit, for example, might focus only on emotional support of the parent, as with Beth, a single working mother who called the Warmline after she yelled at her baby. She said, "I'm calling you before I call the adoption agency. I can't do this anymore." She used the home visitor's empathic support over multiple visits to explore her feelings of loss, anger, and shame, having tried for years to have a baby through in vitro fertilization and now wishing that she could give her baby away. As the visitor consistently and empathically understood and accepted her contradictory feel-

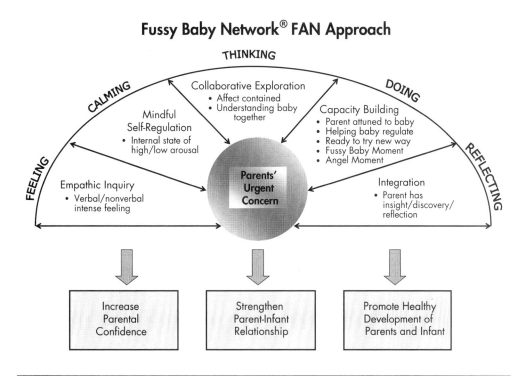

FIGURE 12–1. Fussy Baby Network FAN approach.

Source. Copyright Gilkerson 2010 Erikson Institute Fussy Baby Network.

ings, Beth could begin to integrate the intense and conflicting emotions she often experienced about herself and her baby.

In a contrasting example, multiple core processes were used during one home visit to address the changing concerns. Maria called the Warmline for help with her 5-week-old daughter who would not stop crying and was not sleeping. This was a one-time, 2½-hour visit during which Maria shared that she feared her baby had autism because she had not seen her smile, she did not know how to calm her daughter like her mother did, and she could not tell if her baby was hungry. She reported, "I just feed her whenever she cries." The visit included many moments of empathic inquiry around the mother's overwhelming anxiety and feelings of depression, which, the home visitor learned, began in pregnancy. Mindful self-regulation helped the home visitor slow herself down so she could stay calm and not escalate with the mother's anxiety. Collaborative exploration was used to help find a focus for the visit, which the mother identified as the feeding concern. Capacity building was used at three different points after the baby awoke. First was when the baby woke crying and Maria's doubt set it: "I think she's hungry but I don't know." To help access Maria's intuitive competence, the visitor stated, "She's doing something that makes you feel she's hungry. What are you noticing?" and explored and affirmed the mother's observations. Then, Maria began to share that she could not calm her baby like her mother, who swaddled the baby so expertly. The visitor used the "here and now" moment to ask Maria if she would like to try swaddling her infant. Maria responded excitedly and, with gentle coaching, successfully swaddled her baby herself. Her little girl responded by becoming completely calm and smiling at her mother, who exclaimed, "I've never seen her like this! She smiles. Is that a smile? A real smile?" Maria's anxiety dissolved for a moment and she became calm, lying on the floor looking at her baby and savoring her smiles. During this moment of shared pleasure, the visitor was quiet, protecting the moment for the parent and baby while sharing and affirming it. As more smiles came, Maria said, "I can do this. That was easy. I can do it again!" At the end of the visit, she described her baby as "adorable, hungry, and observant." Among the various things that she and her home visitor had discussed, Maria most wanted to remember that talking to someone helped her understand her baby a little bit better.

Although these descriptions provide a general sense of the FBN approach, the work is entirely individualized. For many families, the short-term intervention is enough to reduce stress and build resilience through coping well with a challenging situation. For other families, in which parental mental health concerns, other contextual factors, and/or infant health or development issues are pressing, FBN serves as a portal of entry to more intensive intervention.

Conclusion

This brief review captures the complexity of early infant crying and the need to expand on the traditional pediatric perspective of the time-limited, benign nature of early crying, after medical problems are ruled out. DeSantis et al. (2004) clearly summarize the current understanding of infant crying: "Spontaneous resolution may occur…, but depending on the intensity, duration, and environmental context, recent research suggests that excessive crying in early infancy may represent a marker of concern for both the child and the family system" (DeSantis et al. 2004, p. 524). We propose that pediatricians and other care providers seeing families with young infants adopt a broader approach for understanding early infant crying that embraces the full spectrum of possibilities, including, but not limited to, medical problems that may contribute to infant crying, heightened parental stress around normal infant crying, parent-infant relationship distress related to mutually interacting infant and parent factors, and emerging infant neurodevelopmental and regulatory differences. Often, these concerns overlap and are quite dynamic in nature. By prematurely closing off one possible contributor, one can oversimplify the complexity of the system and miss potential opportunities to help. The new rule is to support and follow the infant and family until the crying issue has resolved or until further concerns are identified and addressed through a process of listening, observing, differentiating needs, and offering interventions or referrals. The overarching guideline for this infant mental health approach to excessive crying is to maintain an empathic, nonblaming stance toward parents while 1) seeking to understand their experience of the baby, 2) offering supportive collaborative exploration into the causes of the infant's crying and their own distress, and 3) helping them build their parenting capacities to support their infant no matter what the etiology of the crying.

KEY POINTS

- All babies cry, some more than others. Excessive crying is one of the most common presenting complaints for which early pediatric medical care is sought. A troubling association exists between excessive infant crying and shaken baby syndrome (now often called abusive head trauma).

- Increasing evidence suggests that the parent's perception of the crying as problematic, not the actual amount of crying, may predict maternal stress or maternal depression, paternal depression, or later behavioral problems.

- Although more research is needed on the long-term impact of excessive crying on a child's behavior and development, the current clinical understanding is that early infant crying may not be limited to the early months. Interventions to address the complexity of interacting infant, family, and contextual elements may be needed to prevent or ameliorate later behavioral or developmental problems.

- Models of collaborative transdisciplinary care should be available everywhere to address problematic crying concerns quickly and comprehensively, and can include pediatric primary care providers, developmental and behavioral pediatricians, infant and early childhood mental health professionals of all disciplines, psychotherapists, nurses, social workers, early care providers, and early interventionists to appropriately and jointly address the needs of the parents, the child, the family, and the parent-child relationship.

- Erikson Institute's Fussy Baby Network is an innovative model of care that can be replicated in communities everywhere. The approach addresses the parents' urgent concerns about their infant's crying using five core intervention processes that were chosen to promote longer-term parenting capacities: empathic inquiry, mindful self-regulation, collaborative exploration, capacity building, and integration.

References

Abraham S: Mothers' and non-mothers' identification of infant cries. Infant Behav Dev 4:37–40, 1981

Barr RG: The normal crying curve: what do we really know? Dev Med Child Neurol 32:356–362, 1990

Barr RG, Konner R, Bakeman M, et al: Crying in !Kung San infants: a test of the cultural specificity hypothesis. Dev Med Child Neurol 33:601–610, 1991

Barr RG, Trent RB, Cross J: Age-related incidence curve of hospitalized shaken baby syndrome cases: convergent evidence for crying as a trigger to shaking. Child Abuse Negl 30:7–16, 2006

Barr RG, Rivara FP, Barr M, et al: Effectiveness of educational materials designed to change knowledge and behaviors regarding crying and shaken-baby syndrome in mothers of newborns: a randomized, controlled trial. Pediatrics 123:972–980, 2009

Bowlby J: The nature of the child's tie to his mother. Int J Psychoanal 39:350–373, 1958

Brazelton TB, Sparrow J: Touchpoints: Birth to Three. Boston, MA, Perseus, 2006

Craig K, Gilbert-MacLeod C, Lilley CM: Crying as an indicator of pain in infants, in Crying as a Sign, a Symptom, and a Signal: Clinical, Emotional, and Developmental Aspects of Infant and Toddler Crying. Edited by Barr RG, Green JA, Hopkins B. London, MacKeith Press, 2000, pp 23–40

DeGangi GA, Breinbauer C, Roosevelt JD, et al: Prediction of childhood problems at three years in children experiencing disorders of regulation during infancy. Infant Ment Health J 3:156–175, 2000

DeSantis A, Coster W, Bigsby R, et al: Colic and fussing in infancy, and sensory processing at 3 to 8 years of age. Infant Ment Health J 25:522–539, 2004

Douglas PS, Hiscock H: The unsettled baby: crying out for an integrated, multidisciplinary primary care approach. Med J Aust 193:533–536, 2010

Freedman SB, Al-Harthy N, Thull-Freedman J: The crying infant: diagnostic testing and frequency of serious underlying disease. Pediatrics 123:841–848, 2009

Gilkerson L: Fussy Baby Network Core Intervention Processes. Chicago, IL, Erikson Institute, 2009

Gilkerson L: Fussy Baby Network FAN Approach. Chicago, IL, Erikson Institute, 2010

Gilkerson L, Gray L, Mork N: Fussy babies, worried parents and a new support network. Zero Three 25:34–41, 2005

Gilkerson L, Hofherr J, Steier A, et al: Implementing the Fussy Baby Network approach. Zero Three 33:59–65, 2012

Gormally S, Barr RG: Of clinical pies and clinical clues: proposal for a clinical approach to complaints of early crying and colic. Ambulatory Child Health 3:137–153, 1997

Gudmundsson G: Infantile colic: is a pain syndrome. Med Hypotheses 75:528–529, 2010

Hall B, Chesters J, Robinson A: Infantile colic: a systematic review of medical and conventional therapies. J Paediatr Child Health 48:128–137, 2012

Hassall E: Over-prescription of acid-suppressing medications in infants: how it came about, why it's wrong, and what to do about it. J Pediatr 160:193–198, 2012

Hemmi MH, Wolke D, Schneider S: Associations between problems with crying, sleeping and/or feeding in infancy and long-term behavioural outcomes in childhood: a meta-analysis. Arch Dis Child 96:622–629, 2011

Humphry RA, Hock E: Infants with colic: a study of maternal stress and anxiety. Infant Ment Health J 10:263–272, 1989

Jordan B, Heine RG, Meehan M, et al: Effect of antireflux medication, placebo, and infant mental health intervention on persistent crying: a randomized clinical trial. J Paediatr Child Health 42:49–58, 2006

Katch LE: The relationship between infant crying and father well-being. Unpublished doctoral dissertation, Loyola University, Chicago, IL, 2012

Lee C, Barr RG, Catherine N, et al: Age-related incidence of publicly reported shaken baby syndrome cases: is crying a trigger for shaking? J Dev Behav Ped 4:288–293, 2007

Lehtonen L, Gormally SG, Barr RG: Clinical pies for etiology and outcome in infants presenting with early increased crying, in Crying as a Sign, a Symptom, and a Signal: Clinical, Emotional, and Developmental Aspects of Infant and Toddler Crying. Edited by Barr RG, Green JA, Hopkins B. London, MacKeith Press, 2000, pp 67–95

Lester B, Boukydis CZ, Garcia-Coll CT, et al: Colic for developmentalists. Infant Ment Health J 11:321–333, 1990

Long T, Johnson T: Coping with excessive crying. J Adv Nurs 32:155–162, 2001

MacKenzie J, McDonough SC: Transactions between perception and reality: maternal beliefs and infant regulatory behavior, in The Transactional Model of Development: How Children and Contexts Shape Each Other. Edited by Sameroff A. Washington, DC, American Psychological Association, 2009, pp 35–54

Maxted AE, Dickstein S, Miller-Loncar C, et al: Infant colic and maternal depression. Infant Ment Health J 26:56–68, 2005

McCallum SM, Rowe HJ, Gurrin L, et al: Unsettled infant behaviour and health service use: a cross-sectional community survey in Melbourne, Australia. J Paediatr Child Health 47:818–823, 2011

Miller A, Barr R, Eaton W: Crying and motor behavior of six-week-old infants and postpartum maternal mood. Pediatrics 92:551–558, 1993

Nelson SP, Chen EH, Syniar GM, et al: Prevalence of symptoms of gastroesophageal reflux during infancy: a pediatric practice–based survey. Arch Pediatr Adolesc Med 151:569–572, 1997

Papoušek M: Persistent crying, parenting and infant mental health, in WAIHM Handbook of Infant Mental Health, Vol 4. Edited by Osofsky JD, Fitzgerald HE. New York, Wiley, 2000, pp 419–447

Papoušek M, von Hofacker N: Persistent crying in early infancy: a non-trivial condition of risk for the developing mother-infant relationship. Child Care Health Dev 24:395–424, 1998

Pauli-Pott U, Mertesacker B, Bade U, et al: Contexts of relations of infant negative emotionality to caregiver's reactivity/sensitivity. Infant Behav Dev 23:23–29, 2000

Poole SP: The infant with acute, unexplained, excessive crying. Pediatrics 3:450–455, 1991

Räihä H, Lehtonen L, Korvenranta H: Family context of infantile colic. Infant Ment Health J 16:206–217, 1995

Rao MR, Brenner RA, Schisterman EF, et al: Long term cognitive development in children with prolonged crying. Arch Dis Child 89:989–992, 2004

Rautava P, Lehtonen L, Helenius H, et al: Infantile colic: child and family three years later. Pediatrics 96:3–47, 1995

Reijneveld SA, Brugman E, Hirasing RA: Excessive infant crying: the impact of varying definitions. Pediatrics 108:893–897, 2001

Reust CE, Blake RL: Diagnostic workup before diagnosing colic. Arch Fam Med 9:282–283, 2000

Salisbury AL, High P, Twomey JE, et al: A randomized control trial of integrated care for families managing infant colic. Infant Ment Health J 33:110–122, 2012

Schmitt BD: Seven deadly sins of childhood: advising parents about difficult developmental phases. Child Abuse Negl 11:421–432, 1987

Sherman P, Hassall E, Fagundes-Neto U, et al: A global, evidence-based consensus on the definition of gastroesophageal reflux disease in the pediatric population. Am J Gastroenterol 104:1278–1295, 2009

Stifter CA: "Life" after unexplained crying: child and parent outcomes, in New Evidence on Unexplained Early Infant Crying: Its Origins, Nature, and Management. Edited by Barr RG, St. James-Roberts I, Keefe MR. Skillman, NJ, Johnson & Johnson Pediatric Institute, 2001, pp 273–288

Stifter CA, Braungart J: Infant colic: a transient condition with no apparent effects. J Appl Dev Psychol 13:447–462, 1992

Vandenplas Y, Rudolph CD, Di Lorenzo C, et al: Pediatric gastroesophageal reflux clinical practice guidelines: joint recommendations of the North American Society for Pediatric Gastroenterology, Hepatology, and Nutrition (NASPGHAN) and the European Society for Pediatric Gastroenterology, Hepatology, and Nutrition (ESPGHAN). J Pediatr Gastroenterol Nutr 49:498–547, 2009 van der Pol RJ, Smits MJ, van Wijk RP, et al: Efficacy of proton-pump inhibitors in children with gastroesophageal reflux disease: a systematic review. Pediatrics 5:925–935, 2011

Wade S, Kilgour T: Extracts from "clinical evidence": infantile colic. BMJ 323:437–440, 2001

Wake M, Morton-Allen E, Poulakis Z, et al: Prevalence, stability, and outcomes of cry-fuss and sleep problems in the first 2 years of life: prospective community-based study. Pediatrics 117:836–842, 2006

Wessel MA, Cobb JC, Jackson EB, et al: Paroxysmal fussing in infancy, sometimes called "colic." Pediatrics 14:421–434, 1954

Wolke D, Rizzo P, Woods S: Persistent infant crying and hyperactivity problems in middle childhood. Pediatrics 109:1054–1060, 2002

Wurmser H, Laubereau B, Hermann M, et al: Excessive infant crying: often not confined to the first 3 months of age. Early Hum Dev 64:1–6, 2001

Wurmser H, Papoušek M, von Hofacker N: Long-term risks of persistent excessive crying in infants (2004), in Disorders of Behavioral and Emotional Regulation in the First Years of Life: Early Risks and Intervention in the Developing Parent-Infant Relationship. Edited by Papoušek M, Schieche M, Wurmser H. Translated by Kronenberg K. Washington, DC, Zero to Three, 2008, pp 273–298

Ziegler M, Wollwerth de Chuquisengo R, Papoušek M: Excessive crying in infancy, in Disorders of Behavioral and Emotional Regulation in the First Years of Life. Edited by Papoušek M, Schieche M, Wurmser H. Washington, DC, Zero to Three, 2004, pp 85–116

CHAPTER 13

Developmental and Dyadic Implications of Challenges With Sensory Processing, Physical Functioning, and Sensory-Based Self-Regulation

Marie E. Anzalone, Sc.D., O.T.R./L., F.A.O.T.A.

Margaret Ritchey, M.A., R.P.T., D.P.T.

Sensory input is omnipresent. People are constantly receiving input from the environment, relating it to prior experiences, and using it to learn about and interact with the environment—and to use their bodies. A primal merging of the sensory system and the motor system begins in utero and continues throughout life. However, at birth the sensory-motor system is potentiated by the social-relational component. The sensory-motor system invites people into social interaction, and social interaction enhances sensory-motor development.

Sensory integration, a process first described by A. Jean Ayres (1972), an occupational therapist, is one way to understand how humans organize and use sensation. It also provides a way of understanding the challenges faced as individuals interact with their physical and social environments. Of particular interest is the development of this process in infants and young children. Sensory integration theory is a brain-behavior theory, first applied to school-age children by occupational therapists but now widely used with children of all ages. Discussion of the hypothesized neurobiological basis of sensory integration is beyond the scope of this chapter; interested readers can find more information elsewhere (Bundy et al. 2002; Lane and Schaaf 2010). The intent of this chapter is to consider 1) ways in which sensory processing and physical functioning impact the infant-parent relationship; 2) the unique opportunities for the occupational therapist and physical therapist to support dyadic relationships and therapeutically address dyadic functioning in their work; and 3) ways in which all infant mental health clinicians, regardless of discipline, can enhance their dyadic work by incorporating sensory processing, self-regulation, and physical functioning observations and concepts into their encounters with families. Appreciating these opportunities is vital given that challenges with sensory processing, physical functioning, and regulation can be construed as mental health conditions, complicate or exacerbate existing mental health challenges, and/or disrupt dyadic functioning.

Sensory integration theory provides a way of understanding individual differences that derives from the ways in which sensory information from various modalities is used within physical and social environments. Sensory integration is a temperament-related process and one of the ways in which individual differences in personality can be understood (Fox and Polak 2004). While all aspects of the sensory integrative process can contribute to dyadic interaction and mental health, the one most often identified as problematic in young children is the initial step: *sensory registration* (DeSantis et al. 2004).

Kim, born at 34 weeks gestational age, is now 22 weeks adjusted age (28 weeks since birth minus the 6 weeks that she arrived prior to her due date). She is being seen in occupational therapy with her mother, Carol. Carol is asked to play with Kim as she typically would. During play, Carol brings her face close to Kim and engages in animated "motherese" with exaggerated facial expressions, frequently touching Kim on the face and trunk, and eventually picking her up and swinging her. Although most babies would enjoy this kind of sensory-motor play, Kim does not seem to be enjoying it. As Carol increases the sensory yield of her activities, Kim becomes more distressed and irritable; her state of arousal is labile, rapidly cycling between a stressed active alert state to drowsy, with no quiet alert availability present.

When Carol is asked to just be present for her baby but not to interact with her, the situation changes significantly. As soon as Carol becomes quiet and still, Kim brightens up and brings her hands to the midline and to her mouth. She quickly downregulates from crying into a quiet alert state and begins to make excellent eye contact with Carol, eventually breaking into a smile and cooing. Carol seems to have difficulty remaining still, but then she begins to smile, hides her face, and exhibits ambivalent emotions about the social engagement she is seeing in Kim. This is very different from Kim's typical behavior.

After a few minutes of remaining still, Carol begins to play again. She immediately brings her face closer to Kim's (visual looming) and begins talking to her in high-frequency baby talk. Kim remains in quiet alert state momentarily; she looks away briefly but then brings her hands to the midline and kicks as if to calm herself down, then returns to look at her mother. Carol interprets Kim's looking away as a cue to increase the intensity of sensory input that she is providing to Kim in order to reengage Kim's attention. She brings her face closer and talks with greater intensity and volume. She begins to touch and move Kim in her infant seat. As the sensory input increases, the self-regulation and engagement apparent during the quiet play begin to disappear. Kim is now crying again and unable to soothe herself. Carol looks to the therapist, confused. She cannot figure out why her baby was available when she was not playing with her but becomes upset when she does. It seems to her that Kim does not like her or even need her. She describes Kim as a very "independent" baby who does better when left alone. When Kim's behavior is viewed from a sensory integrative perspective, a very different way of interpreting this dyadic interaction becomes apparent.

Kim tends to overregister sensory input provided in the course of typical sensory play. The messages she is giving her mother are confusing and do not seem to make sense to this new mom. Kim is easily overwhelmed by the sensory input from her mother and as a result is fussy, inattentive, and unable to participate in social play. If this session is typical for them, their interactions can lead to continued stressful dyadic interactions and developmental challenges for both mother and baby—and their relationship—as layers of meaning making and interactional patterns are created in the baby and the mother, and embedded in their ways of being together.

In this chapter, we explore ways in which developmental, sensory processing, physical functioning, and self-regulatory challenges can be understood, and how they can enhance or perturb social-emotional development, dyadic functioning, and core infant-parent mental health. A useful construct for inclusion of sensorimotor awareness into mental health assessment can be derived from the description by Zero to Three (2002) of infant mental health as the developing capacity of infants to experience, regulate, and express emotions; to form close and secure interpersonal relationships; and to explore their environment and learn. This construct provides a natural collaborative foundation for transdisciplinary infant mental health work informed by sensory-motor development professionals (e.g., physical and occupational therapists) as they work to foster developmental and dyadic functioning.

Among the first to integrate these concepts into infant mental health were DeGangi and colleagues (1991). Their focus on the regulatory or sensory affective disorders was later integrated into the *Diagnostic Classification of Mental Health and Developmental Disorders of Infancy and Early Childhood* (DC:0-3 and DC:0-3R; Zero to Three 1994, 2005). The challenge is to understand the contribution of somatic factors, such as motor capacity and sensory processing, to the regulatory processes essential for forming relationships and exploring the environment. The infant-parent relationship, core infant-parent mental health, regulatory processes, and sensory-motor function are inextricably linked in that they develop simultaneously and are expressed together. Somatic factors are the mechanisms through which children take in the information that prompts interaction, and the mechanisms through which the interaction is expressed. An important consideration is how challenges in somatic processing and expression influence dyadic interaction.

Sensory Integration

Sensory integration is the organization of sensory information for use. First developed by Ayres (1972), the theory of sensory integration 1) helps describe and explain individual differences in humans, 2) is a way of conceptualizing dysfunction in children, and 3) supports a method of intervention. In this chapter, we focus primarily on the first two components of the theory (Ayres 1972). All individuals take in and experience sensation while interacting with their environment. The way they do this varies widely, but the process consists of four basic steps: intake, attention, interpretation, and using the input expressed as an end product (Figure 13–1).

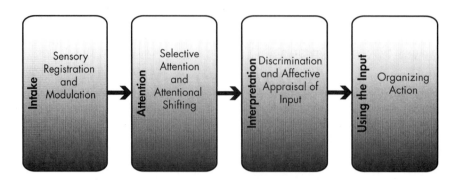

FIGURE 13–1. The four-step process of sensory integration.

The first step, *intake,* involves the initial registration of the sensory event and modulating, or grading, of reaction and response to sensory events occurring in the environment. The second step, *attention,* involves selective attention to events in the foreground while ignoring irrelevant background stimuli, as well as shifting the focus between and within sensory modalities. The third step, *interpretation,* is the most cognitive and affective component. From the perspective of this chapter, the affective appraisal inherent in this step is dependent on the intake step and is central to the formation of adaptive dyadic interactions. Finally, the fourth step involves *using the sensory input.* Use of sensation is variable and can be expressed in the range of end products from motor to cognitive, including behavioral self-regulation, motor coordination and action, and cognitive processing and learning.

Properties of Sensation

Before discussing sensory processing in more detail and presenting a taxonomy of dysfunction in sensory processing disorder, we focus a bit more on what is known about sensation (Kandel et al. 2000). The most obvious way to describe sensation is in terms of *sensory modalities.* Of particular import in sensory integration theory are the somatic senses: vestibular, tactile, and proprioceptive. Proprioceptive input is a type of sensation that is often overlooked, but it is particularly important in the sensory integrative process. Proprioception is sensory input from the muscles and joints that is generated during active movement. For example, sensory input is a major factor that contributes to the effects of exercise, which include neuromuscular and cardiovascular effects, influences on energy, behavioral organization, and even improved mood and attention.

In addition to sensory modalities, one must also consider the *intensity* of the input. Tactile input is a useful example: Touch your arm very lightly and very firmly. For most people, light touch is much more intense than firm touch. Also, a touch to the palm or face is more intense than a touch on the back of the hand. Intensity is also influenced by whether the sensory input is self-generated or imposed. If imposed, it is perceived as more intense than if it is self-generated. In self-generated touch, some sensory input is generated by the movement itself, and the resulting feedback has a modulating influence on the sensory yield (think about tickling yourself vs. being tickled by somebody else). Perceived intensity is highly subjective. What one person considers to be intense may be perceived very differently by another. This speaks to the fact that a parent may intend a touch to be calming or nurturing, but how it will actually be perceived by the child cannot be predicted.

The final property of sensation that should be considered is *duration*. It is important to recognize that the absolute duration of the stimulus within the environment is not the same as the effect of that stimulus within the child's central nervous system. Sensory input is best understood in a summative framework (Kandel et al. 2000). Some stimuli (e.g., light touch or rotary vestibular stimulation) tend to have a sustained effect within the central nervous system (i.e., it takes longer to recover from the sensory event). For example, after a person spins in a circle for a minute, the sustained effect can leave the person dizzy for some time after the input has ended. When the rate of recovery from a sensory event is long, a child may experience an additive effect of sensory experiences over time. This can result in overresponsivity and behavioral dysregulation. This may be the case with Kim in the vignette above. The infant is highly reactive and is getting a lot of intense sensory input from her mother without the opportunity to return to baseline and recover before getting more stimulation. In this case, there is a poor "goodness of fit" between the physical and social environments during free play and Kim's underlying capacities. During free play, the environment is highly stimulating (i.e., high-intensity input at a rapid rate without support) and overwhelms Kim's sensory integrative capacity and tolerance for stimulation (i.e., overregistration of sensory input with a slow recovery rate, limited motor capacity to support self-regulation, and difficulty grading reactivity), resulting in sensory-based dysregulation with irritability and fussiness, while Carol tends to provide too much high-intensity input without reading Kim's behavioral cues of overstimulation.

The situation is very different during the "still face" section of the case study, when Carol begins to hold a neutral face and not interact with Kim for a short time. At this point, Kim opens up and is responsive and playful. Paradoxically, this low-stimulus environment offers a better goodness of fit with Kim's capacity for regulation, and her readiness for interaction emerges. Kim's reaction to her mother's still face is atypical. Most children are upset when their parent is present but not interactively available. In this case, because of Kim's overresponsivity to sensation, the opposite is true.

One thing that is clear from this case study is that the outcome of the sensory integration process is not only about what is occurring within the child, but also about the physical and social environment generating the sensory input. The unique aspect of the play episode described is that there is goodness of fit when Carol is present but not interactive, and Kim is able to maintain a sustained quiet alert state and attend to and make several social overtures to her mother. Kim also evidences good self-regulatory abilities, including being able to actively kick and bring her hands to the midline to calm herself. Unfortunately, rather than learning from Kim's increased responsiveness during the quiet episode, her mother returns to high-intensity play after a brief break. This type of sustained mismatch, in which the child is providing cues that do not seem to affect her mother's behavior, can have a significant effect on the developing dyadic relationship. The cause may be somatic (in this case, sensory), but the outcome can be affective or communicative. If Carol interprets Kim's behavior as "independence" or as Kim not needing her, she may tend to interact with her less rather than modifying her interactions to reciprocally interact with Kim. This misinterpretation may result in derailment in the developmental trajectory of their dyadic interactions, and neither child nor mother will trust the relationship. Similarly, if Kim continues to provide communicative cues (e.g., turning away) that are not responded to, she may eventually stop providing those cues, further disrupting the developmental transactions within the dyad (Sameroff and Chandler 1975). Language and communication may even be disrupted long before the first words begin.

Sensory Processing Disorder

Sensory integration is the term used for the process of taking in and using input. This knowledge can help in understanding children who may not carry a diagnosis or have clear deficits in sensory processing, but who have preferences that help to explain some of their temperamental characteristics or their preferred environments. Kim most likely fits this description. She has the capacity, and given a good fit, she will thrive. Helping her mother learn how to interpret Kim's cues and how to provide responsive and less intense input should help the dyad move forward. Other children, however, may require more than parent coaching to progress, and may have sensory processing disorder, resulting in extreme irritability or fussiness and more developmental challenges. Sensory processing disorder is not a diagnostic category within DSM-IV or DSM-5, but it is comparable to regulatory disorders of sensory processing as described in DC:0-3R (Zero to Three 2005; see Chapter 11, "DC:0-3R: A Diagnostic Schema for Infants and Young Children and Their Families").

Miller et al. (2007) proposed a taxonomy of sensory processing disorders that is useful in this context and describes three major types: 1) sensory modulation disorder, 2) sensory-based motor disorder, and 3) sensory discrimination disorder. Only the first two, sensory modulation disorder and sensory-based motor disorder, will be discussed in this chapter.

Sensory Modulation Disorder

A *sensory modulation disorder* is a disorder in grading responsivity and reactivity to sensory stimuli. It is a problem of registration during the first step (intake) of the sensory integration process (see Figure 13–1). One way to think of sensory modulation disorder is that the magnitude of the response is in line with the perceived intensity of the stimulus to the child. Therefore, if a touch is intended to be gentle but the reaction is as if the touch was painful, the magnitude of the response indicates that to this child, the touch was aversive. There are two primary sensory modulation disorders: sensory overresponsivity, and sensory underresponsivity. These disorders can be understood in terms of the upper and lower thresholds to organized behavior (Figure 13–2).

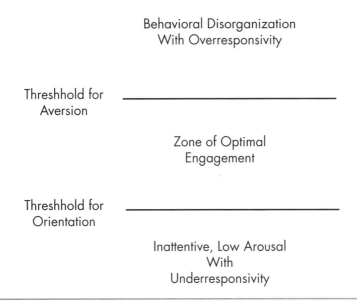

FIGURE 13-2. Zone of optimal engagement.

Sensory modulation disorder is best understood in terms of an upper and lower threshold for optimal arousal and attentiveness. In this figure these thresholds define a zone of optimal engagement. Too much or too little sensory input can lead to the child's being inattentive or disorganized. Social interaction and learning occur in the zone of optimal engagement.

The lower threshold is the point of initial registration and orientation. For heuristic purposes, we think about the distribution of initial thresholds in terms of the normal curve, with most people in the middle range. Most people notice the sound of a clock ticking but do not notice the tags on their clothes. There are individual differences, but most individuals are able to work and play in typical environments. Children with sensory modulation disorder tend to be too overreactive or underreactive in typical environments, to the degree that their responsivity limits their ability to engage in age-appropriate daily living or social activities. Children whose activities are limited by their sensory thresholds are those identified as having sensory modulation disorder. Other terms applied to overresponsivity include *tactile or sensory defensiveness, sensory hyperreactivity, gravitational insecurity,* and *sensory sensitivity.*

The initial threshold helps to identify those children who may have a tendency to be overresponsive or underresponsive, some of whom seem to have difficulty maintaining engagement regardless of what amount of sensory input they are receiving. In this case, the upper limit of organized behavior (threshold of aversion) helps to explain the challenge. In a child who is overresponsive, there is a tendency to overregister sensation (i.e., have a low threshold to initial reaction) or to have a narrowed zone of optimal engagement. In the case of a child with initial underresponsivity, the child may not recover to baseline after a sensory event, resulting in summation of input over time. Summation without recovery may result in behavioral disorganization (i.e., reaching the threshold of aversion) even in a child who is initially underresponsive. Overresponsivity has been documented in electrophysiological research (Mangeot et al. 2001; Miller et al. 1999). Typical behavior in an overresponsive child is characterized by high arousal, decreased attention and distractibility, negative affect due to unpredictable and overwhelming input from the environment, and reactive behavior that may seem impulsive. This is the type of behavior that was reported in Kim. In contrast, the underresponsive child is often unaware of sensory input from the environment. Experiences that are typical in the environment may not be adequate for the underresponsive child to reach threshold and begin to register and orient to salient aspects of the environment. The effect of this underresponsivity is seen not only in attention but also in arousal and affect. The child may seem sleepy or disinterested. His or her behavior is characterized by low arousal, diffuse inattention, decreased or flattened affect, and passivity or decreased activity (Anzalone and Lane 2012).

Although these profiles are described in terms of somatic sensory reactivity, the resulting behavior of children with sensory modulation challenges can have a profound effect on the developing capacity for self-regulation and the formation of dyadic relationships. Self-regulation is often discussed in terms of regulation of emotions or relationships, but early research suggests a somatic core and foundation for the process of self-regulation—with initial regulation of arousal, then attention, then emotions, and finally relationships. For an infant to begin to engage in relationships, he or she must first develop the somatic foundations that enable the child to achieve the attentional and state demands of the zone of optimal engagement. Kim illustrates the challenges faced by dyads that include a child with overresponsivity. In contrast, underresponsive children will often not provide interactive cues, and they request less yet require more support from their caregivers. If one assumes a transactional model of development (Sameroff and Chandler 1975), these children are not able to participate equally in interactive episodes. They need help to reach threshold before they are available for interaction. Helping them to reach threshold for orientation requires that caregivers provide adequate sensory input that is not too complex or intense.

Helping a child achieve and maintain the zone of optimal engagement poses many multidimensional challenges and opportunities for providers. For many parents and providers, becoming aware of behavioral cues and then knowing how to moderate (downregulate or upregulate) the sensory input provided by interaction and the physical environment is a complex and nonintuitive process. Supporting parents in "seeing" behavioral cues is only the initial challenges for providers and may require both regulatory and attentional work on the part of the parent to remain calm enough to attend, watch, and register what is seen. Providers may need first to employ such strategies as coregulatory support for the parent, informational guidance, description, education, watching together, and wondering. Next, they help parents learn to use interpretation and meaning making to make sense of the child's behavior. This may require substantial discussion to build the awareness and understanding through which new meaning can be made. Simple narrative interpretation, education, or reframing, or more complex interventions such as Video Intervention Therapy (see Chapter 17) or psychotherapy, can be used. Finally, providers can help the parent to see the child's cues, make functional meaning of the cues, and then choose a supportive response to the cues (e.g., slowing the pace or sensory yield of the interaction). At this point, providers may need to observe and narrate the effect of strategies the parent tries, offer suggestions, model, reflect on the range of options, or use other coaching supportive strategies. Such supportive interaction is offered in service to the dyadic relationship, and done in the context of the clinician's own reflection-in-action on his/her skills, motivations, and emotional state, and the affect of the interactive process on the parent-provider and parent-child relationships (K. Brandt, personal communication, October 2012).

Sensory-Based Motor Disorder

There are two types of sensory-based motor disorder: dyspraxia and vestibular-proprioceptive postural disorders (Miller et al. 2007). *Dyspraxia* is an impairment in the ability to formulate, plan, and execute unfamiliar goal-directed behavior. Ayres (1972) considers praxis as comparable to language, in that it enables interaction between the child and the physical environment, just as language enables interaction between the child and the social environment. We posit that interaction with the physical environment is one of the foundations for interaction with social partners.

Praxis is best thought of in three phases: ideation, motor planning, and execution. The first phase, ideation, involves figuring out what one wants to do. This phase is the most cognitive component and involves creativity and flexibility as the child perceives the affordances in the current environment and flexibly forms a goal based on the possibilities for action in that environment. The second phase is motor planning or the ability to use a sensory map of the body and, through premotor processes, figure out a plan of action. The sensory map of the body (usually referred to as a *body schema*) is an important aspect of sensory integration. The body schema is formed as a result of feedback from executed movement and serves as a component of feed-forward planning for subsequent movements. Children who are underresponsive or who have sensory discrimination disorders often have impairment in body schema and motor planning. The final phase, execution, is the observable motor component. Children with dyspraxia appear to be clumsy, but the clumsiness is hypothesized to be related to underlying sensory processing and planning deficits rather than a simple developmental motor coordination delay or a neurological diagnosis such as cerebral palsy (Cermak and Larkin 2002).

Vestibular-proprioceptive postural disorders are also a result of underlying sensory processing deficits, even though the manifest behavior is motor and postural. Children with a sensory-based postural disorder have difficulty processing information about body movements or the body in space. Often, this difficulty is seen in children who have an intolerance of prone positioning work or any postural changes. These children tend to be fussy and very cautious in how they negotiate their physical environment. Related motor problems seen in these children may include decreased postural tone, difficulty crossing the midline, bilateral coordination, and an avoidance of postural challenges.

The types of social or dyadic challenges faced by children with either sensory-based motor disorder are similar. These children tend to be cautious and/or inflexible, to avoid interaction with peers as they move into toddler and preschool phases, and to avoid physical activities, preferring instead to direct others or engage in sedentary play. Another challenge faced by these children, especially those with dyspraxia, is that they tend to require maximum attention to the execution of motor activities rather than attention to the goal of the activity. Attentional automaticity, which usually occurs once an individual masters a skill, tends to come late if at all for these children. As a result, there is often inconsistency in motor performance because the motor demands of a task frequently constrain the cognitive and affective demands of the task. Dyspraxia is often seen in conjunction with verbal apraxia, although this connection has not been empirically validated.

While sensory and sensory-based motor processes are important, in the following section we discuss motor factors without a clear sensory etiology: central somatic factors to consider in dyadic interaction, motor delay or deficit.

Motor Delay or Deficit

Sensory challenges are not the only somatic limitations influencing dyadic interaction. Sensory and motor systems are interwoven at a primal level. In utero, a bright light on the mother's abdomen (visual stimulation) results in the baby's head turning. At birth, a loud auditory stimulation leads to a Moro reflex with full motor involvement, and the tactile sensation of something in the palm leads to closing of the fingers in a grasp reflex. Conversely, the motor system supports sensory exploration as the infant reaches at birth to touch the mother's face, or the toddler walks to, squats in, and touches sand. Quickly, sensory processing challenges can become motor deficits or motor deficits can become sensory issues, and both have reverberations in the relationship as baby and mother are influenced in their own ways by these challenges.

Porges (2011) suggests that embryological connections support the integration of motor and relationship development, identifying the social engagement system's cortical associations with brain stem nuclei–controlled functions such as "eyelid opening (e.g., looking), facial muscles (e.g., emotional expression), middle ear muscles (e.g., extracting human voice from background noise), muscles of mastication (e.g., ingestion), laryngeal and pharyngeal muscles (e.g., prosody), and head tilting and turning muscles (e.g., social gesture and orientation)" (p. 189). This muscular activity is necessary for the infant's early survival, which is dependent on access to adequate nutrition, protection, nurturance, and social engagement.

The well-contained in utero environment supports the neuromusculoskeletal system with proprioception and sensory input that shapes tone, strength, form, function, and postural control. Prematurely interrupted physiological development creates motor imbalance at many levels and can contribute to hypotonia, muscle fatigue, respiratory efforts, and inability to sustain antigravity postures (Sweeney and Gutierrez 2010, p. 238). The disruption of motor development due to premature birth subjects an infant to the effects of gravity when in a relatively weak condition, immobilized due to periods of sedation, and restricted in movement due to life-saving medical practices. These physical experiences can alter body alignment and biomechanics, as well as place unexpected demands on the infant's neurological and physiological systems (Sweeney and Gutierrez 2010, p. 239). Similar challenges face the child born with physical malformations or neurological abnormalities that alter physical functioning, and thereby influence social dyadic development.

Children who are born preterm or who have neuromotor impairment also have limited ability to interact flexibly with the physical environment and, as a result, with the social environment. Often, a parent's misperception of the differences between motivation, developmental achievement, and motor capacity can lead to misinterpretation of the child's ability or willingness to meet parental dreams.

> Six-month-old (corrected age) Joshua retained legs and low trunk in extension due to tightness in the posterior trunk, pelvic, and leg muscles, making it difficult to place him in an erect sitting posture. He fussed with the physical therapist's preparatory attempts—no doubt because of the muscular tightness. He had not elevated his legs to bring his hands down for developmentally appropriate exploration of his thighs and knees in the previous months, and the important abdominal muscle activation necessary for postural control was missing. The father insisted that Joshua was fussing because he did not want to sit; "he only wanted to stand." The father's disregard of the physical therapist's description of biomechanical interruption of appropriate developmental milestones due to the tight musculature meant that the therapeutic recommendations would not be implemented by the family. Both father and son were experiencing inflexibility (albeit for different reasons) that would ultimately affect the dyadic relationship.

The physical therapist struggled to understand this parent's interpretation of his baby's communication through his motor and regulatory behavior. The father viewed his 6-month-old (corrected age) son as a chronological 10-month-old and desperately wanted him to be typical. In the father's mind, 10-month-olds should be standing. Joshua enjoyed being supported in stance, and this conformed with the father's image of his son as healthy. He had dreams about his son being involved in sports. However, as Joshua struggled to gain control of his body in his environment, his father struggled with the infant's physical control and his imagined or hoped-for dreams for the baby. On a superficial level, the father was able to resolve these struggles by focusing on the future. One way for the physical therapist to tackle the impasse with Joshua's father was to meet him around his projected image of his son and to discuss the muscular flexibility and balance of muscle power required for athletics. Now was the time to help Joshua gain efficient control of his body, before the substitutions he was beginning to use led to further musculoskeletal problems and injuries, later sidelining him as an athlete. (See Chapter 1, "Core Concepts in Infant-Family and Early Childhood Mental Health," for a discussion of therapeutic gateways; this situation demonstrates entering the system through the explicit gateway while temporarily delaying working in the implicit gateway.)

The physical therapist recognized that getting the parent to see the baby required first that she see the baby the father saw, so that the two "saw the same baby" (Seligman 2000, p. 213). Understanding what is behind the parent's interpretation is accomplished through

a therapeutic alliance that creates a parallel process in which support of the parent translates into the parent's supporting the child, and often means exploring the "messy" origins
of a parent's meaning making. Through an application of the concepts of mentalization
and reflective capacity (Fonagy et al. 2002; Slade 2005), or the ability to imagine what the
"other" (the infant, in this case) is experiencing physically, emotionally, and relationally, the
physical therapist invited the parent to experience the very physical biomechanics confront-
ing the infant. In the case of Joshua, the physical therapist approached the situation through
a behavioral-somatic (explicit) gateway by asking Joshua's father to do a few sit-ups and
thus experience how the sedentary lifestyle–induced tightness in his own hamstring muscles and weakness in his abdominal muscles interfered with his ability to do a long-leg sit
(something that most infants do at Joshua's age), even though it did not interfere with his
ability to stand. While working in this case, the physical therapist became aware of the
expanded parallel process: The baby's body was rigid and inflexible. The physical therapist
perceived the father as rigid and unable to see his "real" baby. Through reflective work, she
became aware of her own rigidity and inflexibility in wanting the father to accept his child
at the level she determined to be adequate or healthy.

Conclusion

Sensory and motor foundations of regulation and behavior are central to the developing capacity of children to interact with their physical and social environments. If a child cannot
make sense of the world, interacting adaptively and flexibly within it is difficult. When that
disruption persists, it can interfere with all aspects of development. The provider working
with a child with sensory processing disorder or motor impairment will need to address somatic concerns concurrently with affective concerns, treating the presenting condition in
tandem with attending the other "patient"—the dyadic relationship. Similarly, the mental
health professional should consider potential somatic bases for dyadic disruption. Intervention is best when it addresses parent understanding, goodness of fit across environments, and
underlying sensory integration capacity (Williamson and Anzalone 2001).

KEY POINTS

- Sensory integration—the organization and use of sensory information—can help
  explain individual differences in how children, especially young children, engage
  in social interaction.
- When a child is inflexible and avoidant, the practitioner should consider sensory
  or motor factors as an alternative to willfulness or affectively driven behavior.
- Challenges in taking in sensory information can lead to underregistration or overregistration of input, and children with these challenges may appear disinterested
  in or overwhelmed by social engagement. Similarly, the altered ability of infants
  or children to age-appropriately use their motor systems in an easy, smooth, and

predictable way can impede their ability for self-protective or regulatory strategies, and the support of caregivers is necessary to help them achieve these and other immediate motor, engagement, and interactive goals.

- Both the child and parent are making meaning of altered sensory and motor capacities, and the meaning plays out in the relationship in ways that occupational therapists, physical therapists, and other professionals can explore with parents in supporting optimal mental and relational health.

- Helping families to understand the sensory or motor foundations of challenging behavior can help improve dyadic interaction.

- Modifying environments to create a better sensory or motor goodness of fit can decrease demands on some children and enable more adaptive engagement, which in turn can support and contribute to the quality of the child-parent relationship and the child's social-emotional development.

References

Anzalone ME, Lane SJ: Sensory processing disorder, in Kids Can Be Kids: A Childhood Occupations Approach. Edited by Lane SJ, Bundy AC. Philadelphia, PA, FA Davis, 2012, pp 437–459

Ayres AJ: Sensory Integration and Learning Disorders. Los Angeles, CA, Western Psychological Services, 1972

Bundy AC, Lane SJ, Murray EA (eds): Sensory Integration: Theory and Practice, 2nd Edition. Philadelphia, PA, FA Davis, 2002

Cermak SA, Larkin D: Developmental Coordination Disorder. San Diego, CA, Singular Publishing Group, 2002

DeGangi GA, DiPietro JA, Greenspan SI, et al: Psychophysiological characteristics of the regulatory disordered infant. Infant Behav Dev 14:37–50, 1991

DeSantis A, Coster W, Bigsby R, et al: Colic and fussing in infancy, and sensory processing at 3 to 8 years of age. Infant Ment Health J 25:522–539, 2004

Fonagy P, Gyorgy G, Elliot J, et al: Affect Regulation, Mentalization, and the Development of Self. New York, Other Press, 2002

Fox NA, Polak CP: The role of sensory reactivity in understanding infant temperament, in Handbook of Infant, Toddler, and Preschool Mental Health Assessment. Edited by DelCarmen-Wiggins R, Carter A. New York, Oxford University Press, 2004, pp 105–119

Kandel ER, Schwartz JH, Jessell TM: Principles of Neural Science, 4th Edition. New York, McGraw-Hill, 2000

Lane SL, Schaaf RC: Examining the neuroscience evidence for sensory driven neuroplasticity: implications for sensory-based occupational therapy for children and adolescents. Am J Occup Ther 64:375–390, 2010

Mangeot SD, Miller LJ, McIntosh DN: Sensory modulation dysfunction in children with attention-deficit-hyperactivity disorder. Dev Med Child Neurol 43:399–406, 2001

Miller LJ, McIntosh DN, McGrath J, et al: Electrodermal responses to sensory stimuli in individuals with fragile X syndrome: a preliminary report. Am J Med Genet 83:268–279, 1999

Miller LJ, Anzalone ME, Lane SJ, et al: Concept evolution in sensory integration: a proposed nosology for diagnosis. Am J Occup Ther 61:135–140, 2007

Porges SW: The Polyvagal Theory: Neurophysiological Foundations of Emotions, Attachment, Communication, and Self-Regulation, New York, WW Norton, 2011

Sameroff AJ, Chandler MJ: Reproductive risk and the continuum of caretaking casualty, in Review of Child Development Research. Edited by Horowitz FD, Hetherington M, Scarr-Salapatek S, et al. Chicago, IL, University of Chicago Press 1975, pp 187–244

Seligman S: Clinical interviews with families of infants, in Handbook of Infant Mental Health, 2nd Edition. Edited by Zeanah CH. New York, Guilford, 2000, pp 211–221

Slade A: Parental reflective functioning: an introduction. Attach Hum Dev 7:269–281, 2005

Sweeney J, Gutierrez T: The dynamic continuum of motor and musculoskeletal development: implications for neonatal care and discharge teaching, in Developmental Care of Newborns and Infants: A Guide for Health Professionals, 2nd Edition. Edited by Kenner C, McGrath JM. Glenview, IL, National Association of Neonatal Nurses, 2010, pp 235–248

Williamson GG, Anzalone ME: Sensory Integration and Self-Regulation in Infants and Toddlers: Helping Very Young Children Interact With Their Environment. Washington, DC, Zero to Three, 2001

Zero to Three: Diagnostic Classification of Mental Health and Developmental Disorders of Infancy and Early Childhood (DC:0-3). Washington, DC, Zero to Three, 1994

Zero to Three: What Is Infant Mental Health? Washington, DC, Zero to Three, 2002

Zero to Three: Diagnostic Classification of Mental Health and Developmental Disorders of Infancy and Early Childhood, Revised (DC:0-3R). Washington, DC, Zero to Three, 2005

CHAPTER 14

Autism Spectrum Disorders

The Importance of Parent-Child Relationships

Mary Beth Steinfeld, M.D.

Ruby Moye' Salazar, L.C.S.W., B.C.D.

Sensitive, responsive caregiving is essential to optimal child development, and caregiver attunement is at the heart of such caregiving. Before the emergence of speech, behavior is the infant's primary means of communicating emotional experience and sharing affective states. These emotional exchanges or "conversations" are transactional (Tronick 1989) and depend on each partner's ability to clearly signal, understand, and respond to the other (Bornstein et al. 2012). When repeated over time, they become the organizing substrate for the developing relationship, as well as for the experience-dependent development of the brain.

Infants and young children with an autism spectrum disorder (ASD) present a particular challenge to infant-caregiver attunement (the sharing of affective states). Difficulty in co-orientation—perceiving, processing, and responding to social experience—and the emergence of unusual behaviors, interests, and reactions interfere with the child's development of social, emotional, and communication skills. Meanwhile, the caregiver struggles to understand the child's intentions and respond with confidence. Parents of a child with an ASD need help finding ways to join their child at an emotional level. From there, they need help learning to build the many, varied interpersonal experiences that allow a child to become aware of himself or herself in relation to others and thus develop self-awareness and an adaptive subjective sense of self-with-other (Greenspan and Wieder 1998; Hobson 2010; Sanders 2002; Stern 1985). Within the context of ASDs, intervention to promote this knowing and being known (affective connectedness) among all involved family members is essential for the optimal development of the child and family.

Because a broad variety of professionals are typically involved in the support and treatment of children with ASDs and their families, managing their child's care can be overwhelming and confusing for parents. The key to reducing parents' stress—and improving therapeutic effectiveness—is a family-focused transdisciplinary approach, with all involved professionals working together to maintain a well-integrated, coherent program of care that can respond flexibly to developmental progress and change (Greenspan and Wieder 1998; Osborne et al. 2008).

At the center of care, the family needs a "secure-base" professional, a person they can rely on over time—someone who knows the child, the parents, and other family members, and who can provide support, continuity, and guidance as the family navigates the child's life changes and developmental trajectory. Infant and early childhood mental health practitioners are in a good position to fulfill this role.

Following a brief overview of the biological aspects of autism, we present an infant mental health approach to working with children with ASDs and their families. We emphasize the impact that the ASD has on the developing relationships in a young child's life and how relationship-based approaches can contribute to improved outcomes. Our aim is to expand the growing awareness in the field of ASD treatment that attuned child-parent relationships in the first years of life are crucial and that strengthening close family relationships should be a lifetime endeavor.

Background

Since publication of DSM-5, discrete subtypes along the autism spectrum (e.g., Asperger's syndrome, autism, pervasive developmental disorder not otherwise specified) have been subsumed under the broader term *autism spectrum disorder*. ASD refers to the etiologically and clinically heterogeneous group of neurodevelopmental disorders characterized by persistent deficits in reciprocal social communication and social interaction, and restricted, repetitive patterns of behavior, interests, or activities, as defined by DSM-5 (American Psychiatric Association 2013, pp. 50–59). Underlying neurobiology affects the way the brains of individuals with ASD process, respond to, and organize experience, leading to atypical neurological, developmental, and behavioral trajectories. Evidence-based behavioral interventions are effective in improving developmental, behavioral, and adaptive skills in children with autism (Lord and McGee 2001; National Autism Center 2009; Rogers and Vismara 2008). Although the condition is lifelong in most cases, early intervention holds the potential for significant improvement and, in some cases, for resolution of symptoms and possibly even prevention or cure (Dawson 2008).

Epidemiology

The prevalence of autism continues to rise, with the most recent estimates suggesting that 1 of every 88 children in the United States has an ASD, with boys about 5 times more likely to have the diagnosis (1 in 54) than girls (1 in 252) (Centers for Disease Control and Prevention 2012). Possible reasons for the large increase over the past couple of decades include the expansion of diagnostic criteria to a spectrum disorder, improved screening and diagnostic tools, improved access to services, and greater clinician and public awareness, as well as a genuine rise in incidence, of unknown cause (Ozonoff and Rogers 2003; Rutter 2005). The public health implications of this increase for educational, medical, and adult services are tremendous.

Etiology

Most cases of ASDs are idiopathic and are believed to be the result of unknown environmental exposures within the context of genetic vulnerability (Muhle et al. 2004). Monozygotic twins are more likely to be concordant for ASD than dizygotic twins, at rates of 36%–95% and 0%–31%, respectively (Centers for Disease Control and Prevention 2012). Concordance for subthreshold levels of social and communication difficulty, known as the broader autism phenotype, is also more common in monozygotic than dizygotic twins (Bailey et al. 1995). These statistics support the view that although ASD is highly genetic, more than one gene is involved in idiopathic ASD, and suggest that epigenetic processes and environmental modifiers likely contribute to the variable expression of the ASD phenotype (Muhle et al. 2004).

The recurrence risk for autism in simplex families (having one child with an ASD already) is 13.5%, whereas the risk in multiplex families (having more than one child with an ASD) is 32.3%, with a higher recurrence risk for male (25.9%) than female (9.6%) infants (Ozonoff et al. 2011). Nonautistic members of multiplex families have increased rates of the broader autism phenotype.

A genetic etiology can be identified in 10%–20% of cases (Abrahams and Geschwind 2008). ASDs occur in several identifiable genetic syndromes, such as fragile X, tuberous sclerosis, and 15q deletion and 22q deletion syndromes (Hansen and Hagerman 2003). Copy number variants and de novo nucleotide mutations are increasingly implicated (Abrahams and Geschwind 2008; Sanders et al. 2012). Abnormalities have been found on every chromosome (Gillberg 1998), and more than 100 candidate genes and susceptibility loci have been identified. Abnormalities in genes with roles related to brain development are under investigation (Dawson 2008), including genes associated with neurotransmitter functions and synaptic binding neuroligins (Rutter 2011; Zoghbi 2003). Thalidomide and valproate are teratogenic for ASDs (Hansen and Hagerman 2003). More recently, maternal autoantibodies to fetal brain tissues involved in neuron development have been associated with development of autism (Braunschweig et al. 2013).

Neurobiology

Neuroimaging studies have documented abnormalities in the timing of growth and organizational patterns in both gray and white matter. White matter underconnectivity between distant temporal, parietal, and associated cortical regions has been found, as have areas of overconnectivity between cortical and subcortical regions and within primary sensory cortices (Anagnostou and Taylor 2011). Because many of these studies involve older individuals, it is likely that some of these differences are the result of ASD rather than the cause. However, Wolff et al. (2012) prospectively found abnormal white matter pathways in infants ages 6–24 months who developed autism, suggesting that abnormal connectivity may be present even before behavioral signs are noted. Ongoing studies of infants and toddlers at risk for autism promise new insights.

The "social brain" (Brothers 1990) refers to the structural and functional neural systems underlying human social competencies. Abnormalities have been found in all anatomical areas of the social brain in individuals with autism (Polšek et al. 2011). Pelphrey et al. (2011) provide an excellent overview of the current theories addressing potential neural circuitry abnormalities of the social brain early in life that may result in the clinical features of autism.

How Infants Relate and Learn

In her excellent review about brain plasticity and autism, Dawson (2008) emphasizes the essential role of early parent-infant relationships in the development of social brain circuitry and cortical specialization for language and social learning. Interpersonal engagement is key. Within the context of social interaction, infants use statistical learning to perceive consistencies in their sensory social experiences. They orient to relevant aspects of their environment—faces, voices, and social behaviors—to discern patterns and make predictions (Rogers and Dawson 2009). Kuhl (2007) demonstrated, for example, that infants are born able to perceive the sounds produced in every human language. Over the course of the first year, infants become increasingly competent at analyzing the sound combinations to which they are exposed, but lose the ability to "hear" sounds to which they are not exposed. Passive exposure to a foreign language (e.g., via television) does not protect against this loss. Only within the context of interpersonal interaction does this perceptual capacity remain as a substrate for subsequent language learning.

How ASDs Affect Relating and Learning

At this point, no reliable behavioral signs of emerging autism in infants age 6 months or younger have been identified. Infants developing an ASD may begin to show decreased initiation of and responsiveness to social interaction by age 8–10 months. By age 12 months, they may show decreases in eye contact, directed facial expressions, vocalizations, and response to name, and may exhibit repetitive behaviors that are unusual compared to those of typically developing children (Ozonoff et al. 2008, 2010; Zwaigenbaum et al. 2004). Atypical neurological development and maturation (Pelphrey et al. 2011) set the stage for inefficient and ineffective processing of socially relevant information. Social brain development is further compromised as cycles of underresponsiveness by the infant result in fewer sustained social interactions with the caregiver (each is impacted by the other's difficulty in reading his or her cues). Considering the role that neuroplasticity plays in organizing experience into neural circuitry, the importance of early identification of these atypical patterns and prompt intervention becomes clear.

Because of the way infants developing ASDs respond to their environments (limited interactional play, less initiating, greater fixation), it is very important that reciprocal human interactions be promoted as primary experiences. If day-to-day life is more limited, more insular, and less varied, then the child with an ASD becomes more rigid, more patterned, and more inflexible. Parents may unwittingly allow repetitive, isolated, solitary play in an effort to prevent behavioral outbursts (dysregulation). They may encourage an overfocus on preferred, academic interests (e.g., the alphabet or colors) in a misguided effort to promote cognitive skills. In such situations, both the child and the family need guidance to support the development of flexible social, communication, behavioral, and interpersonal skills so that the child's experiences can be more fully integrated into the world of people and things.

Early Signs and Onset Patterns

Ozonoff et al. (2010) found no difference in the frequency of socially directed behaviors in 6-month-olds who ultimately developed ASDs compared with control subjects. However, these same infants demonstrated a gradual loss of social communication skills beginning between 6 and 12 months of age, and continuing through 36 months. Interestingly, the parents in this study did not report regression in skills at any point during the study (Ozonoff et al. 2010), although ASD-related parent concerns at 12 months did predict those children who later were diagnosed with ASD (Ozonoff et al. 2009). This study suggests that the behavioral onset of ASDs consists of an unrecognized gradual regression in most children rather than lack of social skills development from the outset (the most commonly described onset pattern), or a more abrupt regression at age 18–24 months (as has been described in approximately 30% of cases).

These findings demonstrate that it is possible to identify children at very young ages who are presenting with signs and symptoms of emerging ASDs. Effective treatment programs are available to address the social-communication difficulties in these early-identified children (Dawson et al. 2010; Rogers and Dawson 2009; Rogers et al. 2012). Even before formal diagnosis, interventions to expand social engagement, turn taking, initiation, imitation, joint attention, and communication are recommended, to slow or even reverse gradual regression into autism (Rogers and Dawson 2009).

Consciously noted or unconsciously perceived by the parent, the behaviors and interactional capacities of a child with an ASD are not typical, and this may place the dyad at risk for relational impacts. Although ASDs are not mental health illnesses, they may contribute to, exacerbate, or generate challenges to the overall mental health and well-being of the family and the parent-child relationship, and require therapeutic work to scaffold, advance, and/ or therapeutically treat the child, parent, dyad, and/or family. The impact and risk escalate when the diagnosis is made and new realities emerge, meanings are made, and the inevitable cycle of grieving—even if already in process—is activated around a condition with a name.

Diagnosis

When parents begin to have concerns about a child's relatedness, behavior, or developmental progress, their fears can interfere with timely diagnosis and intervention. Professionals providing primary medical care, as well as those providing child care, should cultivate collaborative relationships with developmental professionals who will be able to partner with them and with families to achieve appropriate intervention services in a timely way.

Current American Academy of Pediatrics guidelines recommend that primary care providers administer an autism-specific screening tool—such as the Modified Checklist for Autism in Toddlers (M-CHAT; Robins et al. 2001)—at ages 18 and 24 months (Johnson and Myers; American Academy of Pediatrics Council on Children With Disabilities 2007). Given the possibility of subtle social regression between 6 and 12 months, pediatricians should monitor infant communicative intent and social interaction, including imitation, gesture games, and response to name, as part of well child visits beginning at age 9–12 months. Primary care providers should err on the side of caution and refer early to infant development providers for early intervention (e.g., speech therapy, occupational therapy, preschool special education) and refer for formal developmental/autism evaluation to developmental pediatricians or multidisciplinary assessment teams, as appropriate, whenever developmental delays or red flags for autism are present. Although formal diagnosis is important, one need not wait for a formal diagnosis before instituting early intervention services, because access to diagnosing professionals may be delayed by long waiting lists.

Formal diagnosis of ASD is based on criteria defined by DSM-5 (American Psychiatric Association 2013), and formerly DSM-IV-TR (American Psychiatric Association 2000). Best practice guidelines emphasize the need for direct observation of the child and caregiver in as natural a setting as possible and the collection of parent information regarding early signs and symptoms (because time limitations make it unlikely that all behavioral signs will be observed during a diagnostic assessment). Unfortunately, current standard practice allows few paid hours for assessment, even though a minimum of 5–10 hours may be needed when presentation of the child or the family is complex. The diagnosis generally includes administration of a standardized structured behavioral observation, a parent interview, and developmental and adaptive skills testing. The Autism Diagnostic Observation Schedule, Second Edition (ADOS-2; Lord et al. 2012a, 2012b), and Autism Diagnostic Interview—Revised (ADI-R; Lord et al. 1994) are considered the current gold standard assessment tools; they systematically review the diagnostic criteria (ADI-R) or provide repeated opportunities to observe clinical features (ADOS-2). It is important that the parents participate during young children's assessments, because observing a child with a familiar caregiver will provide a more accurate picture of both strengths and areas of challenge. By gently highlighting the child's specific capacities and difficulties with social communication as well as the child's unusual interests and behaviors during the observation, the evaluator can help parents better understand developmental patterns unique to their child and the basis for diagnosis and need for intervention. Following formal diagnosis, a more extensive assessment will yield further data for developing a comprehensive intervention plan.

The time of diagnosis is typically a time of great disequilibrium for the family. Although it is crucial for the evaluator to join the family where they are in terms of their ability to hear and process realities, it is also important to explain clearly the ASD world they are entering. The expert ASD evaluator will have accessible a range of services and support materials to draw from as evaluator and family together determine a specific plan for next steps.

Family-Focused Assessment

A family-focused approach to formal diagnosis and subsequent in-depth assessment by a "secure base" professional or team are often the family's entry into the world of ASDs, so this is an important time for the practitioner to join with the child and parent (or other family members) to build their understanding of the road ahead, to assess their capacities, to strengthen their confidence, to help them understand their child's needs (and their own), and to build their communicative competence with their child. The practitioner is modeling—by how he or she relates to everyone in the family—the philosophy of encouraging, the effectiveness of coaching, and the benefits of curiosity, reflection, and discussion as a pattern of communication in moving forward to build capacities and solve problems. Assessment is an essential step in bringing the parents and their child into better attunement. A family-centered, transdisciplinary assessment enables evaluators and parents to learn together about the child and also about the family's emotional and learning styles. The goal is to establish both a comprehensive constitutional profile of the child and a compatible intervention plan for the family. This approach requires a paradigm shift. Instead of viewing behavioral symptoms as core deficits, the focus is on interactional and behavioral symptoms as indicators of deeper, more complex issues. By allowing a generous span of time for the assessment, evaluators can experience a fuller range of the child's developmental patterns and the caregivers' capacities and concerns, and thereby set the stage for building a strong working alliance with the family.

Several steps are involved in the family-focused assessment process. In a welcoming environment, the clinician(s) sensitively coaches family members to demonstrate the deeper realms of their relatedness as they share play and interact with their child. This respectful observing and gentle coaching serves as the beginning of the clinician-family partnership and the process of understanding the family's skills, strengths, and challenges. This first step in intervention allows the clinician(s) and family to design a clinical program best fitted for all.

Some parents will choose to come without their child for the first visit so they can talk about themselves and check out their fit with the practitioner(s). Others will be eager to have the clinician meet their child because they are looking for immediate relief in answers, advice, and assurances. Every step in the process—even the first conversation with office staff—requires sensitivity. Paperwork should be designed with consideration of the new world the family is entering and may need to be optional or assisted if the parents are unable (for either literacy or emotional reasons) to provide the requested information.

A quality assessment process involves skilled clinical observation of both spontaneous and coached interactions; shared information regarding engaging, joint attention, and problem solving; and discussions of family practices across multiple contexts and within all significant relationships. When an in-person visit is not possible, videotaped observations may substitute. If the child is older, clinical observations and caregiver or teacher reports from home, school, and other settings are important. By collecting a broad range of behavioral observations across multiple environments, the clinician(s) will discern the child's unique constitutional profile, as well as the conditions under which the child is optimally intentional, interactive, and developmentally integrated. The framework offered in the Developmental, Individual-Difference, Relationship-Based model (Greenspan and Wieder 1998) is a reasonable construct for organizing an understanding of how the child can become a developmentally integrated, functional person. The components of this model (Wieder et al. 2008) are summarized in Table 14–1.

When parents actively participate in the assessment, the clinician(s) can use shared observations and experiences to clarify the parents' understanding of the child's constitutional profile, and can partner with the parents to discern ways to support the child's progress.

Intervention and Treatment

Current best practice guidelines call for intensive individualized intervention of at least 25 hours per week focused on promoting social skills, functional communication, and developmentally appropriate play, among other skills (Lord and McGee 2001; National Autism Center 2009). The central role of family is stressed, but specific implementation guidelines related to the family's role are not established. Excellent reviews of available evidence-based behavioral treatments for children with ASDs are available (National Autism Center 2009; Rogers and Vismara 2008) and are not addressed here.

Lovaas's (1987) study showed that intensive, systematically administered discrete trial training, based on principles of applied behavior analysis, resulted in improved IQ and adaptive skill acquisition in young children with autism, and increased the ability to mainstream them at school. Subsequently, developmental skill-building programs led by behaviorists and administered by trained tutors became widely available. Overall, the prognosis of early identified autism has improved. The majority of children with ASDs no longer have intellectual disability (Chakrabarti and Fombonne 2001), due, at least in part, to intensive early intervention, as well as to diagnosis of more children on the milder end of the spectrum.

Improved understanding of the kinds of social-communication and regulatory difficulties faced by people with ASDs has led to a broader range of services. Developmental-relational interventions that emphasize child initiation and joint attention are increasing (Casenhiser et al. 2013; Kasari et al. 2008; Rogers and Dawson 2009; Solomon et al. 2007), and more speech-language pathologists are seeking training on the treatment of pragmatic language problems. Occupational therapists work with children to improve attention and processing capacities, motor planning and sequencing, and sensory regulatory modulation.

TABLE 14–1. Components of the Developmental, Individual-Difference, Relationship-Based model

I. Functional emotional developmental capacities	How the child integrates all core developmental capacities (motor, cognitive, language, spatial, sensory) to reach emotionally meaningful goals: regulation and joint attention, engagement, reciprocity in intentional two-way communication, social problem solving, creating and using ideas as the basis for creative thinking and giving meaning to symbols (using words and ideas), logic, emotional thinking, and judgment by building bridges between ideas and feelings.
II. Individual differences in sensory, modulation, processing, and motor planning	Biologically based differences that support—or challenge—the core developmental capacities described above. Differences result from genetic, prenatal, perinatal, and maturational variations and/or deficits.
III. Relationships and interactions	Developmentally appropriate, or inappropriate, interactive patterns with parents and other primary caregivers. These patterns are influenced by the child's biology and contribute to how child and parent navigate the child's developing functional capacities. Appropriate interactions mobilize the child's intentions and affects and enable a broader range of experiences that propel the developmental continuum forward.

Source. Adapted from Greenspan and Wieder 1998; Wieder et al. 2008.

Curriculum-based social skills programs provide opportunities to work on a variety of skills, including conversation, friendship, safety awareness, and theory of mind. Long-term friendship groups run by experienced autism specialists provide a safe haven in which children can build lasting relationships and an important sense of belonging.

Family Relationship–Focused Intervention

Currently, autism intervention for young children predominantly uses intensive behavioral strategies to build skills. A philosophy that embraces relationships as the foundation of meaningful learning, however, allows intensive practice of concepts in naturalized relational interactions and play, thereby building skills by using shared affect as the central organizer of experience. The relationship-focused practitioner helps parents recognize and prioritize interpersonal connection in all interactions and interventions, thereby nurturing the integration of experience across developmental domains (motor, cognition, communication, social, emotional). The practitioner's goal is to provide guidance and continuity as parents (and family) learn how to best be together and how to enable their child to be ever more present in the world.

Processing the Diagnosis

When their child is diagnosed with autism, parents inevitably experience feelings of anxiety, confusion, and profound loss as they reconcile the child they have imagined with this new diagnostic perspective. This loss generates a grieving process, which, although difficult, is the road to healing for the parents individually and as a couple, and for the family.

The loss-grief cycle (Foley 2006) begins with disorientation and disequilibrium. The parents will be in a state of disbelief. They must aim for regulation and reestablishment of homeostasis, often by using their usual, but taxed coping styles. Professionals must be especially sensitive, allowing parents to process and to make sense of what they are experiencing. They will need help in embracing the importance of early and intensive intervention.

Once a relative emotional equilibrium has been established, the searching phase in the loss-grief cycle begins. Parents may tend to deny the magnitude and intractability of the autism and/or search for alternative opinions. Practitioners must not rush this phase, because it allows parents to move from passive to active, and to strengthen feelings of purpose, determination, empowerment, and hope—qualities essential for the long haul of autism. Practitioners can provide a secure base to help parents explore in appropriate ways and not veer into distortions of reality or endless seeking of the impossible. As the family moves from assessment to intervention, parents will be looking for recommendations in establishing services. They will want to combine their child's early intervention services and other individual and family counseling and support in ways that will work for them. This may be a very good time for them to become engaged in parent-to-parent networking.

It is best practice for professionals to listen to the parents' concerns and to suggest specific resources, rather than to hand out generic lists or booklets. Being able to establish services is an indication that parents are moving into the acknowledgment phase of the loss-grief cycle, redefining themselves individually, their child with autism, and their family as a unit. The practitioner offers support as parents share their feelings and experiences, discover their child's capacities for connection, and learn how to shape unwanted behaviors, establish personal and family balance in day-to-day living, and keep up hope for the future.

The "aging out" or transition of children from early intervention at age 3 years to school-based services can be challenging, and parents may require assistance in negotiating the public school's individualized education program (IEP) process. The practitioner can help parents recognize and use the knowledge, experience, confidence, and reflective skills they have gained to navigate the transition and advocate for best practices for their child.

As parents gain perspective and redefine themselves and their family, their relationships deepen. The family will gain more stability, and move into the recovery phase of the loss-grief cycle, coming to some sense of acceptance. Key aspects of recovery include fewer intrusive thoughts and fears, less numbing, better mood, more energy, a more realistic view of themselves and their child, and increased ability to handle their child in a greater range of situations; their daily life begins to normalize, and there is more thinking about the future (Foley 2006).

Recovery can extend over a long period of time and slowly gives way to the maintenance phase of the loss-grief cycle. In this phase, the family system has more balance, the child is less the center of energy, and both child and parents gain more independence. Family members are able to expand their own interests and experience new areas of growth. In this phase, internalized coping strategies and adaptive mechanisms allow for realistic relationships and normative perspectives.

Importance of Active Family Involvement

Because active family involvement is essential for best outcomes, the practitioner should take seriously the parents' perspectives. These can range from extreme denial or irrational concerns to availability and good intuitiveness and insight. Discussing in detail the family's quality of life, aspirations, realities and dreams, daily routines, and relationships will engender professional-parent trust and a true partnership. By discerning ecological factors—ages and stages of family members, family processes and patterns, sibling and extended family characteristics, needs and roles of family members, connectedness in the community, and realistic and potential supports—the practitioner will be better able to offer insights and guidance. Respect for issues of ethnicity, culture, and individuality is fundamental. All these are the building blocks of a strong alliance that will enable the professional to help parents to fulfill their hopes for themselves, their children, and their family.

No matter what point a practitioner enters or reenters the life of a child with autism and the lives of his or her family, it is important to take a life-span perspective. Life will bring uncontrollable and unexpected events. The practitioner's goal is to identify what can be done to enhance relationships, nurture growth, and establish a sustainable, ever-improving quality of life for all.

KEY POINTS

- Infants and young children with autism spectrum disorders (ASDs) present a particular challenge to infant-caregiver attunement. Difficulty in co-orientation and the emergence of unusual behaviors, interests, and reactions tend to interfere with the child's development of social, emotional, and communication skills.
- The prevalence of ASD continues to rise, and many families are facing related concerns.
- At this point, no reliable behavioral signs of emerging ASD in infants age 6 months or younger have been found. Infants developing ASD may begin to show decreased initiation of and responsiveness to social interaction by age 8–10 months. By age 12 months, they may show decreases in eye contact, directed facial expressions, vocalizations, and response to name, and may exhibit repetitive behaviors that are unusual compared to those of typically developing children.
- When their child is diagnosed with ASD, parents inevitably experience feelings of anxiety, confusion, and profound loss as they reconcile the child they have imagined with this new diagnostic perspective. This loss generates a loss-grief cycle that, although difficult, is the road to healing for the parents and family, and to helping the child.
- Although ASDs are not mental health illnesses, they may contribute to, exacerbate, or generate challenges to the overall mental health and well-being of the family and the parent-child relationship. Therefore, therapeutic work is needed to scaffold, advance, and/or therapeutically treat the child, parent, dyad, and/or family. The impact and risk escalate when the diagnosis is made and new realities emerge, meanings are made, and the inevitable cycle of grieving—even if already in process—is activated around a condition with a name.
- The child and family are best treated by a "secure base" professional who, with the team, supports integrated functional development.

References

Abrahams BS, Geschwind DH: Advances in autism genetics: on the threshold of a new neurobiology. Nat Rev Genet 9:341–355, 2008

American Psychiatric Association: Diagnostic and Statistical Manual of Mental Disorders, 5th Edition. Arlington, VA, American Psychiatric Association, 2013

Anagnostou E, Taylor MJ: Review of neuroimaging in autism spectrum disorders. Mol Autism 2:1–9, 2011

Bailey A, Le Couteur A, Gottesman I, et al: Autism as a strongly genetic disorder. Psychol Med 25:63–77, 1995

Bornstein M, Suwalsy J, Breakstone D: Emotional relationships between mothers and infants. Dev Psychopathol 24:113–123, 2012

Braunschweig D, Krakowiak P, Duncanson P, et al: Autism-specific maternal autoantibodies recognize critical proteins in developing brain. Transl Psychiatry 3:e277, 2013

Brothers L: The social brain. Concepts in Neuroscience 1:27–51, 1990

Casenhiser D, Shanker S, Stieben J: Learning through interaction in children with autism: preliminary data from asocial-communication-based intervention. Autism 17:220–241, 2013

Centers for Disease Control and Prevention: Prevalence of autism spectrum disorders. MMWR Surveill Summ 61:1–19, 2012

Chakrabarti S, Fombonne E: Pervasive developmental disorders in preschool children. JAMA 285:3093–3099, 2001

Dawson G: Early behavioral interventions, brain plasticity, and the prevention of autism spectrum disorders. Dev Psychopathol 20:775–803, 2008

Dawson G, Rogers S, Munson J, et al: Randomized, controlled trial of an intervention for toddlers with autism: the Early Start Denver Model. Pediatrics 125:e17–e23, 2010

Foley G: The loss-grief cycle: coming to terms with the birth of a child with disability, in Mental Health in Early Intervention: Achieving Unity in Principles and Practice. Edited by Foley GM, Hochman JD. Baltimore, MD, Paul H Brookes Publishing, 2006, pp 227–243

Gillberg C: Chromosomal disorders and autism. J Autism Dev Disord 28:415–425, 1998

Greenspan SI, Wieder S: The Child With Special Needs: Encouraging Intellectual and Emotional Growth. Reading, MA, Addison-Wesley, 1998

Hansen RL, Hagerman RJ: Contributions of pediatrics, in Autism Spectrum Disorders: A Research Review for Practitioners. Edited by Ozonoff S, Rogers SJ, Hendren RL. Washington, DC, American Psychiatric Publishing, 2003, pp 87–109

Hobson P: Explaining autism: ten reasons to focus on the developing self. Autism 14:391–407, 2010

Johnson CP, Myers SM, American Academy of Pediatrics Council on Children With Disabilities. Identification and evaluation of children with autism spectrum disorders. Pediatrics 120(5):1183–1215, 2007

Kasari C, Paparella T, Freeman S, et al: Language outcome in autism: randomized comparison of joint attention and play interventions. J Consult Clin Psychol 76:125–137, 2008

Kuhl P: Is speech learning "gated" by the social brain? Dev Sci 10:110–120, 2007

Lord C, McGee JP (eds): Educating Children With Autism. Washington, DC, National Research Council, National Academy Press, 2001

Lord C, Rutter M, Le Couteur AM: Autism Diagnostic Interview–Revised: a revised version of a diagnostic interview for caregivers of individuals with possible pervasive developmental disorders. J Autism Dev Disord 24:659–685, 1994

Lord C, Rutter M, DiLavore PC, et al: Autism Diagnostic Observation Schedule, 2nd Edition (ADOS-2) Manual (Part I), Torrance, CA, Western Psychological Services, 2012a

Lord C, Rutter M, DiLavore PC, et al: Autism Diagnostic Observation Schedule, 2nd Edition (ADOS-2) Manual (Part II): Toddler Module. Torrance, CA, Western Psychological Services, 2012b

Lovaas O: Behavioral therapy and normal educational and intellectual function in young autistic children. J Consult Clin Psychol 55:3–9, 1987

Muhle R, Trentacoste S, Rapin I: The genetics of autism. Pediatrics 113:e472–e486, 2004

National Autism Center: National Standards Report. 2009. Available at: http://www.nationalautismcenter.org./nsp. Accessed March 30, 2013.

Osbourne L, McHugh L, Saunders J, et al: Parenting stress reduces the effectiveness of early teaching interventions for autism spectrum disorders. J Autism Dev Disord 38:1092–1103, 2008

Ozonoff S, Rogers SJ: From Kanner to the millenium, in Autism Spectrum Disorders: A Research Review for Practitioners. Edited by Ozonoff S, Rogers SJ, Hendren RL. Washington, DC, American Psychiatric Publishing, 2003, pp 3–36

Ozonoff S, Macari S, Young G: Atypical object exploration at 12 months of age is associated with autism in a prospective sample. Autism 12:457–472, 2008

Ozonoff S, Young G, Steinfeld MB, et al: How early do parent concerns predict later autism diagnosis? J Dev Behav Pediatr 30:367–375, 2009

Ozonoff S, Iosif AM, Baguio F, et al: A prospective study of the emergence of early behavioral signs of autism. J Am Acad Child Adolesc Psychiatry 49:256–266, 2010

Ozonoff S, Young G, Carter A, et al: Recurrence risk for autism spectrum disorders. Pediatrics 128:e488–e495, 2011

Pelphrey K, Shultz S, Hudac C: Research review: constraining heterogeneity: the social brain and its development in autism spectrum disorder. J Child Psychol Psychiatry 52:631–644, 2011

Polšek D, Jagatic T, Capanec M, et al: Recent developments in neuropathology of autism spectrum disorders. Transl Neurosci 2:256–264, 2011

Robins D, Fein D, Barton M, et al: The Modified Checklist for Autism in Toddlers: an initial study investigating the early detection of autism and pervasive developmental disorders. J Autism Dev Disord 31:131–144, 2001

Rogers SJ, Dawson G: Early Start Denver Model for Young Children With Autism. New York, Guilford, 2009

Rogers SJ, Vismara LA: Evidence-based comprehensive treatments for early autism. J Clin Child Adolesc Psychol 37:8–38, 2008

Rogers SJ, Dawson G, Vismara LA: An Early Start for Your Child With Autism. New York, Guilford, 2012

Rutter ML: Incidence of autism spectrum disorders: changes over time and their meaning. Acta Paediatr 94:2–15, 2005

Rutter ML: Progress in understanding autism 2007–2010. J Autism Dev Disord 41:395–404, 2011

Sanders L: Thinking differently: principles of process in living systems and the specificity of being known. Psychoanal Dialogues 12:11–42, 2002

Sanders S, Murtha M, Gupta A, et al: De novo mutations revealed by whole-exome sequencing are strongly associated with autism. Nature 485:237–241, 2012

Solomon R, Necheles J, Ferch C, et al: Pilot study of a parent-training program for young children with autism: the PLAY Project Home Consultation program. Autism 11:205–224, 2007

Stern D: The Interpersonal World of the Human Infant. New York, Basic Books, 1985

Tronick E: Emotions and emotional communication in infants. Am Psychol 44:112–119, 1989

Wieder S, Greenspan S, Kalmanson B: Autism, assessment, and intervention. Zero Three 28:31–37, 2008

Wolff J, Gu H, Gerig G, et al: Differences in white matter fiber tract development present from 6 to 24 months in infants with autism. Am J Psychiatry 169:589–600, 2012

Zoghbi H: Postnatal neurodevelopmental disorders. Science 302:826–830, 2003

Zwaigenbaum L, Bryson S, Rogers T, et al: Behavioral manifestations of autism in the first year of life. Int J Dev Neurosci 23:143–152, 2004

CHAPTER 15

Touch in Parent-Infant Mental Health

Arousal, Regulation, and Relationships

Mark Ludwig, M.S.W., L.C.S.W.
Tiffany Field, Ph.D.

In this chapter, we highlight the case for presenting touch and other nonverbal interactions as essential areas for infant research and intervention. Most parent-infant research has focused on nontactile forms of nonverbal communication, including gaze, prosody of speech and "motherese" (Stern 1985), and parent-infant communication rhythms (Beebe et al. 2000). Although attention has been given to the effects of touch and touch deprivation on infant regulation and social-emotional development (Stack and Jean 2011), basic touch research and touch intervention remain underdeveloped (Field 2000, 2001; Hertenstein 2011).

The Context of Touch: Regulatory Processes in Dynamic Developmental Systems

A central premise of parent-infant mental health theory is that human behavior and development can best be understood in terms of dynamic bioregulatory, neurological, psychological, cognitive, motoric, and relational systems in complex interaction (Fogel 2011; Sander 2008; Tronick 2007). Infant behavior in particular is a meaningful, organized "assembly of functional organizations" (Rochat 2001). The nonverbal nature of this earliest developmental period highlights the centrality of touch in communication and regulation at all levels: touch and touch interactions are crucial at these various organizational levels during the critical period from birth to age 3 years. Much research has focused on state regulation processes in the infant-parent relationship: during this early period, the dynamic, fundamental triad of *arousal-regulation-relationship* is at the core of development. In adequate infant care, arousal is regulated as the infants' psychobiological systems are collaboratively supported by the sensitive ministrations and attuned attention of the caregivers. In the first 6 months and throughout the early years, touch is the most potent form of arousal regulation (Feldman et al. 2010; Ferber et al. 2008).

First Sense That Organizes Self, Other, and World

Touch is the human infant's first learning modality, shaping experience even during the prenatal period. The infant's tactile sense develops from the first gestational week onward, and is the most advanced sense at birth. It underlies the organism's growing awareness of itself and the environment. Prenatal sensorimotor, proprioceptive, and tactile discrimination systems are thought to develop through the touch stimulation provided by fetal movement, push-back pressure from the elastic uterine wall, self-contact between body parts requiring coordinated movements of the limbs and head, and touching of the pulsing umbilical cord (Mori and Kuniyoshi 2010; Sann and Streri 2008). Body learning, self-organizing schemata, and behavioral patterns may first emerge from the dynamic interaction of the developing fetal nervous systems and the uterus, fluid movement, and self-touch.

Importance of Touch for Adequate Development

The human infant cannot develop adequately without receptive and active touch experience. The parent–infant "love affair" that guarantees early survival and stimulates and supports subsequent development is rooted in the mutual attraction and gratification of babies' and caregivers' feeling each other's skin, warmth, movements, and the like. This mutuality has an intrinsic, evolutionary underpinning. For example, the particularly smooth and soft skin of the infant is universally perceived as a pleasant tactile experience for the toucher (Guest et al. 2009). The skin and body of the neonate are richly endowed with touch and pressure receptors whose stimulation begins a cascade of healthful, interrelated biological and psychological processes (Field 2001).

Physiological Benefits of Touch Interaction in Early Development

Numerous studies indicate both the healthful benefits of touch and the effectiveness of touch in relieving psychological and physiological distress. Extensive animal studies with mammals (Suchecki et al. 1993) have explored the long-term social and neurological benefits of adequate contact, grooming, and licking. Suchecki et al. (1993) found that maternal regulation of the infant's hypothalamic-pituitary-adrenal axis through touch and nursing occurred at multiple levels. Other studies have documented positive physiological and biochemical effects of touching (Weiss 2000), including decreases in infant blood pressure and heart rate, as well as decreased cortisol levels and increased oxytocin and prolactin levels (Feldman et al. 2007; Uvnas-Moberg and Peterson 2005). In a study comparing skin-to-skin sleeping with maternal separation sleeping, Morgan et al. (2011) used heart rate variability data monitoring with full-term neonates and reported "a 176% increase in autonomic activity and an 86% decrease in quiet sleep duration during separation compared with skin-to-skin contact" (p. 817).

Neurological, Neuroendocrinological, and Autonomic Aspects of Touch

Humans are genetically and biologically organized to seek, exchange, process, and use touch interactions to establish relationships, for regulation, and for social and personal communication. Regarding the role of behavioral chemistry in parent-infant touch interaction, Weller and Feldman (2003) surveyed the role of cholecystokinin and opioid peptides in early contact interactions and bonding in animals and the suspected role of these touch-induced agents in emotion regulation in infants in the context of separation, contact, and attachment processes. They found that postnatal touch was a crucial factor in maintaining regulatory balance and helped to reduce risk factor–induced emotional dysregulation.

The work of Stephen Porges (2001, 2011) has generated a great deal of interest in the functional evolution and developmental complexity of the vagal systems by showing how social engagement is an evolving, active force in interpersonal neurobiological regulation. Notably, low vagal tone has been found to be associated with impaired post-stress re-regulation (Degangi et al. 1991). However, proximity, cuddling, touch, and safe interpersonal interactions support vagal tone regulation. Vagal tone increases immediately after massage therapy sessions and across repeated sessions of massage therapy (Diego et al. 2007). This likely happens via the stimulation of dermal and subdermal pressure receptors that are innervated by vagal afferent fibers, which ultimately project to the limbic system in the brain, including hypothalamic structures involved in autonomic nervous system regulation and cortisol secretion. This vagal activity–touch interaction likely coordinates touch-based forms of interactive psychobiological regulation with eye contact, auditory communication, emotional matching, and other forms of rhythmic caregiver-infant interactions (Tronick 2007).

Psychological and Emotional Functions of Interactive Touch

Adequate and attuned touch provides a regulatory foundation for early psychological and social-emotional development (Barnard and Brazelton 1990). As Feldman (2011) notes,

"Maternal touch…is not just one more thing mothers do: It is the basic channel for the expression of parenting and serves as the bedrock to the individual's future capacity to provide love and nourishment to future attachment relationships" (p. 374). Touch constitutes the most effective single component (Stack and Jean 2011) of the complex interpersonal, nonverbal communication system (touch, gaze, vocalizations, movement, positioning) that underlies attachment and regulation in early life. Touch alone is as effective as facial and vocal communication in calming and regulating infants in mother-infant interactions (Stack and Muir 1992).

Emotional Communication Via Touch

A growing body of research supports the innate evolutionary wisdom and parental intuition that touch communicates emotional experiences and intentions (Muir 2002). Hertenstein et al. (2002, 2006) and others have established that in adults, emotion of the toucher can be identified correctly from the simple experience of a stranger touching you on your arm. These experiments with adults found that the emotions of anger, fear, disgust, love, gratitude, and sympathy could be understood nonverbally through touch alone. More emotions could be conveyed when the senders were allowed to touch any appropriate part of the human body to convey a specific emotion (Hertenstein et al. 2009). Such innovative experiments are establishing that humans receive a great deal more emotional information through touch than was previously known (Jean et al. 2009). If caregivers are communicating their emotional states to children through touch, the necessity of heightened caregiver awareness is quite clear. If children are also communicating emotions nonverbally through their own acts of caregiver touching, then recognition and response to these communications should enhance the child's sense of himself or herself as a competent communicator. On the other hand, touch that communicates the caregiver's negative emotional states or overlooks the child's responses to touch may degrade the vitality of the child's response to touch and the child's belief in himself or herself as an effective emotional communicator via touch.

Touch Sensitivity and Touch Aversion

Touch interaction is an essential lifelong behavior that is adapted to changing human needs across the lifespan. In the beginning, touch and holding provide essential care, security, and regulation. As the child grows, touch and holding become less frequent (Green et al. 1980), are ritualized, or are sought and provided on an ad hoc basis in response to distress or as an expression of affection. Attuned bodily interactions meet the child at the somatic level and provide congruence for the earliest senses of an embodied self (Stern 1985). Although touch patterns change rapidly across the first year as the child engages the world more actively and becomes mobile, an early history of attuned touch appears to be part of an implicit relational substrate that is sustained and reflected in the reciprocity in later communication, a feature highly correlated with effective social-emotional and affect regulation (Lyons-Ruth et al. 1990).

Research over many decades has drawn the association between affectionate and tender touch and attachment security (Ainsworth et al. 1978; Leyendecker et al. 1997). On the other hand, caregivers' or infants' touch aversions or avoidance early in life can have a profound effect on the bonding and attachment relationship with primary caregivers. When touch aversion is present, an essential and potent resource of early interactive regulation is unavailable and the child must adapt, often with some developmental cost. Genetic and constitutional factors such as temperament and parent-infant temperament "fit" may give rise to touch-aversive behaviors when there is an unfulfilled parental touch expectation for reciprocity from more apprehensive and reactive children. Preterm infants are known to develop highly sensitive sensory response schema and sensory processing disorders that may develop into lasting tactile hypersensitivities (Case-Smith et al. 1998). Touch aversion and touch sensitivity are common features of sensory integration dysfunction (Ayres 2005) and autism spectrum disorders (Tomchek and Dunn 2007), in which modulation and regulation of sensory inputs are impaired.

Feldman et al. (2004) found that children with infant eating disorders had less affectionate and more negative touch interactions and more touch rejection. Touch responses can also be affected by transitory and chronic traumatic experiences, such as early intrusive medical procedures associated with the neonatal intensive care unit (NICU) (Weiss and Wilson 2006), prolonged experience of pain, or stressful caregiving practices such as repeated use of enemas, or through milder insensitivities such as the pinching, poking, prodding, shaking, and jiggling associated with the caregiving of mothers with depressive symptoms (Malphurs et al. 1996). Finally, a robust research literature links maternal depression (Herrera et al. 2004; Weinberg and Tronick 1998) and insecurity of attachment (Ainsworth 1979) to learned touch aversion, touch avoidance, and touch deprivation.

Benefits to the Toucher in Parent-Infant Touch Interaction

Mutual physical, psychological, and emotional benefits occur for all partners in touch interactions. As stimulation of pressure receptors mediates the positive effects of massage on its "recipient" (Field 2001; Field et al. 2010), these pressure receptors are also stimulated in the hands of the person providing the massage or touch. Demonstrating the mutual or reciprocal effects of touch is a complex problem, but this coregulation paradigm may be a model for further research. Neu et al. (2009) found that the cortisol levels of mothers who held their premature infants decreased while they were holding their babies. The infants also had lowered cortisol levels after being held. Regular massage also reduced heart rate and anxiety levels in both parents and child cancer patients (Post-White et al. 2009). Parents' effective use of touch for coregulation of affect in their children may build competency and confidence in the parents and increase their sensitivity to the infants' cues (Clausen et al. 2012).

Touch Interventions

The quality and impact of touch often lie outside the toucher's immediate awareness. Parents and caregivers may touch as they were touched as children. Parent-infant mental health practitioners are keenly attentive to such nonverbal communication of transgenerational styles with caregiver-infant dyads in treatment (Champagne 2008; Fraiberg et al. 1975). In parent-infant mental health training, considerable attention is given to tracking the strength and style of dyadic nonverbal cueing and whole-body expressions of arousal states and affective tone. Methods for evaluating infant-parent interactions often include observations of patterns of touch both explicitly and implicitly. For example, the NCAST Parent-Child Interaction Feeding and Teaching Scales (Barnard 1994) represent a detailed and well-researched program that looks at infant engagement and disengagement cues and infant states that support readiness for contact, and provides a tracking system to identify parents who may be having difficulty maintaining connection to their young child's internal state and needs.

At times, parents need assistance and feedback to be able to coordinate their touch sensitively with the needs of the child. For example, Tronick (2007) found that poking, pinching, prodding, and other forms of touch are associated with misattuned parenting and chronically dysregulated dyads. Interventions that reflect current interest in parental reflective functioning (Fonagy et al. 2005; Slade 2002) and mindfulness (Siegel 2001) consider the qualities, timing, and appropriateness of touch, as well as parents' awareness of the impact of all their engagements on their child's regulation and affect in real time.

Infant-parent touch-focused interventions have been most developed in cases demonstrating a high risk of problematic medical, developmental, or psychological outcome. Parent-infant touch interventions have been used in medical and mental health centers serving families with young children (Feldman 2011; Field 2011); generally, however, pediatricians and popular parenting manuals, with few exceptions (Brazelton 1992), offer little guidance on everyday touch sensitivity to the normative parenting population.

In contrast, the potent positive impacts of sensitive and timely touch for children at risk and the negative consequences of misattuned or insufficient touch interaction have been given considerably more attention. With regard to touch with preterm and NICU babies, the Touch Research Institute (Field 2001) has conducted an active program of touch research and intervention since 1992. Preterm infant massage has been an area of special focus. Preterm infants receiving moderate-pressure massage may show fewer stress behaviors, as was noted in a study by Field et al. (2006). Compared with the light-pressure massage group, the moderate-pressure group gained significantly more weight per day and, during the behavior observations, showed significantly lower increases in 1) active sleep, 2) fussing, 3) crying, 4) movement, and 5) stress behavior (hiccupping). Babies in the moderate-pressure group also showed a smaller decrease in deep sleep, a greater decrease in heart rate, and a greater increase in vagal tone. All of these changes suggest a decrease in general arousal, which, in turn, may explain improved immune function in preterm neonates. When conducted by parents, these early touch experiences support the development of attachment and bonding, connection points that are often stressed when parents cannot find direct means to help their hospitalized children.

There have also been noteworthy interventions targeting attachment and interpersonal regulation in the parent-infant dyad. Touch interventions that support emotional attunement and secure attachment patterns target the development of the sensitive interpersonal skill thought to be essential in the parent's scaffolding of a child's long-term achievement of affect and impulse regulation. The Fostering Mindful Attachment program (Cooper et al. 2008) was designed to bring infant-parent mental health services to children from birth to age 1 year and their parents in residential substance abuse treatment using parent-infant massage as a platform for supporting attunement and early attachment processes. In this program, caregivers learn to track their infant's response to qualities of touch interactions and develop new capacities to recognize and attend to their own internal states of arousal. Facilitators' interventions are aimed at cognitive, emotional, sensory, relational, motor, and arousal patterns. Ongoing research (Clausen et al. 2012) shows trends toward higher knowledge of infant development and lower parenting stress after completion of the intervention program. Following the intervention, participants more often perceived their children as less difficult and easier to understand.

Conclusion

In this chapter, we have presented an integrated perspective on touch and touch-focused interventions in early development and on current infant-parent mental health clinical theory and practice. Current research is beginning to call attention to what human bodies have always known: touch is an essential element in shaping development, including neurophysiological functioning and the overall sense of self. Still, insufficient attention has been paid to the meaning and effects of touch. Touch still appears to be "the neglected sense" relative to the other senses.

We have looked at the physiological, neurological, and endocrinological benefits of touch interaction in early development, along with the consequences of touch deprivation and the possible mechanisms behind touch aversion. Finally, we have discussed general principles for working with touch in parent-infant dyads and, more specifically, touch interventions for infants and parent-infant dyads at risk. The emerging evidence indicates that continued efforts to understand the foundational effects of touch and touch interactions and to develop interventions based on these understandings may be very fruitful. Practice models that understand the complex tactile needs of the child should be considered as part of holistic professional interventions and parenting education programs.

KEY POINTS

- Touch is the human infant's first learning modality, shaping experience even before birth. Caregiver-infant touch is a complex psychophysiological interaction that impacts multiple neurological and biological systems in both the child and the caregiver. Touch is the most effective single intervention for regulating the neurological and affective systems of infants and young children.

- Affectionate and tender touch is associated with attachment security, whereas caregivers' or infants' touch aversions or avoidance early in life can negatively impact the dyadic relationship with primary caregivers (including attachment). When touch aversion is present, an essential and potent resource of early interactive regulation is unavailable and the child must adapt, often with developmental cost.

- Touch aversion, touch avoidance, and touch deprivation in children have been associated with insecure attachment, maternal depression, preterm birth, transitory and chronic traumatic experiences (e.g., intrusive medical procedures, neonatal intensive care, prolonged pain, repeated enemas), and insensitive caregiving (e.g., pinching, poking, prodding, shaking, jiggling).

- Positive physical, psychological, and emotional benefits occur for both partners in touch interactions, including lower cortisol levels, reduced heart rate, and lower anxiety levels. Parents' effective use of touch for coregulation of affect in their children may build competency and confidence in the parents and increase their sensitivity to the infants' cues.

- Parents and parent educators may want to focus on the development of caregiver reflective capacity regarding their own emotional and autonomic arousal during touch interactions, because recent research indicates that touch may communicate emotional experiences and intentions.

References

Ainsworth M: Infant-mother attachment. Am Psychol 34:932–937, 1979

Ainsworth M, Blehar M, Waters E, et al: Patterns of Attachment: A Psychological Study of the Strange Situation. Hillsdale, NJ, Erlbaum, 1978

Ayres J: Sensory Integration and the Child: Understanding Hidden Sensory Challenges. Los Angeles, CA, Western Psychological Services, 2005

Barnard K: NCAST Caregiver/Parent-Child Interaction Teaching Manual. Seattle, University of Washington, School of Nursing, 1994

Barnard K, Brazelton TB: Touch: The Foundation of Experience. Madison, CT, International Universities Press, 1990

Beebe B, Jaffe J, Lachmann F, et al: Systems models in development and psychoanalysis: the case of vocal rhythm coordination and attachment. Infant Ment Health J 21:99–122, 2000

Brazelton TB: Touchpoints: The Essential Reference—Your Child's Emotional and Behavioral Development. Boston, MA, Addison-Wesley, 1992

Case-Smith J, Butcher L, Reed D: Parents' report of sensory responsiveness and temperament in preterm infants. Am J Occup Ther 52:547–555, 1998

Champagne F: Epigenetic mechanisms and the transgenerational effects of maternal care. Front Neuroendocrinol 29:386–397, 2008

Clausen JM, Aquilar RM, Ludwig ME: Fostering healthy attachment between substance dependent parents and their infant children. J Infant Child Adolesc Psychother 11:376–386, 2012

Cooper A, Ludwig M, Heineman T: Fostering Mindful Attachment: a relational approach to infant-parent massage. The Source: Newsletter of the National Abandoned Infants Assistance Resource Center 18:16–18, 2008

Degangi G, Dipietro J, Greenspan S, et al: Psychophysiological characteristics of the regulatory disordered infant. Infant Behav Dev 14:37–50, 1991

Diego M, Field T, Hernandez-Reif M, et al: Preterm infant massage elicits consistent increases in vagal activity and gastric motility that are associated with greater weight gain. Acta Paediatr 96:1588–1591, 2007

Feldman R: Maternal touch and the developing infant, in The Handbook of Touch: Neuroscience, Behavioral, and Health Perspectives. Edited by Hertenstein MJ, Weiss SJ. New York, Springer, 2011, pp 373–408

Feldman R, Keren M, Gross-Rozval M, et al: Mother-child touch patterns in infant feeding disorders: relation to maternal, child, and environmental factors. J Am Acad Child Adolesc Psychiatry 43:1089–1097, 2004

Feldman R, Weller A, Zagoory-Sharon O, et al: Evidence for a neuroendocrinological foundation of human affiliation: plasma oxytocin levels across pregnancy and the postpartum period predict mother-infant bonding. Psychol Sci 18:965–970, 2007

Feldman R, Singer M, Zagoory O: Touch attenuates infants' physiological reactivity to stress. Dev Sci 13:271–278, 2010

Ferber S, Feldman R, Makhoul I: The development of maternal touch across the first year of life. Early Hum Dev 84:363–370, 2008

Field T: Infant massage therapy, in Handbook of Infant Mental Health. Edited by Zeanah C. New York, Guilford, 2000, pp 494–500

Field T: Touch. Cambridge, MA, MIT Press, 2001

Field T: Massage therapy: a review of recent research, in The Handbook of Touch: Neuroscience, Behavioral, and Health Perspectives. Edited by Hertenstein MJ, Weiss SJ. New York, Springer, 2011, pp 469–498

Field T, Diego M, Hernandez-Reif M: Moderate versus light pressure massage therapy leads to greater weight gain in preterm infants. Infant Behav Dev 29:574–578, 2006

Field T, Diego M, Hernandez-Reif M: Preterm infant massage therapy research: a review. Infant Behav Dev 33:115–124, 2010

Fogel A: Theoretical and applied dynamic systems research in developmental science. Child Dev Perspect 5:267–272, 2011

Fonagy P, Gergely G, Jurist E, et al: Affect Regulation, Mentalization, and the Development of Self. New York, Other Press, 2005

Fraiberg S, Adelson E, Shapiro V: Ghosts in the nursery: a psychoanalytic approach to the problems of impaired infant-parent relationships. J Am Acad Child Adolesc Psychiatry 14:387–421, 1975

Green J, Gustafson G, West M: Effects of infant development on mother-infant interactions. Child Dev 51:199–207, 1980

Guest S, Essick G, Dessirier JM, et al: Sensory and affective judgments of skin during inter- and intrapersonal touch. Acta Psychol (Amst) 130:115–126, 2009

Herrera E, Reissland N, Shepherd J: Maternal touch and maternal child-directed speech: effects of depressed mood in the postnatal period. J Affect Disord 81:29–39, 2004

Hertenstein M: Touch: its communicative functions in infancy. Hum Dev 45:70–94, 2002

Hertenstein MJ, Weiss SJ: The Handbook of Touch: Neuroscience, Behavioral, and Health Perspectives. New York, Springer, 2011

Hertenstein M, Keltner D, App B, et al: Touch communicates distinct emotion. Emotion 6:528–533, 2006

Hertenstein M, Holmes R, McCullough M, et al: The communication of emotion via touch. Emotion 9:566–573, 2009

Jean A, Stack D, Fogel A: A longitudinal investigation of maternal touching across the first 6 months of life: age and context effects. Infant Behav Dev 32:344–349, 2009

Leyendecker B, Lamb M, Fracasso M, et al: Playful interaction and the antecedents of attachment: a longitudinal study of Central American and Euro-American mothers and infants. Merrill Palmer Q (Wayne State Univ Press) 43:24–27, 1997

Lyons-Ruth K, Connell DB, Grunebaum HU, et al: Infants at social risk: maternal depression and family support services as mediators of infant development and security of attachment. Child Dev 61:85–98, 1990

Malphurs J, Raag T, Field T, et al: Touch by intrusive and withdrawn mothers with depressive symptoms. Early Development & Parenting 5:111–115, 1996

Morgan B, Horn A, Bergman N: Should neonates sleep alone? Biol Psychiatry 9:817–825, 2011

Mori H, Kuniyoshi Y: A human fetus development simulation: self-organization of behaviors through tactile sensation. From IEEE 9th International Conference on Development and Learning. August 2010. Available at: http://ieeexplore.ieee.org/xpl/articleDetails.jsp?reload=true&arnumber=5578860&contentType=Conference+Publications. Accessed March 31, 2013.

Muir D: Adult communications with infants through touch: the forgotten sense. Hum Dev 45:95–99, 2002

Neu M, Laudenslager M, Robinson J: Coregulation in salivary cortisol during maternal holding of premature infants. Biol Res Nurs 10:226–240, 2009

Porges SW: The polyvagal theory: phylogenetic substrates of a social nervous system. Int J Psychophysiol 42:123–146, 2001

Porges SW: The Polyvagal Theory: Neurophysiological Foundations of Emotions, Attachment, Communication, and Self-Regulation. New York, WW Norton, 2011

Post-White J, Fitzgerald M, Savik K, et al: Massage therapy for children with cancer. J Pediatr Oncol Nurs 26:16–28, 2009

Rochat P: The Infant's World. Cambridge, MA, Harvard University Press, 2001

Sander L: Living Systems, Evolving Consciousness, and the Emerging Person: A Selection of Papers From the Life Work of Louis Sander. Edited by Amadei G, Bianchi I. New York, Analytic Press, 2008

Sann C, Streri A: Intermanual transfer of object texture and shape in human neonates. Neuropsychologia 46:698–703, 2008

Siegel DJ: The Developing Mind: How Relationships and the Brain Interact to Shape Who We Are. New York, Guilford, 2001

Slade A: Keeping the baby in mind: a critical factor in perinatal mental health. Zero Three 22:10–16, 2002

Stack D, Jean A: Communicating through touch: touching during parent-infant interactions, in The Handbook of Touch: Neuroscience, Behavioral, and Health Perspectives. Edited by Hertenstein MJ, Weiss S. New York, Springer, 2011, pp 273–298

Stack D, Muir D: Adult tactile stimulation during face-to-face interactions modulates five-month-olds' affect and attention. Child Dev 63:1509–1525, 1992

Stern D: The Interpersonal World of the Human Infant. New York, Basic Books, 1985

Suchecki D, Rosenfeld P, Levine S: Maternal regulation of the hypothalamic-pituitary-adrenal axis in the infant rat: the roles of feeding and stroking. Brain Res Dev Brain Res 75:185–192, 1993

Tomchek SD, Dunn W: Sensory processing in children with and without autism: a comparative study using the Short Sensory Profile. Am J Occup Ther 61:190–200, 2007

Tronick E: The Neurobehavioral and Social-Emotional Development of Infants and Children (Norton Series on Interpersonal Neurobiology). New York, WW Norton, 2007

Uvnas-Moberg K, Petersson M: Oxytocin, a mediator of anti-stress, well-being, social interaction, growth, and healing [in German]. Z Psychosom Med Psychother 51:57–80, 2005

Weinberg K, Tronick E: Emotional characteristics of infants associated with maternal depression and anxiety. Pediatrics 102:1298–1304, 1998

Weiss SJ, Wilson P: Origins of tactile vulnerability in high-risk infants. Adv Neonatal Care 6:25–36, 2006

Weiss S, Wilson P, Hertenstein M, et al: The tactile context of a mother's caregiving: implications for attachment of low birth weight infants. Infant Behav Dev 23:91–111, 2000

Weller A, Feldman R: Emotion regulation and touch in infants: the role of cholecystokinin and opioids. Peptides 24:779–788, 2003

CHAPTER 16

Developmental Psychopathology

Core Principles and Implications for Child Mental Health

Stephen P. Hinshaw, Ph.D.

Cassandra L. Joubert, Sc.D.

Our goal in this chapter is to introduce readers to the discipline of developmental psychopathology (DP), which emerged in the 1970s and 1980s as a means of integrating child and adolescent psychology and psychiatry with the principles of developmental science (Cicchetti 1984; Sroufe and Rutter 1984). Since that time, DP has contributed a rich account of the etiology and underlying mechanisms of behavioral and emotional disorders of youth. The DP model aims to transcend a categorical diagnostic approach by accounting for continuities and discontinuities in the development of pathology over the lifespan. After our review of basic principles, we briefly discuss sex differences in developmental disorders, the stigma that still attends mental illness, and implications for intervention, three crucial topics that follow from DP models. Although each of these areas could yield book-length coverage, our intent is to provide a cogent summation. For longer coverage, from which the material below on DP is adapted, see the review chapter by Hinshaw (2013). For a larger "status report" on the advances made via DP, see the volume edited by Cicchetti and Cohen (2006) and the review article by Cicchetti and Toth (2009).

Rationale for a Developmental Psychopathology Approach

To understand why DP models are needed, one must first consider the high levels of suffering and impairment involved in child and adolescent psychopathology, from depression's link to hopelessness and despair through the association of attention-deficit/hyperactivity disorder (ADHD) with major academic and social deficits, and the relation between eating disorders and major disruptions in physical well-being as well as healthy self-image. Although resilience can and does occur in some cases (Luthar and Brown 2007), the risk of lingering impairment from mental disturbance is real. Furthermore, not only do behavioral, emotional, and developmental disturbances in childhood and adolescence usually persist into adulthood, but what are considered to be adult mental disorders typically reveal precursors in the early years of development (Kessler et al. 2005). Symptoms and impairments typically start early and remain problematic for years to follow.

Traditional efforts in psychology and psychiatry are too static to account for the complex, underlying developmental processes that fuel risk and protection. In other words, the reciprocally deterministic nature of development is not well captured in yes/no diagnostic systems. Moreover, 1) clinical conditions result from multiple pathways and trajectories, signaling equifinality, and 2) youth with similar risk factors or vulnerabilities early in development diverge markedly in their later outcomes, a process known as multifinality (Cicchetti and Rogosch 1996). Both processes signal that linear models and simple diagnostic categories are not sufficiently explanatory. Furthermore, the sheer magnitude of neuronal development during prenatal and neonatal time periods, coupled with the complex interactions taking place with ever-widening social environments across development, means that single-variable accounts of both normal and atypical development are doomed to be overly reductionistic. The multilevel, transactional approach of DP is needed to deal with the complex phenomena at hand.

Despite the scientific and clinical urgency surrounding this topic, huge barriers prevent full understanding and full access to evidence-based treatment. A primary reason is that mental disturbance is still highly stigmatized (Hinshaw 2007). Such intense stigma and shame often prevent help-seeking and serve to make mental health a lower priority than physical health, despite the inextricable linkages between the two. After a review of core DP principles and sex differences in child and adolescent psychopathology, we return to stigmatization.

Developmental Psychopathology Concepts and Principles

What characterizes a truly developmental view of psychopathology, as opposed to the kinds of descriptive, symptom-focused presentations that still dominate most classification systems? Several core points are commonly viewed as central. At the outset, we note that a core ramification of DP is that the typical variable-centered approach to studying behavioral and emotional disorders—which focuses on effects of one or more risk or protective variables across an entire sample—must be bolstered by consideration of unique subgroups. Such groups may be defined by genotypes, personality variables, socialization practices, neighborhoods, or other key factors, and their unique developmental journeys require "person-centered" research methods (Bergman et al. 2006). Even with more traditional, variable-centered approaches, moderator and mediator variables must always be considered (Hinshaw 2002; Kraemer et al. 2001).

Normal and Atypical Development: Mutually Informative

DP models emphasize that phenomena defined as abnormal represent aberrations in normal developmental pathways and processes. That is, these conditions are not qualitatively distinct, separate from normative development. Rather, they signify that core developmental tasks and milestones may not be achieved, with negative consequences for later hurdles in life. Without a full understanding of typical development, the study of pathology remains incomplete and decontextualized. For example, illuminating the nature of ADHD requires a thorough understanding of the normative development of attention, impulse control, and self-regulation (Nigg 2006). Similarly, investigations of autism must be fully integrated with understanding of the development of interpersonal awareness and empathy, which typically takes place over the first several years of life (Dawson and Toth 2006). The process is a two-way street, however, in that it requires the complementary view that investigations of pathological conditions provide a valuable perspective on normal developmental mechanisms. In other words, the study of disrupted developmental progressions illuminates understanding of what is normative. Neurology abounds with relevant examples. "Split-brain" patients (i.e., those who have had their cerebral hemispheres separated to provide relief from specific neurological disorders) provide unprecedented insights into normative brain processes. Famous case studies of individuals who had key brain structures or regions surgically removed (e.g., Henry Molaison, long known as HM, whose hippocampus was removed) greatly facilitate knowledge about human memory systems (see Gazzaniga et al. 2009).

But does the same reasoning apply to child and adolescent mental disorders, which are far more complex than single neurological aberrations or specific surgical procedures? We argue that it does. For instance, in high-functioning autism, intelligence is normal but social interactions are compromised, presumably because of deficits in the development of what is called "theory of mind," the ability to register false beliefs and understand that others have differing perspectives from one's own (Baron-Cohen 2000). Nearly all typically developing 4-year-olds can master theory-of-mind tests (and some false-belief detection begins far earlier, even in infancy), suggesting that basic social understanding is undergirded by a domain-specific cognitive module that operates almost automatically. Some individuals with high-functioning autism can learn to "pass" the kinds of experimental tests used to appraise theory of mind via effortful processing, but their social interactions usually do not become smooth and effortless. Thus, disruptions in social cognition and social performance in persons with autism may help to clarify the automatic and highly developed nature of the skilled interpersonal performance in normal development.

Another example pertains to the horrifying "experiments of nature" that occur when infants and toddlers are subjected to brutal institutionalization and lack of human contact during the earliest years of development (O'Connor 2006). Examining rates of recovery during placement into stable homes (even experimentally; Nelson et al. 2007) is extremely informative about the normative development of secure relationships and cognitive performance (see McLaughlin et al. 2012 regarding implications for attachment theory).

Continuities and Discontinuities

DP models emphasize both continuous and discontinuous processes at work in the development of pathology. For example, antisocial behavior is stable over time, meaning that the most aggressive and antisocial preschoolers tend to become the most aggressive and antisocial children and adolescents. However, the precise forms of externalizing/antisocial behavior shift: those children with extremes of temper tantrums and defiance during the toddler and preschool years have a high likelihood of displaying physical aggression in grade school, covert antisocial behaviors in preadolescence, various forms of delinquency by their teen years, and partner abuse in their 20s and beyond. In short, heterotypic continuity is present, meaning that the specific form of the underlying antisocial trait changes with development.

Another important consideration is that patterns of continuity may differ considerably across distinct subgroups that display different developmental trajectories. Not all highly aggressive or antisocial children remain so: some are prone to desist with the transition to adolescence. Others—composing the so-called early starter or life-course-persistent subgroup—maintain high rates through at least early adulthood. In addition, a large subset does not display major externalizing problems in childhood but instead shows a sharp increase with adolescence (Moffitt 2006). Understanding such discontinuous subgroups yields greater understanding than do overall curves of "growth" across the population.

Multiple Levels of Analysis

The greatest potential for progress (and for complexity) in the DP field is present when investigators traverse micro and macro levels to understand mechanisms underlying the development of adjustment and maladjustment. Linking events at the level of the gene (e.g., genetic polymorphisms; transcription and translation) to neurotransmission and neuroanatomical development, and subsequently to individual differences in temperament, social cognition, and emotional response patterns, is essential (Cicchetti 2008). At the same time, such bottom-up conceptions must be supplemented by top-down understanding of the ways in which family interaction patterns, peer relations, school factors, and neighborhood/community processes influence the developing, plastic brain, even at the level of gene expression, invoking the concept of epigenetic influences. Progress in understanding pathology requires multidisciplinary efforts involving investigators ranging from geneticists and biochemists, to clinicians focusing on individual pathology, experts on family and neighborhood processes, investigators of clinical service systems, and public health officials and policy makers. Such large-scale research necessitates collaboration across traditional academic boundaries, leading to major payoffs (Caspi et al. 2010).

Risk and Protective Factors

Risk factors (and constitutional vulnerabilities) are those antecedent variables that predict dysfunction. The ultimate goal is to discover those variables that are both malleable and potentially causal of the disorder in question (Kraemer et al. 2001). Yet, disordered behavior is not uniform, and risk factors are not inevitable predictors. For example, being female is a protective factor against most forms of psychopathology in the first decade of life but serves as a risk factor for severe internalizing conditions during adolescence (Hinshaw 2009). Maltreatment is a risk factor for later pathology, but not in every case. *Resilience* is the term used to define unexpectedly good outcomes, or competence, in the presence of adversity or risk (Sapienza and Masten 2011). DP is centrally involved in the search for protective factors, those variables and processes that mitigate risk and promote more-successful outcomes than would be expected. The processes involved in promoting competence and strength rather than disability and despair must be discovered, because they can be harnessed for prevention efforts. In short, a crucial goal is to understand why some children born into poverty fare well in adolescence and adulthood, why some individuals with alleles that tend to confer risk for pathological outcomes do not evidence psychopathology, why some youth with difficult temperaments develop into highly competent adults, and why some children who lack secure attachments or enriching environments during their early years nonetheless show academic and social competence later on.

Reciprocal, Transactional Models

Pathways from childhood to adolescent and adult functioning are marked by reciprocal patterns or chains, in which children influence parents, teachers, and peers, who in turn shape the further individual development of the child. Such mutually interactive processes themselves reverberate over time, leading to what are termed *transactional models*. Relatedly, developmental processes often operate via cascading, escalating chains (Masten et al. 2006); in other cases, however, buffers or protective factors may "break the chain." In an elegant musical metaphor, Boyce (2006) presents the notion of "symphonic causation" to illustrate the confluence of biological and contextual influences on development.

A great many cognitive and personality outcomes are at least moderately heritable, meaning that genetic factors explain a sizable proportion of individual differences in the trait, attribute, or disorder in question. However, via gene-environment correlations, contexts (genetically associated with the trait in question) may passively amplify the expression of the trait. Furthermore, individuals may seek or evoke environmental responses that further promote the trait's unfolding. Finally, certain genotypes may become expressed only in the context of certain environmental factors, signifying the operation of gene-environment interactions (Dodge and Rutter 2011; Rutter et al. 2006). In short, linear models and single-variable influences now yield to broader, more complex conceptions of causal pathways. Neither biological predisposition nor early environment is a sufficient explanation; understanding their integration is essential.

Context and Culture

A key tenet of DP is that family, school-related, neighborhood, and wider cultural contexts are central for the unfolding of aberrant as well as adaptive behaviors. Across the life span of the human species, what may have served as adaptive behaviors at certain points in human evolutionary history may be maladaptive in current times, given the major environmental and cultural changes that render certain genetically mediated traits far less advantageous than previously. Two relevant examples are 1) the storage of fat in times of uncertain meals and sudden need for survival-related activity, now leading to obesity in sedentary individuals, and 2) the presence of undue anxiety in relation to certain feared stimuli (e.g., snakes), which was undoubtedly adaptive in earlier times but is now termed "specific phobia." There are few absolutes in terms of either behavior patterns that are inherently maladaptive or risk factors that inevitably yield dysfunction. Cultural settings, as well as contexts, are all-important for shaping and even defining healthy versus unhealthy adaptation. Similarly, key environmental factors (such as parenting styles) are neither always uniformly positive nor uniformly negative in terms of their developmental effects. In short, effects of risk or protective factors may differ markedly depending on developmental timing, the family and social contexts in which they are experienced by the developing child, and the niche that exists in a given culture for their expression and resolution (Serafica and Vargas 2006). According to the DP perspective, setting and context are essential (Cicchetti and Cohen 2006).

Along this line, current models are moving away from the idea that certain genotypes are inevitably risk factors for psychopathology. Some "risk" alleles, in fact, may yield better than expected outcomes in optimal contexts, serving as "plasticity" factors, yielding differential susceptibility to both positive and negative environmental settings (Belsky and Pluess 2009). Overall, DP emphasizes malleability and plasticity. Through what is termed "probabilistic epigenesis" (Gottlieb and Willoughby 2006), genes do not provide a one-way causal influence on neural structures and behavior, because interactive, reciprocal, and bidirectional influences occur with other brain structures and products, behavioral patterns, and environmental influences.

Overall, the development of psychopathological functioning is multidetermined, complex, transactional, and, in many instances, nonlinear. It would be nearly impossible to imagine otherwise, given the staggering complexity of the brain and the multiple influences, ranging from the microsocial to the macrosocial, that impinge on the developing infant, toddler, and child. Longitudinal, multilevel investigations are needed to understand psychopathology and competence from a developmental perspective, with the potential for high-yield prevention and intervention efforts. Giving up the simplicity of categorical diagnoses in favor of complex, multidetermined pathway models may not be simple, but DP models are bound to convey greater explanatory power.

Sex Differences

During the first decade of life, the major forms of psychopathology predominate in boys. In fact, autism, aggressive conduct disorder, and ADHD occur at male-to-female ratios ranging from 3:1 to 5:1, even in community samples where referral bias is not an issue. Even major depression is slightly more likely to appear in boys than girls prior to adolescence. For complex reasons, only some of which are known, boys are more vulnerable than girls not only to mental disorders but also to the effects of a range of physical and social stressors (Hinshaw 2009).

Starting around age 11, however, girls catch up quickly in terms of the onset of serious psychopathology. By mid-adolescence, they display all but the most violent forms of conduct problems to nearly the extent that boys do. Crucially, girls have skyrocketed above their male counterparts with respect to rates of depression, eating disorders, and self-injurious behavior (Hinshaw 2009). Furthermore, by adulthood, women appear at ADHD clinics at the same rates as men. In short, something occurs during early to mid-adolescence, undoubtedly a combination of pubertal hormones, sex-role expectations, and tendencies to ruminate—as well as modeling for aggression in both sexes—propelling girls into major pathology.

Adolescence constitutes a paradox in and of itself: it is the time of the greatest physical and cognitive skills of one's entire lifetime, yet it is simultaneously an era of high risk for sensation seeking, physical injury, and serious mental disturbance. Voluminous research on relevant mechanisms is under way (Romer and Walker 2007; Steinberg 2010). Demands on girls for academic prowess, empathy and compassion, a sexualized "look," and endless perfection all conspire to up the ante for serious conflict in teenage girls, particularly for those with underlying vulnerabilities or a history of trauma (Hinshaw 2009).

Investigations of the sex with the lower prevalence of a given condition (e.g., girls with autism, boys with eating disorders) may be quite informative. Indeed, according to the "gender paradox," the sex with the lower prevalence is posited to have more of the relevant genetic, biological, or psychosocial risk factors that conspire to push the individual into the realm of pathology (Eme 1992). As a result, research on DP should include both studies directly comparing the sexes plus within-gender investigations that provide rich detail on either male or female manifestations.

Stigma

From all appearances, Western culture seems to be far more open and accepting regarding mental disorder and mental health than half a century ago. In fact, public knowledge of mental illness has grown considerably since the 1950s. Paradoxically, however, the American public is more likely to link mental illness with dangerousness, and desires greater social distance from those with mental disorders than in the past (Phelan et al. 2000). Why? Perhaps it is because of the increased numbers of seriously impaired individuals on the streets, out of psychiatric hospitals but without needed community services and resources. Or maybe it is because of increased public awareness that "dangerousness" is one of the few remaining reasons for involuntary commitment. Alternatively, although biogenetic ascriptions to mental illness (i.e., that mental illness is a "brain disease," a "disease like any other") have been touted as the solution for stigma—such that blame should be reduced if these are truly illnesses as opposed to weak character or moral flaws—the evidence is not clear in this regard (Jorm and Griffiths 2008; Martinez et al. 2011; Pescosolido et al. 2010).

Stigma may be internalized as "self-stigma," eroding self-image and dampening motivation to seek help. Furthermore, stigma and shame are experienced intensely by families, in part because of lingering models of mental disturbance that explicitly lay the blame for mental illness on faulty parenting, serving to dissuade parents from seeking assessments or intervention for their offspring (Heflinger and Hinshaw 2010). The ultimate paradox and ultimate tragedy are that many forms of pharmacological and psychosocial treatment "work" for child and adolescent psychopathology, so delays in seeking care are likely to lead to enhanced suffering and impairment. When the impairment becomes chronic, stigma intensifies and a vicious cycle is in place. Reducing stigma requires multiple levels of intervention (e.g., increased public education, far greater personal contact, different media images, enforcement of antidiscrimination laws) and has the potential to enhance the public image of people with mental disorders (Hinshaw 2007).

Implications for Intervention

The DP perspectives noted in this chapter suggest strongly that treatment for mental disorders can and should be directed at multiple targets: underlying biological tendencies (e.g., impulsivity, activity level, inhibition) via medications, psychological processes (e.g., internalization, rumination, anxiety) via treatment such as cognitive-behavioral or other forms of individual therapy, parental factors (e.g., overly close or distant boundaries, coercive discipline) via family therapy, or school contextual variables (e.g., higher frequency of reward, appropriate consequences, accommodations) via teacher consultation and school-wide interventions. Neighborhood-level interventions may facilitate reductions in property crime and posttraumatic stress disorder, as well. Indeed, the transactional models discussed herein mean that changes at one level of the child's or adolescent's system are likely to reverberate through other levels. Multimodal therapy, combining biological and psychosocial intervention, often yields the largest gains (see Hinshaw 2002).

Still, core questions remain. Are there sensitive or even critical periods for treatment? In other words, is it always the case that earlier intervention will be superior to later treatment? How can various treatments be sufficiently manualized and standardized for viable research evaluations, still maintaining sufficient individualization and clinical tailoring to help each individual case? If the child's symptoms and impairments are part of a reciprocal/transactional web, where should intervention begin: bottom-up, focusing initially on the child, or top-down, starting with families, schools, or communities? Despite the advances made in many forms of treatment for a number of child and adolescent disorders, the answers to these questions are not entirely clear.

Perhaps the largest need lies in the areas of 1) prevention and 2) promotion of protective factors (for discussion, see Howe et al. 2002; Tremblay 2010). If basic research can identify, with increasing specificity, those factors that antecede and causally relate to the emergence of psychopathology, truly preventive measures can be put into place. Yet, can any universal preventive strategies help to stop serious psychopathology in the most vulnerable cases? (By analogy, can fluoridation work for those at genetic risk for the worst tooth decay?) Or, if prevention is targeted to those at risk for mental disorders, how can one be sure that those in "high-risk" groups are not false-positives (i.e., those predicted to have later problems who would have desisted in any event)? And would such high-risk designation incur labeling and potential stigmatization? Is enough known about protective factors that are not just the polar opposites of risk factors—for example, high versus low IQ or nurturing versus neglectful families—to put such factors into practice for those at risk? Intervention science has much to learn from DP, and vice versa.

Conclusion

The study of atypical development is complex, multilevel, and transactional, with the potential for revealing processes through which normal development gets sidetracked. By viewing child and adolescent psychopathology as a richly layered set of psychobiological and contextual processes, investigators and clinicians can realize the utter heterogeneity inherent in current classification systems, inquire about transactional pathways, and direct treatment efforts toward both physiological/neural and contextual factors that may steer the individual in question to a more productive and meaningful life course. Sex differences in presentation of mental disorder yield opportunities for greater scientific enlightenment. The rampant stigmatization that still surrounds mental illness presents significant but surmountable barriers. Overcoming stigma may actually be the key to better science and better practice.

To our minds, the questions we have posed in this brief chapter are among the most important issues in all of science, requiring expertise that spans genes, brains, individuals, families, schools, communities, and society at large. Given the untold suffering and impairment accruing from child and adolescent psychopathology, the stakes are high. We urge new generations of scientists, practitioners, and policy makers to join relevant efforts of translating basic science into improved treatment and prevention.

KEY POINTS

- Developmental psychopathology (DP), which emerged as a means of integrating child and adolescent psychology and psychiatry with the principles of developmental science, has contributed to the understanding of the etiology and underlying mechanisms of behavioral and emotional disorders of youth, and aims to transcend a categorical diagnostic approach by accounting for continuities and discontinuities in the development of pathology over the lifespan.

- High levels of suffering and impairment occur in child and adolescent psychopathology. Although resilience can and does occur in some cases, the risk of lingering impairment from mental disturbance is real. Not only do behavioral, emotional, and developmental disturbances in childhood and adolescence usually persist into adulthood, but what are considered to be adult mental disorders typically reveal precursors in the early years of development.

- DP models emphasize both continuous and discontinuous processes at work in the development of psychopathology. Some children experience early negative interactive processes with parents and teachers that lead to problematic transactional patterns, whereas other children experience buffers or protective factors that can break these patterns.

- Key environmental factors, including parenting styles, are neither always uniformly positive nor uniformly negative in terms of their developmental effects. The effects of risk or protective factors may differ markedly depending on developmental timing, the family and social context in which they are experienced by the child, and the niche that exists in a given culture for their expression and resolution. According to the DP perspective, setting and context are essential.

- Families experience intense stigma and shame, in part because of lingering models of mental disturbance that lay blame for mental illness on faulty parenting and serve to dissuade parents from seeking assessment or intervention for their child. Pharmacological and psychosocial treatments "work" for child and adolescent psychopathology, so delays in seeking care lead to needless suffering and impairment. Overcoming stigma may actually be the key to better science and better practice.

References

Baron-Cohen S: Theory of mind and autism: a fifteen-year review, in Understanding Other Minds: Perspectives From Developmental Cognitive Neuroscience. Edited by Baron-Cohen S, Tager-Flusberg H, Cohen D. Oxford, UK, Oxford University Press, 2000, pp 3–20

Belsky J, Pluess M: Beyond diathesis stress: differential susceptibility to environmental influences. Psychol Bull 135:885–908, 2009

Bergman LR, von Eye A, Magnusson D: Person-oriented research strategies in developmental psychopathology, in Developmental Psychopathology, 2nd Edition, Vol 1: Theory and Method. Edited by Cicchetti D, Cohen DJ. Hoboken, NJ, Wiley, 2006, pp 850–888

Boyce T: Symphonic causation and the origins of childhood psychopathology, in Developmental Psychopathology, 2nd Edition, Vol 1: Theory and Method. Edited by Cicchetti D, Cohen DJ. Hoboken, NJ, Wiley, 2006, pp 797–817

Caspi A, Hariri AR, Holmes A, et al: Genetic sensitivity to the environment: the case of the serotonin transporter gene and its implications for studying complex diseases and traits. Am J Psychiatry 167:509–527, 2010

Cicchetti D: The emergence of developmental psychopathology. Child Dev 55:1–7, 1984

Cicchetti D: A multiple-levels-of-analysis perspective on research in development and psychopathology, in Child and Adolescent Psychopathology. Edited by Beauchaine TP, Hinshaw SP. Hoboken, NJ, Wiley, 2008, pp 27–57

Cicchetti D, Cohen DJ (eds): Developmental Psychopathology, 2nd Edition. Hoboken, NJ, Wiley, 2006

Cicchetti D, Rogosch F: Equifinality and multifinality in developmental psychopathology. Dev Psychopathol 8:597–600, 1996

Cicchetti D, Toth SL: The past achievements and future promises of developmental psychopathology: the coming of age of a discipline. J Child Psychol Psychiatry 50:16–25, 2009

Dawson G, Toth K: Autism spectrum disorders, in Developmental Psychopathology, 2nd Edition, Vol 3: Risk, Disorder, and Adaptation. Edited by Cicchetti D, Cohen DJ. Hoboken, NJ, Wiley, 2006, pp 317–357

Dodge KA, Rutter M: Gene-Environment Interactions in Developmental Psychopathology. New York, Guilford, 2011

Eme RF: Selective female affliction in the developmental disorders of childhood: a literature review. J Clin Child Psychol 21:354–364, 1992

Gazzaniga MS, Ivry RB, Mangun GR: Cognitive Neuroscience: The Biology of the Mind, 3rd Edition. New York, WW Norton, 2009

Gottlieb G, Willoughby MT: Probabilistic epigenesis of psychopathology, in Developmental Psychopathology, 2nd Edition, Vol 1: Theory and Method. Edited by Cicchetti D, Cohen DJ. Hoboken, NJ, Wiley, 2006, pp 673–700

Heflinger C, Hinshaw SP: Stigma in child and adolescent mental health services research: understanding professional and institutional stigmatization of youth with mental health problems and their families. Adm Policy Ment Health 37:61–70, 2010

Hinshaw SP: Intervention research, theoretical mechanisms, and causal processes related to externalizing behavior patterns. Dev Psychopathol 14:789–818, 2002

Hinshaw SP: The Mark of Shame: Stigma of Mental Illness and an Agenda for Change. New York, Oxford University Press, 2007

Hinshaw SP: The Triple Bind: Saving Our Teenage Girls From Today's Pressures. New York, Ballantine, 2009

Hinshaw SP: Developmental psychopathology as a scientific discipline: relevance to behavioral and emotional disorders of childhood and adolescence, in Child and Adolescent Psychopathology, 2nd Edition. Edited by Beauchaine TP, Hinshaw SP. Hoboken, NJ, Wiley, 2013, pp 3–26

Howe GW, Reiss D, Yuh J: Can prevention trials test theories of etiology? Dev Psychopathol 14:673–694, 2002

Jorm AF, Griffiths KM: The public's stigmatizing attitudes towards people with mental disorders: how important are biomedical conceptualizations? Acta Psychiatr Scand 118:315–321, 2008

Kessler RC, Berglund P, Demler O, et al: Lifetime prevalence and age-of-onset distributions of DSM-IV disorders in the National Comorbidity Survey Replication. Arch Gen Psychiatry 62:593–602, 2005

Kraemer HC, Stice E, Kazdin A, et al: How do risk factors work together? Mediators, moderators, and independent, overlapping, and proxy risk factors. Am J Psychiatry 158:848–856, 2001

Luthar SS, Brown PJ: Maximizing resilience through diverse levels of inquiry: prevailing paradigms, possibilities, and priorities for the future. Dev Psychopathol 19:931–955, 2007

Martinez A, Piff PK, Mendoza-Denton R, et al: The power of a label: mental illness diagnoses, ascribed humanity, and social rejection. J Soc Clin Psychol 30:1–23, 2011

Masten AS, Burt KB, Coatsworth JD: Competence and psychopathology in development, in Developmental Psychopathology, 2nd Edition, Vol 3: Risk, Disorder, and Adaptation. Edited by Cicchetti D, Cohen DJ. Hoboken, NJ, Wiley, 2006, pp 696–738

McLaughlin KA, Zeanah CH, Fox NA, et al: Attachment security as a mechanism linking foster care placement to improved mental health outcomes in previously institutionalized children. J Child Psychol Psychiatry 53:46–55, 2012

Moffitt TE: Life course persistent versus adolescence limited antisocial behavior, in Developmental Psychopathology, 2nd Edition, Vol 3: Risk, Disorder, and Adaptation. Edited by Cicchetti D, Cohen DJ. Hoboken, NJ, Wiley, 2006, pp 570–598

Nelson CA, Zeanah CH, Fox NA, et al: Cognitive recovery in socially deprived young children: the Bucharest Early Intervention Project. Science 318:1937–1940, 2007

Nigg JT: What Causes ADHD? Understanding What Goes Wrong and Why. New York, Guilford, 2006

O'Connor TG: The persisting effects of early experiences on psychological development, in Developmental Psychopathology, 2nd Edition, Vol 3: Risk, Disorder, and Adaptation. Edited by Cicchetti D, Cohen DJ. Hoboken, NJ, Wiley, 2006, pp 202–234

Pescosolido BA, Martin JK, Long JS, et al: "A disease like any other?" A decade of change in public reactions to schizophrenia, depression, and alcohol dependence. Am J Psychiatry 167:1321–1330, 2010

Phelan JC, Link BG, Stueve A, et al: Public conceptions of mental illness in 1950 and 1996: what is mental illness and is it to be feared? J Health Soc Behav 41:188–207, 2000

Romer D, Walker EF (eds): Adolescent Psychopathology and the Developing Brain. New York, Oxford University Press, 2007

Rutter M, Moffitt TE, Caspi A: Gene-environment interplay and psychopathology: multiple varieties but real effects. J Child Psychol Psychiatry 47:226–261, 2006

Sapienza JK, Masten AS: Understanding and promoting resilience in children and youth. Curr Opin Psychiatry 24:267–273, 2011

Serafica FC, Vargas LA: Cultural diversity in the development of child psychopathology, in Developmental Psychopathology, 2nd Edition, Vol 1: Theory and Method. Edited by Cicchetti D, Cohen DJ. Hoboken, NJ, Wiley, 2006, pp 588–626

Sroufe LA, Rutter M: The domain of developmental psychopathology. Child Dev 55:17–29, 1984

Steinberg L: A dual systems model of adolescent risk-taking. Dev Psychobiol 52:216–224, 2010

Tremblay RE: Developmental origins of disruptive behavior problems: the "original sin" hypothesis, epigenetics, and their consequences for prevention. J Child Psychol Psychiatry 51:341–367, 2010

CHAPTER 17

Video Intervention Therapy for Parents With a Psychiatric Disturbance

George Downing, Ph.D.
Susanne Wortmann-Fleischer, M.D.
Regina von Einsiedel, M.D.
Wolfgang Jordan, M.B.A., M.I.M.
Corinna Reck, Ph.D.

When an adult with a serious psychiatric disorder also happens to be the parent of an infant or small child, a double therapeutic task is indicated. Both the adult and the parent-child relationship are in need of help.

Although no statistics are available, psychiatric disorder in parents is clearly a worldwide problem of stunning proportions. Broad treatment concepts are lacking for working with such patients. Some excellent literature exists, but it mainly concerns mothers with depression and/or posttraumatic stress disorder (e.g., Beebe et al. 2012; Lieberman and Van Horn 2008; Reck 2012; Reck et al. 2011). Discussions of other disorders can be found (e.g., Downing et al. 2008; Reck 2012; von Einsiedel et al. 2012; Wan and Green 2009; Wortmann-Fleischer et al. 2005), but much more research is needed. Information about fathers with psychiatric disorders is particularly lacking.

On a positive note, effective cognitive-behavioral therapy (CBT) approaches, with solid empirical support, have been developed for almost every specific psychiatric disturbance. These psychotherapy methodologies are often used to supplement medication. However, these approaches also have paid little attention to parent-infant and parent-child relationships. When programs do include attention to family relationships, the emphasis is usually on how the other family members can better support the patient (e.g., with reduced hostility and criticism). Although this perspective is useful, it leaves untouched the crucial question of how the patient can give more of what is needed to an infant or child.

In this chapter, we discuss the basics of Video Intervention Therapy (VIT) and operationalize this therapeutic approach in the context of working with parents who have psychiatric disturbances. VIT works in any number of clinical circumstances, but in this chapter we focus on vignettes related to parents with psychiatric disturbances, because in such situations, addressing relational and behavioral systems is both critical and urgent.

The Challenges

Given a parent with a psychiatric disturbance, special obstacles may be encountered in the treatment of the parent-child relationship. From a psychiatric diagnosis alone, one cannot predict with any certainty what the relationship between parent and child (or infant) will be like. One cannot tell how good or bad the relationship will be, or what its strengths and weaknesses will be. Although there is a great deal of variability, some overall tendencies can be pointed out. Table 17–1 itemizes some typical problems that affect the relationships of patients with psychiatric disturbance.

The challenges described in Table 17–1 are formidable, and therapists might wonder how they can help these patients. VIT has proven to be a useful therapeutic technique. VIT begins with a recording of a parent-infant interaction. The therapist and patient or patients (e.g., mother and father, mother and grandmother who share caretaking) look at the video together. They regard the interactional exchange with care and at whatever level of detail best fits the counseling or therapy, and an array of new therapeutic opportunities is made possible. Although there are many different ways to work with video in a therapy or counseling context, what will obviously help most in work with parents who have psychiatric disturbances is a methodology that 1) directly addresses the obstacles listed in Table 17–1 and 2) lends itself to tight coordination with any concurrent psychotherapy for the disorder.

The VIT approach described in this chapter uses a cognitive-behavioral methodology and was originally designed to deal with interactions between parents with psychiatric disturbances and their children.[1] Attention to the details of what is seen in a video allows a parent to learn to observe better, to better interpret what he or she sees, and to better men-

---

[1]There exist today a number of different video methodologies. VIT has been especially influenced by the approaches of Beatrice Beebe (2003, 2005) and Mechtild Papousek (2000; Papousek and Wolwerth de Chuquisengo 2003), as well as, for the first author (G.D.), years of exchange with Ed Tronick (2007) about early interaction. Some other approaches of interest are those of Aarts (2000); Benoit (Benoit et al. 2001); Bernstein (1997); Erikson and Durz-Reimer (1999); Fivaz-Depeursinge, Corboz-Warnery, and Keren (2004); Juffer, Bakermans-Kranenburg, and van Ijzendoon (2008); Marvin, Cooper, Hoffman, and Powell (2002; Cooper et al. 2005); McDonough (2004); Schechter (Schechter et al. 2006); and Zelenko and Benham (2000).

TABLE 17–1. Typical problems affecting the relationships of patients with psychiatric disorders

1.	Lack of cognitive availability	Many patients with psychiatric disorders have a lot going on in their minds: anxieties, preoccupations, unpleasant images, stark criticisms of self, stark criticisms of others, rumination about what happened an hour ago, rumination about what may happen tomorrow, meta-rumination about the rumination, and worry about their state of mind. For some patients, overall mental processing is slowed down, independent of content.
2.	Reduction of cognitive resources	The lack of cognitive availability can have a negative impact on relationships. It can especially affect the relationship with an infant or small child, because caretaking demands so much moment-by-moment attention.
3.	Poor noticing of interpersonal cues	This is a natural spinoff of reduced cognitive resources. In some cases, another factor may also be present: a weak mobilization of what Porges (2011) calls the "social engagement system," a component of autonomic functioning. Trauma-based dissociation is one known version (Porges 2011).
4.	Information processing biases with regard to interpersonal cues	Poor overall noticing can go together, for some patients, with a hypervigilant alertness to certain types of signal (e.g., signals of hostility).
5.	Poor interpretation of interpersonal cues	One issue is noticing too few cues and/or having excessive alertness for one type of cue. Another issue is to misinterpret when one does in fact notice the cues.
6.	Poor mentalization of the other person	This includes how a patient interprets cues, but much more as well. It concerns the overall capacity to imagine the other's mental universe (Fonagy et al. 1991).
7.	Pessimism about the capacity for change	The more serious their psychiatric disorder, the more doubtful patients tend to be about their ability to make significant personal changes. This form of suffering—a feeling of being deficient in a fundamental way—is a natural consequence.
8.	Poor medication compliance	This is a problem with a certain subgroup. When present, it can have obvious implications not only for the patient but also for the relationship with the child.

talize about the child in a broader sense. Work with these modes of understanding is then coupled with work with new behavioral competencies. Critically, a therapeutic focus is also brought to the parent's inside states: to thoughts, emotions, and body registrations as they are experienced during interaction. This focusing process in turn sets the stage for finding new strategies for coping with rumination, upsetting intrusive images, auditory hallucinations, hard-to-regulate negative feelings, and so on. Detailed work with negative self-attributions, pessimism about change, and motivation for medication compliance can also be useful. VIT has psychotherapy, counseling, and mental health coaching variants, each with a different degree of complexity. Both the psychotherapy and counseling variants emphasize such attention to inside states.

Given the cognitive-behavioral framework of VIT, and given that almost all forms of psychotherapy for psychiatric disorders today are CBT variants, a close fit on a practical level is easily achieved. Explorations during video sessions can be tied to themes discussed in the adult psychotherapy, and vice versa, such that the patient experiences a productive continuity of therapeutic work.

VIT can be done individually or in group formats, or can even be directly integrated into a standard cognitive-behavioral group therapy for a particular disorder (Wortmann-Fleischer 2012; Wortmann-Fleischer et al. 2005). Most parents with psychiatric disturbances are capable of making rapid improvement in their interactional and caretaking skills with a child, but require therapeutic assistance that reaches them on the right level. A small minority of parents, however, make too little progress despite appropriate therapeutic support. Hard decisions then have to be made, including whether the parent may retain custody of a child. Often, after losing custody, a parent continues to have a relationship with the child, maintaining contact through visits. In such cases, any positive changes in the relationship brought about by VIT will still have considerable value. If the visits take place in the context of a professionally supervised format, a practitioner may even be able to continue to aid the dyad and their shared destiny. Some agencies and teams use VIT for just this purpose.

Overview of Video Intervention Therapy

VIT was first developed in psychiatric settings and has since been put to use in many other contexts. The psychiatric settings include several parent-infant inpatient units in Europe, where a mother (or occasionally a father) in psychiatric difficulty can be hospitalized together with the infant (von Einsiedel et al. 2012; Wortmann-Fleischer et al. 2005). At the University of Heidelberg, Germany, for example, one such unit has been in operation for over 10 years (Reck 2012). In another such unit, at the Nordbaden Psychiatric Center, also in Germany, empirical confirmation of the effectiveness of the method has been shown. Among the outcome measures was blind coding of pretreatment and posttreatment interaction videos, demonstrating that positive change occurred not only in the mother's state of being but also in the relationship (Hornstein et al. 2007).

Other settings include a treatment program for young children with autism at the University of Basel, Switzerland; support programs for the parents of premature infants, at the

University of Bologna and the University of Cesena, Italy; and a program for adolescent mothers at the University of Milan–Bicocca, Italy. Still other applications have been used in treatment centers for substance abuse; institutions for both children and parents with developmental disabilities; support programs for families who adopt; centers for supervised parental visits with children in out-of-home placement; home-visiting programs for high-risk families with low socioeconomic status; private practice settings; and a variety of family counseling centers. VIT is used by counselors, psychotherapists, social workers, nurses, physicians, early interventionists, educators, and others.

VIT puts more emphasis on behavior than do some CBT approaches. This is to be expected because patient and therapist alike are confronted throughout the session by actual behavior as observed in the video. Extensive investigation of inner states can also take place.

Most often VIT functions as a module within a broader treatment program. During a video session, a standardized procedure (described in the section "The Standard Protocol" later in this chapter) is employed. This procedure remains constant, regardless of the wider program in which it is embedded. What varies are the number of video sessions, their frequency, and how they are linked to other treatment components.

VIT is a mentalization-based approach that fits quite comfortably with a CBT perspective (Bjoegvinnson and Hart 2006). It draws on both mentalization techniques as described by Fonagy and his colleagues (Allen et al. 2006; Fonagy 2008; Slade 2005, 2008; Steele and Steele 2005, 2008) and other techniques developed within VIT itself. Most of the institutions using VIT integrate it within programs organized according to CBT principles.

Benefits of Using Video in Therapy

Sessions with video provide a fast, efficient way to help. A video is filmed of a parent-child interaction that is relevant to the problems the parent is having and the age of the child. The video does not include the professional using VIT with the family. The video can be of the parent and child involved in playing, nursing or feeding, a bath, a diaper change, bedtime rituals, mealtime, preparing to leave for school, a conflict or boundary-setting situation, or another activity. For VIT work with older children or adolescents, or with an adult couple relationship, other kinds of activities are selected. The video should be 5–10 minutes in length and can be filmed in the practice setting or in the family home using a tripod or other means to capture the video. Good sound quality is vital for analysis and use of the video.

Ideally, the therapist will have an opportunity to view the video prior to the session, in order to analyze behavioral patterns and select specific portions of the video that may be the most useful for the session. In the VIT session, one or both parents look at the video with the therapist, following the six-step protocol described below in the section "The Standard Protocol." Built into this procedure is a series of branching options. As a session unfolds, two general sorts of therapeutic focus become possible. One is a concentration on what in VIT is called the *outer movie* or behavior—that is, the visible actions of both parent and child. The other is on the *inner movie*—that is, what each participant subjectively experienced during the interaction. Although the inner movie cannot be seen, it can be accessed with the therapist's support. For example, the therapist might say, "Imagine that you are right there, in what we are seeing. Imagine you are experiencing it as it happens. Can you imagine this?" Adults and older children almost always can. The therapeutic investigation then moves to subjective thoughts and feelings. Contact can be made with body experience also and, to a degree, with an awareness of how a person is organizing his or her body in the interaction (e.g., gestures, movements, shifts of posture). VIT therapists must take into account a number of factors when choosing where to concentrate. Attention might be given chiefly to the outer movie, the inner movie, or an interweaving of the two.

Analysis of the Video

VIT therapists use a specific set of categories when looking at a video in preparation for a session. This grid, or "scanning map," can be quickly learned. The scanning map was developed by the first author (G.D.) in collaboration with Ed Tronick (2007). It is based on attachment, video microanalysis, and several other forms of developmental research. Space does not permit a detailed discussion in this chapter; briefly, however, this scanning map includes assessment of nine interaction categories: 1) connection, 2) organization of space, 3) organization of time, 4) discourse development, 5) autonomy, 6) boundaries, 7) negotiations, 8) collaboration, and 9) creativity. A clinical analysis of a video can be accomplished by an experienced therapist in about 15 minutes.

The Standard Protocol

The six-step procedure used in VIT is summarized in Table 17–2. The clinical examples provided below demonstrate the steps in more detail. Most of the examples are from actual cases, and a few are composites. To help readers learn the VIT fundamentals, we have kept references to diagnoses simple, with infrequent mention of comorbidities, special symptoms, and the like.

For the six-step procedure, a 50-minute session will typically suffice, although longer sessions may be useful in some situations. Normally this six-step procedure is followed just as described below, but there can be exceptions. VIT is meant to be genuinely collaborative, with the patient's input and thinking central to the process. As a result, a patient's ideas now and then spark a creative turn, and the therapeutic exchange veers away from its planned direction. Whenever such a shift appears productive, the therapist can set aside the typical procedure.

Step 1

In Step 1, the therapist shows a selected part of the video, and the patient is asked to comment. The patient or patients (e.g., a parental couple) are encouraged to share what they have found of interest in the video. Discussion based on these remarks may ensue. Usually at this point the exchange remains short. In the following dialogue, the video being dis-

---

TABLE 17–2. **Summary of the six-step intervention procedure**

Step 1	Therapist shows selected part of video and asks patient to comment.
Step 2	Therapist points out one or more positive aspects of interaction seen in video (e.g., evidence of behavioral change discussed in a previous visit, positive exceptions to negative patterns) and shares reasons for seeing them as positive. (Some sessions end after this step.)
Step 3	Therapist makes a transition to discussion of negative pattern in video interaction.
Step 4	Negative pattern just highlighted is explored in depth, and a variety of techniques can be introduced (e.g., mentalization, emotional exploration, body techniques, parent's childhood past).
Step 5	Therapist and patient reflect together on one or more new actions that patient can take at home, and focus shifts concretely to the when, where, and how of behavioral change.
Step 6	Therapist summarizes main points elaborated in session. Therapist and patient discuss arrangements for making of new video, and schedule next session.

---

cussed is of a face-to-face interaction between a mother with a diagnosis of psychosis (symptoms in remission) and her 4-month-old son.

> THERAPIST: What do you find interesting in what we just saw?
> PATIENT: I see I'm doing too much. Roberto was looking at me in that nice way, and then I started touching him and making all those cooing sounds, and then he turned away. It was too much for him.
> THERAPIST: That's a nice observation. How do you feel, saying this?
> PATIENT: A little embarrassed. But not too much. It's good to be able to see it all this way, like looking in a window.
> THERAPIST: Fine. Why don't we come back later to this idea you just had. First, I'd like to show you a couple of things I noticed. Is that OK?

In the above dialogue the patient is genuinely insightful. This is not always the case, and some patients respond in more problematic ways. The next dialogue concerns a video of a mother with a diagnosis of borderline personality disorder who is walking about a room in her home, trying to quiet a 6-month-old (corrected age) infant. The infant, who was born 3 months prematurely and with a very low birth weight, currently has a series of regulation problems.

> THERAPIST: What do you find interesting in what we just saw?
> PATIENT: This is so typical. So typical. Whatever I do seems not to help. His face is so angry. He's criticizing me.
> THERAPIST: Criticizing you?
> PATIENT: All the time. Just like here. He thinks I'm a bad mother.
> THERAPIST: He's certainly crying hard in this segment. What makes you think this means he's criticizing you?
> PATIENT: I just know it. I know my baby.

THERAPIST: OK, well, why don't we come back to this later. First, there a few things in
the video I would like to show you. Is that OK?

The following dialogue is with a mother with a diagnosis of depression who in the
video segment is preparing a meal in her kitchen. The infant, age 23 months, is sitting at
the table drawing.

THERAPIST: What do you find interesting in what we just saw?
PATIENT: That sweater. It's not a good color on me.
THERAPIST: Anything else stand out for you?
PATIENT: No.
THERAPIST: OK, I'd like to show you several things I noticed in the video.

If both parents are present, the therapist will likely begin in another manner. The next
dialogue concerns a video of a mother without any psychiatric diagnosis and a father
diagnosed with bipolar disorder who are playing on the floor with their twin infants, age
14 months.

THERAPIST: Helena, to start off, say a little about what you noticed about yourself in the
video. Don't talk about Giorgo, just yourself. What do you like best about what you
do here? [*Helena answers.*] Is there anything you like less, anything you wish you could
do differently? [*Helena continues.*]
THERAPIST: Thanks. Giorgo, let's hear what stood out for you. Do the same thing: just
talk about yourself, not about Helena. What do you like best about what you do in
the interaction? [*Giorgo answers.*] Is there anything you like less, anything you wish
you could do differently? [*Giorgo continues.*]

The therapist in this example structures the initial questions in this way to make sure that
neither parent uses the video to criticize the other. In later sessions, once a couple has
learned how to give feedback constructively to each other, this constraint may be relaxed.

Step 2

In Step 2, the therapist points out one or more positive aspects of the interaction seen in
the video and shares his or her reasons for seeing them as positive. Some additional discussion may take place. Parents often are unaware of what they are doing well, or have
only a vague notion. The video permits more exact representations to be formed. This is
helpful in many ways, one being that if the patient wants to change elements of his or her
behavior, he or she will benefit from knowing what competencies are already in place.

The following example concerns a video of a father with a diagnosis of borderline personality disorder who is spoon-feeding his infant, age 9 months.

THERAPIST: Look at this. [*Shows a 15-second segment of the video.*] Look at how nicely you
hold the spoon and wait. Then when Ginna signals she is ready, you bring the spoon
to her mouth. You two are learning to coordinate this quite well.

PATIENT: Sometimes I get impatient, I have to admit.

THERAPIST: I can imagine. But you manage to respect her signals anyway.

PATIENT: It seems to me that what you said is right. We are coordinating it.

Sometimes the therapist also inquires about how the parent is reacting to this positive change in behavior—that is, how he or she now feels seeing it along with hearing the therapist's description. The question is added because such images at times have considerable power. They not only transmit information but also may create a strong emotional response.

The next example relates to a video of a mother diagnosed with psychosis (currently asymptomatic) playing on the floor with her 15-month-old. The therapist has just stopped the video on an image where the infant is looking at his mother and smiling broadly.

THERAPIST: Look at this smile on him. Look at how much he wants to share his pleasure with you.

PATIENT: This is good. I hadn't noticed the first time. Real good. [*Begins to cry.*]

THERAPIST: Take your time.

THERAPIST: [*Parent has stopped crying.*] So I see how this touches you. What thoughts does it bring up?

PATIENT: We are making it. We are getting there. Bruno is getting there. I am getting there. [*Cries again briefly.*]

When positive images so forcefully impact a parent, the therapist might also use them for motivation (i.e., for medication compliance, continuation of the therapy, or some specific difficult personal change).

The next dialogue pertains to a video of a mother diagnosed with bipolar disorder who is playing on the floor with her 15-month-old. The therapist has just stopped on an image of the mother smiling broadly at her child.

THERAPIST: I can see how you are taking this in. That is really fine. It is a picture worth putting deep inside you, so that you can remember it.

PATIENT: I'm taking it in, believe me.

THERAPIST: When you see this picture, and you feel inside how important little Fred is to you, what does this mean to you with respect to taking your medication? I know you made your plan in the group, and you have mentioned that you have some mixed reactions to all that. What are your thoughts about it now?

PATIENT: I think I can't fool around with this. I have to think it through better, take it seriously. If it were just me, I don't know. But there is Fred. I need to be serious about it for him.

THERAPIST: If Fred had language for all this, what would he say?

PATIENT: Do it for me, Mom. I need you, Mom.

THERAPIST: That sure sounds right.

A significant aspect of Step 2, when relevant, concerns behavioral change. Suppose that in work with a previous video, a plan was made that a parent (or older child or couple member) would try to implement some new practical action. When a video shows the individual doing the new behavior, in whole or in part, pointing this out is essential. Clients often announce that they were unable to change—that they tried but couldn't do it, or that they forgot to try. Their discouragement is evident. However, a new video may tell an opposite story and demonstrate change moments. Typically, these change events are small and fleeting. Because they are so partial and/or infrequent, the person simply did not register them. Hence, the value of the video is that it allows the patient to take in what he or she has in reality accomplished. Acknowledging even a small change can restore motivation and permit investigation of what made the change possible, a valuable piece of information.

The next example relates to a video of a mother diagnosed with adult attention-deficit/hyperactivity disorder and her 22-month-old daughter. The mother has complained in the therapy that the girl habitually ignores parental limits and has much difficulty regulating aggressive impulses. In this video, the girl is screaming provocatively and several times throws toys at the mother.

> THERAPIST: You've said that you see no change at all, but I find something different in the video. Let me show you. [*Replays a 1-minute segment.*] This time, what did you notice?
>
> PATIENT: The same as just before. She's terrible. Whatever I do is useless. And I didn't say things to her the way we practiced in the last session.
>
> THERAPIST: True, you are speaking to her in a complicated way, a little over her head. Short, clear messages might be better for setting a limit. But let's look at the segment again. This time, pay a lot of attention to your voice—to the tone and manner of your voice. [*Shows segment again.*]
>
> PATIENT: Is it different? I guess it is different, somehow.
>
> THERAPIST: Very different. During this entire minute your voice stays calm. It stays respectful. Remember what we saw on the last video? How you were screaming back at her the whole time? Here we see a significant change.
>
> PATIENT: I guess that's right. But it's not getting what I want from Elena.
>
> THERAPIST: No, not yet. That will come soon enough. The key thing is you are changing on your side. How did you do it? What helped you to use a calm voice, even with your daughter being so provoking?

Occasionally during Step 2, a *positive exception* technique is employed if a certain negative pattern shows up pervasively in the video but at one point a positive exception to the pattern can be found. The therapist points out the exception, and suggests that the parent might benefit from doing more of this exception behavior.

In another video, a 13-year-old mother with a diagnosis of depression is changing the diaper of her 6-week-old infant. Throughout the video the mother's face is expressionless. She does not speak, and her movements have a mechanical quality. An exception event occurs at the end of the diaper change, when the mother leans forward, bringing her face to where the infant can better see it. The mother smiles briefly and says, "There we go. All clean and ready."

> THERAPIST: Let me show you something I liked very much. [*Shows the smile event, stopping on an image where the mother's smile, though not large, is clear and evident.*] See how you smile here?

PATIENT: Sure.

THERAPIST: This is a good moment. You smile at Maria Louisa, and you even lean forward so she can see your face well.

PATIENT: Sure, I see.

THERAPIST: It is a good idea. Did you know that Maria Louisa is coming into a period where she can learn to trade smiles back and forth, and trade little voice sounds back and forth?

PATIENT: Yes?

THERAPIST: Yes. This will be very important for her to do. It is a way infants learn how to be social. They learn the nonverbal back-and-forth before they have to worry about putting language into it. You can help her with that.

PATIENT: I can?

THERAPIST: You can…a lot. Smiling at her in this way gives her a kind of demonstration. You could do that now much more. And when she starts to give her own smiles, which is coming soon, you can give smiles in reply. To teach her about the back-and-forth.

PATIENT: I can?

THERAPIST: It would be very helpful for her.

PATIENT: I don't feel so good these days. How do I give her smiles? That sounds hard.

THERAPIST: Of course. But here [*gestures toward the video picture*] you manage to. Here you do it.

PATIENT: True.

THERAPIST: How did you manage it? Imagine you are there, just after the change, giving this smile.

PATIENT: I can a little, I guess.

THERAPIST: How do you get the smile going? What helped you do it? What at this moment is different?

PATIENT: It's like I want to let her know that the change is finished, that we got it done.

THERAPIST: Good. So it's a sense of wanting to communicate something to her.

PATIENT: Right. That sounds right.

THERAPIST: Fine. If you're willing, let's think together about some other kinds of things you might want to communicate to her.

PATIENT: Sure.

For young adolescent parents, video intervention is sometimes the first thing that arouses their interest in therapy. (For an excellent discussion of work with adolescent mothers, including video intervention, see the volume by Riva Crugnola [2012].) There may be times when the therapist works exclusively with Step 2 and goes no further in the VIT process. At the close of Step 2, the session might end, or perhaps the video work ends and some other kind of therapeutic exchange takes place in the time remaining. In VIT, this is called an *abbreviated session*. It might be done with a patient whose motivation is low or one whose trust in the therapist seems problematic. On occasion, an abbreviated session is used with someone who has extreme, unwarranted doubts about herself or himself as a parent ("I am a very bad mother"). The positive patterns provide counterevidence to the negative attributions.

Step 3

In Step 3, the therapist makes a transition to pointing out and speaking about a negative pattern in the video interaction. Most often only one pattern is selected, but two or more may be chosen if they are tightly linked. The therapist must be careful about the words chosen when introducing and describing the pattern. Language should be diplomatic and supportive rather than confrontational.

In the video segment discussed in the following dialogue, a mother with a diagnosis of borderline personality disorder with self-harm symptoms is sitting on a chair while her son, age 18 months, plays on the floor on the other side of the room. At a certain point, the child crosses the room carrying a toy fox, then reaches out and tries to hand the fox to the mother. The mother appears not to notice this and begins adjusting the child's clothing.

> THERAPIST: So, we have seen several things you do quite nicely in the interaction.
> PATIENT: I'm surprised. This is stuff I wasn't aware of, not very clearly anyway.
> THERAPIST: Well, as I explained, these are all things that for sure are helping Tom with his development. I also noticed something else—something that, if you changed a little what you do, could be another way to help Tom with his development. Would you like me to go into that?
> PATIENT: OK, sure.
> THERAPIST: Look at this part again. [*Again shows the infant crossing the room and trying to hand the fox to the mother.*] Did you see what happened?
> PATIENT: Not really.
> THERAPIST: Look again. [*Shows in slow motion the infant trying to hand over the fox.*] See how he is trying to give you the toy? This is something we want him to learn in his development: handing things to other people, gestures of giving things to other people.

Step 4

In Step 4, the negative pattern just highlighted is explored in depth. Usually, this is the heart of the session. It is also the step to which the most time is dedicated. Any of a variety of techniques can now be introduced, such as mentalization, increased contact with emotion, or investigation of a parent's childhood past. Often, body techniques are also used to clarify and/or regulate emotion (Downing 2008, 2011; Downing et al. 2008). The previous example, of the mother who needs to learn how to reinforce her child's giving gestures, continues in the following dialogue.

> PATIENT: So what can I do?
> THERAPIST: You can notice when he wants to give you something, and then let him hand it to you. And you can give a nice response back, something that makes him feel good about giving something to someone.
> PATIENT: All right, I'll try. But I don't know quite what I should do. What would "give a nice response" be?
> THERAPIST: If you want, let's role-play this a few times. I'll play Tom and I'll hand you something. Then we can think together about some different alternatives of how you could respond.
> PATIENT: OK.

This exchange demonstrates one way to structure the Step 4 exploration. The therapist started right off with a focus on behavioral change. If, as here, the parent understands what is intended quickly enough, then new options open up. There are many opportunities for further work in Step 4, with several branchings available. For example, the therapist might branch off to work with "other-mentalization," the capacity to mentalize about the other's subjective experience. In VIT, a number of techniques can be used for this, including a simulation technique, as demonstrated in the following continuation of the previous dialogue.

THERAPIST: Let's go back to the video. Can we look again at that same part where Tom brings you the toy?

PATIENT: Again. Well, all right.

THERAPIST: We don't have to.

PATIENT: No, it's OK.

THERAPIST: Here we go. But this time, imagine you are Tom in the video. Try to imagine what he might be thinking and feeling at each moment.

PATIENT: OK.

THERAPIST: [*Stops on a picture of Tom halfway across the room, heading toward the mother.*] As Tom, what are you thinking here?

PATIENT: I like this fox. It is a cute fox. I'm going to show it to Mom.

THERAPIST: What is the feeling with that?

PATIENT: A good feeling. Fun.

THERAPIST: [*Plays a little more of the video, stopping it on a picture of Tom holding the toy out to the mother as she in turn is reaching for his shirt, to adjust it.*] And here? What are you thinking, as Tom?

PATIENT: She's not interested. She doesn't even see it. She's just interested in making my shirt look right.

THERAPIST: Emotionally, what is this like?

PATIENT: Disappointing, and a little confusing. Like I want to do something to connect with her, and it's not working.

THERAPIST: OK, that's really good, how you are making guesses at what might be going on in Tom. As yourself now, what do you think about all this?

PATIENT: If he wants to connect with me, I really want to encourage that.

To hypothesize in this manner about the child's experience is only one type of entry into the so-called inner movie. More commonly, the therapist can move directly to the parent's own inner experience, as in the following dialogue with a mother diagnosed with panic disorder. In the video the mother is putting some toys out on the floor, and the infant, who is age 13 months (adjusted age after being born 2 months preterm), is following her. At one point the infant loses his balance, staggers a bit, then actually falls to the floor. The mother instantly lets out a loud "Ooooh!" and sweeps him up into her arms. Her face looks very frightened. The infant appears quite unbothered by the experience.

THERAPIST: Let's again go over the part where Federico falls. OK?

PATIENT: Well, I do get the point. In the video I make too big a deal about it, as if something dramatic or dangerous has happened.

THERAPIST: Yes, you seem very clear about it now. Clear that he in fact was fine, was not hurt, and was ready to get right back up. But if you are willing, let's look at it again, and see if we can better understand what is going on for you at that moment.

PATIENT: All right, that might be interesting. I think I get into that frame of mind a lot.

THERAPIST: This time imagine you are there, in the interaction. Can you imagine that?

PATIENT: I'll try.

THERAPIST: [*Again shows a few seconds of the sequence, stopping on a picture where the boy first begins to stagger.*] So there you are in the interaction, and you see this. How do you first react? What do you feel? What thoughts come to mind?

PATIENT: It's a not very rational feeling. Like "Danger! Do something! He will get hurt! Stop him from hurting himself."

THERAPIST: Those are the thoughts. What are the emotions with them?

PATIENT: Afraid, almost panicky, and a little sense of guilt, as if, if he falls, then I'm a bad mother.

THERAPIST: Stay with the panic. Where do you feel it in your body?

PATIENT: In my chest. My chest is all tight and at the same time my breath wants to speed up. If I let it, it might go out of control.

THERAPIST: Stay a little with this. What other thoughts come?

PATIENT: An image. One I hate. It was the day in the unit when the nurse saw something was wrong with Federico's heart rate. She saw the monitor, her whole face changed, and she right away called a colleague to help. They asked me and my husband to leave Federico's area for the moment. We were beside ourselves.

THERAPIST: That was a hard moment.

PATIENT: I start to tremble just thinking about it.

THERAPIST: Many parents have these kinds of experiences in the neonatal intensive care unit. It is very common, as you know.

PATIENT: That's right.

THERAPIST: How would it be if we made a plan for how you can get freer of these frightening memories?

PATIENT: Definitely. Yes.

THERAPIST: OK, we will come back to that at the end of the session. If it's all right, let's stay now with this moment in the video when Federico starts to fall. Let's go to a very practical level. We can explore what you could do inside, in such moments, to hold back the overprotective behavior.

PATIENT: I like that idea.

In VIT work with parents with psychiatric disorders, it is common to come across trauma flashbacks, hyperarousal, states of dissociation, and the like. During the session the therapist will likely use cognitive techniques, distancing techniques (Hayes et al. 1999), and brief body techniques (Downing et al. 2008; Morlinghaus 2012) to help the parent learn how to reduce the intensity of these symptoms.

If warranted, more direct therapeutic work with trauma will also be recommended to a parent. This might be done parallel to the video sessions, or at a later point. For example, in the parent–infant unit at the University of Heidelberg, a body-oriented form of trauma work is offered as a separate module for some severely traumatized parents (Morlinghaus 2012).

Sometimes in Step 4 a shift is made to discussing the parent's own childhood to promote insight or augment motivation. In the video discussed in the next vignette, a 23-

month-old is playing at home with her 4-year-old sister and 6-year-old brother. The children are squabbling and arguing. As their exchange escalates, the 6-year-old hits the 4-year-old, who begins crying, and then pushes the 23-month-old, who falls and also begins crying. Their mother, who has a diagnosis of substance abuse disorder, then enters the scene and yells at them all to stop making so much noise.

THERAPIST: So we agree that this is not good of Gianni, how he hits and pushes the others.

PATIENT: Right, he shouldn't do it. I've told him. On the other hand, I don't think it's so serious. Children fight. It's natural. Later they grow out of it.

THERAPIST: I'm not so sure. There's research about this. When siblings have a lot of physical violence, it can be very wounding, traumatizing even, for whoever has the violence inflicted on them.

PATIENT: If you say so. I am not so sure.

THERAPIST: When you were a child, was there any physical violence in the family?

PATIENT: Was there ever. My mom and dad. Some of the nights when he was drinking…wow.

THERAPIST: What was that like for you?

PATIENT: Terrible.

THERAPIST: Was anyone violent with you?

PATIENT: Not often. My mother once in a while. And my younger brother and I sometimes were into it. We fought a lot, actually.

THERAPIST: How much younger?

PATIENT: Two years. But he was strong as a kid.

THERAPIST: Think back to that. What was it like for you?

PATIENT: Pretty ugly, really. I don't like thinking about it.

THERAPIST: Well, this is good, how right now you are in fact letting yourself think about it, even if the memories are painful. Tell me, do you really want to let your own children go through the same thing?

PATIENT: I see what you mean.

THERAPIST: Imagine your youngest daughter as an adult. Imagine her looking back at her childhood. Do you want her to have the same kind of bad memories?

PATIENT: No, no. I don't want that. But I don't see how I can to stop the three of them. They go out of control. They do what they want.

THERAPIST: Let's go back to the video then. I can help you think about some alternative ways to deal with it, if you wish.

Some of the techniques typically used in Step 4 bring patients into contact with emotion. With many patients who have psychiatric disorders, this must be done with considerable delicacy. A paradox is at play: often such patients need more aid with emotion contact and regulation than other kinds of patients. On the other hand, certain emotions (which differ from patient to patient) may quickly frighten them. Emotion-focused and body-focused techniques can then be employed for graduated exposure, thus mobilizing emotion in manageable doses.

Of course, another option during Step 4 is to continue to focus on behavioral change, and nothing more, leaving aside the inner movie, if necessary. However, generally speaking, in working with parents who have psychiatric disorders, a therapist does not want to ignore the inner movie too frequently, because the need for better coping with inner states can be urgent. Occasionally, the therapist will stay with the outer movie for reasons other than a parent's fear of contact with emotions. For example, a prospective change may require a lot of psychoeducation, for which the use of Step 4 is pivotal. One illustration of this is in the case of a child with a serious language delay, where the therapist might want to use the video to help the parents recognize special opportunities for stimulating language development. In this instance, the psychoeducational information has a certain complexity, and use of Step 4 might need to be reserved for this topic alone.

Step 5

In Step 5, the therapist and the patient reflect together on one or more new actions that the patient can take at home, and the focus shifts squarely to the when, where, and how of behavioral change. Arrangements may even be made for keeping some form of daily record.

Often, this step is brief. Until this point in the session, the parent has been immersed in the observed behavior in the video. Even if there has been a strong focus on inner states during Step 4, these states have been tied to the observed interaction. Hence, the parent likely already has a good grasp of the behaviors under discussion by the time Step 5 is reached. Sometimes during Step 4, it happens in a natural fashion that the specifics of behavioral change become an explicit topic. In this case, the move to Step 5 represents a wrapping up of the discussion.

The following dialogue concerns a video of an 18-year-old mother diagnosed with bulimia nervosa and her 5-month-old (corrected age) child in a face-to-face interaction. The infant was born 3 months premature with a very low birth weight.

THERAPIST: I can see that you have really understood what we have been talking about today: that Petra needs a slower rhythm of contact. And that if you watch her signals more carefully, you can let that guide you.

PATIENT: I think it's clear. It was really helpful, seeing those tiny looks and face changes in the video.

THERAPIST: Right. As we saw, Petra's signals are often not so clear. She can be hard to read. It is a frequent enough problem with some preterm babies. So, when do you think would be a good time for you to try this slower rhythm of contact?

PATIENT: Right away. When we are home. No special time.

THERAPIST: That sounds excellent. The more you try it, the better. But it could be helpful also to plan something like a regular 10-minute block of time, maybe two or three times each day this next week, when you could give your full attention to practicing this new way to be with her. And if you are willing, you could even write down a few notes about how it went. What do you think about this idea?

PATIENT: All right, why not. When in the day then?

THERAPIST: Well, let's discuss it. And I can show you how to jot down some notes. You can bring the notes back to the next session, and we can look together briefly at how it all went.

Step 6

In Step 6, the therapist summarizes the main points elaborated in the session. The therapist and patient discuss arrangements for making a new video, and they schedule the next session.

Conclusion

VIT is a six-step process in which the clinician moves deliberately through a series of therapeutic levels in an approach that can be modified to meet the unique therapeutic goals and directions that emerge, as well as the therapist's specific training and discipline.

This chapter has provided a short overview of a large topic. Intervention with video is an extraordinary instrument, and the field is clearly just at the beginning of learning the range and potential for the use of video in psychotherapy, counseling, coaching, and other modalities. One can be confident that the coming years will bring continuing new advancements.

KEY POINTS

- Video Intervention Therapy (VIT) is a variant of cognitive-behavioral therapy, but can be used in psychotherapy, counseling, and coaching situations by clinicians in a variety of disciplines.
- Both outer behavior (the "outer movie") and inner experience (the "inner movie") can be targeted for exploration.
- Across settings, the basic intervention procedure with a video remains largely invariant, whereas numerous options exist for how the video module can be integrated into a treatment program as a whole.
- A beginning version of VIT can be learned very quickly, and then additional skills progressively acquired.

References

Aarts M: Marte Meo Basic Manuel. Harderwijk, The Netherlands, Aarts Productions, 2000

Allen J, Fonagy P, Bateman A: Mentalizing in Clinical Practice. Washington, DC, American Psychiatric Publishing. 2008

Beebe B: Brief mother–infant treatment: psychoanalytically informed video feedback. Infant Ment Health J 24:24–52, 2003

Beebe B: Mother-infant research informs mother-infant treatment. Psychoanal Study Child 60:7–46, 2005

Beebe B, Cohen P, Sossin M, et al: Mothers, Infants, and Young Children of September 11, 2001: A Primary Prevention Project. New York, Routledge, 2012

Benolit D, Madigan S, Lecce S, et al: Atypical maternal behavior toward feeding-disordered infants before and after intervention. Infant Ment Health J 22(6):611–616, 2001

Bernstein V: Using home videos to strengthen the parent-child relationship. IMPrint 20:2–5, 1997

Bjoegvinnson T, Hart J: Cognitive behavior therapy promotes mentalizing, in Handbook of Mentalization-Based Treatment. Edited by Allen J, Fonagy P. West Sussex, England, Wiley, 2006, pp 157–170

Cooper G, Hoffman K, Powell G, Marvin R: The Circle of Security intervention: differential diagnosis and differential treatment, in Enhancing Early Attachments: Theory, Research, Intervention, and Policy. Edited by Berlin L, Ziv Y, Amaya-Jackson L, Greenberg M. New York, Guilford, 2005, pp 127–151

Downing G: A different way to help, in Human Development in the 21st Century: Visionary Ideas From Systems Scientists. Edited by Greenspan S, Shanker S. Cambridge, UK, Cambridge University Press, 2008, pp 200–205

Downing G: Uneasy beginnings: getting psychotherapy underway with the difficult patient. Self Psychology: European Journal for Psychoanalytic Therapy and Research 45:207–233, 2011

Downing G, Buergin D, Reck C, et al: Intersubjectivity and attachment: perspectives on an inpatient parent-infant case. Infant Ment Health J 29:278–295, 2008

Fivaz-Depeursinge E, Corboz-Warnery A, Keren M: The primary triangle: treating infants in their families, in Treating Parent-Infant Relationship Problems: Strategies for Intervention. Edited by Sameroff A, McDonough S, Rosenblum K. New York, Guilford, 2004, pp 123–151

Fonagy P: The mentalization-focused approach to social development, in Mentalization: Theoretical Considerations, Research Findings, and Clinical Implications. Edited by Busch F. New York, Analytic Press, 2008, pp

Hayes S, Strosahl K, Wilson K: Acceptance and Commitment Therapy: An Experiential Approach to Behavioral Change. New York, Guilford, 1999

Hornstein C, Trautmann-Villalba P, Holm E, et al: Interaktionales Therapieprogramm für Mutter mit postpartalen psychischen Storungen: Erste Ergebnisse eines Pilotprojecktes. Nervenarzt 78:679–684, 2007

Juffer F, Bakermans-Kranenburg M, van IJzendoorn M: Methods of the video-feedback programs to promote positive parenting alone with sensitive discipline, and with representational attachment discussions, in Promoting Positive Parenting: An Attachment-Based Intervention. Edited by Juffer F, Bakermans-Kranenburg M, van IJzendoorn M. New York, Erlbaum, 2008, pp 11–22

Lieberman A, Van Horn P: Psychotherapy With Infants and Young Children: Repairing the Effects of Stress and Trauma on Early Attachment. New York, Guilford, 2008

Marvin R, Cooper G, Hoffman K, et al: The Circle of Security project: attachment-based intervention with caregiver-preschool child dyads. Attach Hum Dev 1:107–124, 2002

McDonough S: Interaction guidance: Promoting and nurturing the caregiving relationship, in Treating Parent-Infant Relationship Problems: Strategies for Intervention. Edited by Sameroff A, McDonough S, Rosenblum K. New York, Guilford, 2004, pp 79–95

Morlinghaus K: Körperorientierte Psychotherapie und Tanztherapie auf der Mutter-Kind-Einheit in Heidelberg, in Stationäre Eltern-Kind-Behandlung: Ein interdisziplinärer Leitfaden. Edited by Wortmann-Fleischer S, von Einsiedel R, Downing G. Stuttgart, Germany, Kohlhammer, 2012, pp 157–161

Papousek M: Use of video feedback in parent-infant counseling and psychotherapy [in German]. Prax Kinderpsychol Kinderpsychiatr 49:611–627, 2000

Papousek M, Wollwerth de Chuquisengo R: Auswirkungen mütterlicher Traumatisierungen auf die Kommunikation und Beziehung in der frühen Kindheit, in Bindung und Trauma: Risiken und Schutzfaktoren für die Entwicklung von Kindern. Edited by Brisch KH, Hellbrügge T. Stuttgart, Germany, Klett-Cotta, 2003, pp 75–103

Porges SW: The Polyvagal Theory: Neurophysiological Foundations of Emotions, Attachment, Communication, and Self-Regulation. New York, WW Norton, 2011

Reck C: Zum Einfluss der postpartalen Depressionen und Angststörungen auf die Affektregulation in der Mutter-Kind-Interaktion und Ansätze zu deren behandlung (Heidelberger Therapiemodell), in Stationäre Eltern-Kind-Behandlung: Ein interdisziplinärer Leitfaden. Edited by Wortmann-Fleischer S, von Einsiedel R, Downing G. Stuttgart, Germany, Kohlhammer, 2012, pp 49–58

Reck C, Noe D, Stefenelli U, et al: The interactive coordination of currently depressed inpatient mothers and their infants. Infant Ment Health J 32:542–562, 2011

Riva Crugnola C: La relazione genitore-bambino: Tra adeguatezza e rischio. Bologna, Italy, Mulino, 2012

Schechter D, Myers M, Brunelli S, et al: Traumatized mothers can change their minds about their toddlers: understanding how a novel use of videofeedback supports positive change of maternal attributions. Infant Ment Health J 27:429–447, 2006

Slade A: Minding the baby: enhancing parental reflective functioning in a nursing/mental health home visiting program, in Enhancing Early Attachments: Theory, Research, Intervention, and Policy. Edited by Berlin L, Ziv Y, Amaya-Jackson L., Greenberg M. New York, Guilford, 2005, pp 152–177

Slade A: Working with parents in child psychotherapy: engaging the reflective function, in Handbook of Mentalization-Based Treatment. Edited by Allen J, Fonagy P. London, Wiley, 2008, pp 207–235

Steele H, Steele M: The construct of coherence as an indicator of attachment security in middle childhood: the Friends and Family Interview, in Attachment in Middle Childhood. Edited by Kerns K, Richardson R. New York, Guilford, 2005, pp 137–160

Steele H, Steele M: Ten clinical uses of the Adult Attachment Interview, in Clinical Applications of the Adult Attachment Interview. Edited by Steele H, Steele M. New York, Guilford, 2008, pp 3–90

Tronick E: The Neurobehavioral and Social-Emotional Development of Infants and Children. New York, WW Norton, 2007

von Einsiedel R, Wortmann-Fleischer S, Downing G, et al: Fachliche, wirtschaftliche und räumliche Kriterien einer stationären Mutter-Kind-Behandlung in Kliniken für Erwachsenenpsychiatrie, in Stationäre Eltern-Kind-Behandlung: Ein interdisziplinärer Leitfaden. Edited by Wortmann-Fleischer S, von Einsiedel R, Downing G. Stuttgart, Germany, Kohlhammer, 2012, pp 29–48

Wan MW, Green J: The impact of maternal psychopathology on child-mother attachment. Arch Womens Ment Health 12:123–134, 2009

Wortmann-Fleischer S: Interaktionales therapieprogramm für psychisch kranke mütter, in Stationäre Eltern-Kind-Behandlung: Ein interdisziplinärer Leitfaden. Edited by Wortmann-Fleischer S, von Einsiedel R, Downing G. Stuttgart, Germany, Kohlhammer, 2012, pp 94–99

Wortmann-Fleischer S, Downing G, Hornstein C: Postpartale psychische Störungen: Ein interaktionszentrierter Therapieleitfaden. Stuttgart, Germany, Kohlhammer, 2005

Zelenko M, Benham A: Videotaping as a therapeutic tool in psychodynamic infant-parent therapy. Infant Ment Health J 21:192–203, 2000

CHAPTER 18

Evidence-Based Treatments and Evidence-Based Practices in the Infant-Parent Mental Health Field

Connie Lillas, Ph.D., M.F.T., R.N.

Joshua Feder, M.D.

James Diel, M.Ed., M.F.T.

Kristie Brandt, C.N.M., M.S.N., D.N.P.

Mental health practitioners are increasingly asked to provide evidence-based treatments (EBTs). *Evidence-based treatment* is often used synonymously with *evidence-based practice* (EBP); however, these are different efforts to effectively employ research in the service of rational treatment. Within the infant-family and early childhood field, this confusion may impact services provided for infants, young children, and their families. In this chapter, we review the advantages and limitations of EBT and then discuss how EBP addresses the limitations of EBTs and provides guidance for clinical work as well as policy.

Evidence-Based Treatments

Concerned that clinicians have often provided care without research data to support their interventions, proponents of EBTs offer that rigorous, research-based attention to treatment outcome and efficacy has been an important step forward in health care. Clinical research guides professionals toward effective intervention and away from using resources without reasonable expectation of benefit. EBTs also provide a standardized method for reliably replicating an effective model.

EBT provides a path toward ethical care, balancing competing forces, such as the financial gain of the practitioner, human bias, the entrenchment of practices due to the avoidance of updating one's approach, and contextual demands and availability of resources (e.g., urban vs. rural), all of which can be viewed as traditions that resist change. In parallel, in the mental health field in general and in child diagnosis in particular, specific schemes such as DSM-5 (American Psychiatric Association 2013) and the Diagnostic Classification of Mental Health and Developmental Disorders of Infancy and Early Childhood: Revised Edition (DC:0-3R; Zero to Three 2005) emphasize observable and sometimes measurable diagnostic criteria. Overall, the reliance on randomized controlled trials (RCTs) may well be superseding previously established traditions.

Thus, EBT attempts to move toward optimal intervention grounded in research studies. In general, such studies are evaluated on their design, including clarity of concept, population selection, randomization, blinding, statistical analysis, discussion of limitations, and disclosure of funding sources. What constitutes "evidence" is guided by a hierarchy of scientific evidence (Miller et al. 2005). The strength of the evidence grows with more well-controlled studies, with RCTs being the most highly regarded. Quasi-experimental studies do not have a control group but are still useful, offering guidance for further study without definitive conclusions about outcomes. Correlational studies with systematic review across cases or programs are also valuable in addressing the effects of different levels of treatment duration or intensity, especially when the more systematic clinical trials do not adequately differentiate between those levels. Anecdotal case studies, professional opinion, and best practice guidelines developed by clinical consensus are often starting points for research, but have little data to back them.

Substantial variation exists in how treatments are deemed to be EBTs: "Various authorities have established different and sometimes conflicting standards for when there is *enough* evidence to constitute an EBT" (Miller et al. 2005, p. 269). Some sources distinguish "proven practices" from "promising practices." In general, there has been some uncertainty in drawing "a discrete line (EBT or not) on what is actually a continuous dimension (amount, type, and strength of available evidence)" (Miller et al. 2005, p. 269).

Clearinghouses, including those with an emphasis in the early childhood age range, have been established to deal with the research explosion. Some are driven by diagnostic criteria, such as trauma or substance abuse. Others emphasize delivery of services, such as Early Head Start or home visitation. Some treatments are named on several lists of EBTs; others are named on only a few. The criteria used by clearinghouses differ, and the research "evidence," as in all health-related sciences, is in continuous flux. The Substance Abuse and Mental Health Services Administration's National Registry of Evidence-based Programs and Practices (www.nrepp.samhsa.gov) offers extensive reviews of interventions across age groups. External reviewers judge the quality of research evidence for each intervention, assigning each a score. Scoring is based on six factors: reliability of measures, validity of measures, intervention fidelity, missing data and attrition, potential confounding variables, and appropriateness of analysis. Other factors assessed include readiness for dissemination, costs, replications, and contact information.

State and federal clearinghouses approve specific programs, curricula, and treatments for certain conditions. Some identify the type and strength of research focus, including promising practices, whereas others include the identification of programs that are not recommended. Although a caveat on Web sites may state that the governing body does not "endorse" the treatment list, these clearinghouse lists tend to drive agencies' appraisals of what is acceptable and what is not in the field. Several clearinghouses are currently searchable online (see Seibel et al. 2012, p. 32).

Early childhood EBTs draw on a variety of treatment modalities, including existential, cognitive-behavioral, and psychodynamic treatment approaches. In the early childhood field, many of the EBTs are developed for young children who have experienced abuse or a traumatic event, and this emphasis is reflected in the EBTs reviewed here.

- *Parent-Child Interaction Therapy* (PCIT) is an existential, here-and-now approach that includes coaching parents through a one-way mirror with a "bug-in-the-ear" hearing device. In addition, behavioral elements are included. Parents are taught positive behavioral approaches to engage and nurture their child while discouraging negative behavior and setting age-appropriate limits (Nixon et al. 2003). More than one psychotherapy modality is integrated into PCIT.
- *Trauma-Focused Cognitive Behavioral Therapy* (TF-CBT), reflecting the cognitive-behavioral tradition, is a popular EBT offering free online training, which has been completed by more than 60,000 mental health professionals since 2005. This treatment focuses on the trauma narrative, affective regulation, cognitive coping skills, and caregiver acceptance and participation (Cohen and Mannarino 1996).
- *Child-Parent Psychotherapy* (CPP) comes from a psychodynamic tradition, linking to past relationships. Parents are helped to read the child's cues in real time, understand how their behavior has affected the child, and learn how one's history produces perceptions that interfere with one's availability and responsiveness to the child (Lieberman et al. 2006).

Limitations and Challenges of Evidence-Based Treatments

The rise of the EBT approach has been accompanied by concerns about overreliance on a limited list of treatments. In addition, certain specific risks have been noted, including overlooking cultural variation, the complexity and severity of infant mental health cases, mismatches between EBTs and clinical practice, and the limitations of RCTs (Institute of Medicine 2001; Weisz and Gray 2008).

Cultural Variation

Rote adherence to a treatment manual or fidelity standards required by an EBT can impede a nuanced and culturally responsive approach to treatment. Many EBT models are normed on populations with a limited range of cultural backgrounds and may not take into account the specific differences between, among, and within populations (Gray-Little and Kaplan 2000). "The evidence has not always been gathered from families who match the racial, cultural, social or economic factors that are typical of the families programs are targeting for services (Strain and Dunlop). The circumstances under which studies are done may not match the circumstances in communities that wish to replicate evidence based approaches" (Seibel et al. 2012, p. 30). Cultural subgroup differences are often not accounted for during the development of a specific EBT approach. For example, the Positive Parenting Program (Triple P; Sanders et al. 2000) makes use of a quiet time that serves as a warning and a time-out as a consequence. According to the manual, the parent is to remove the child from the activity and place him or her in a distraction-free setting. In low–socioeconomic status urban communities, many single-parent families live in dwellings that are crowded, without even a separate bedroom. A quiet, separate space is simply not available to implement this technique.

Some EBTs come from non-U.S. populations and cultures. For example, the Triple P EBT was originally normed in Australia on two-parent, middle-income families whose primary clinical concern was noncompliance with family rules and parental direction. This normative population may differ from the families to which the EBT is being applied, such as parents of varied cultural backgrounds, socioeconomic status, and educational levels in the United States. Overall, then, culturally responsive providers may be well advised to defer to the family's cultural norms after conveying to the family the relative risks of violating the cultural norms of their new country (such as the requirement of child abuse reporting for corporal punishment) as well as the benefits involved of retaining the practices from their culture of origin.

Clinical Complexity

EBTs are typically conducted with subjects who have a single diagnosis. These cases often do not match more complex cases, especially in community mental health populations, whose symptoms may cross diagnostic categories. For example, a toddler who is not eating might be suffering from anxiety, depression, socioeconomic stress, chronic illness, or trauma. Because test populations must have a specific diagnosis to exclude confounding variables, they may not reflect clinic populations; therefore, the results may not generalize easily to everyday care (Addis and Kransnow 2000; Weisz and Gray 2008). Inadvertent harm may occur when an EBT is used to treat a singular diagnosis (e.g., separation anxiety) in a child who has also suffered significant trauma. Strict adherence to an EBT does not allow the individualized treatment diversification needed to address multiple issues in one treatment plan (Bonisteel 2009; Upshur and Tracy 2008; Weisz and Gray 2008).

Mismatches Between Evidence-Based Treatments and Clinical Practice

At times, an EBT may overlook other critical elements of the presenting situation. Clinicians should be aware that some treatments require skills that are not developmentally present. EBTs may require capacities on the part of the child or parent that are linked to chronological age, but may neither require nor prepare the provider of the EBT to determine the particular child's or parent's competencies across such domains relevant to the treatment. For example, an EBT may require that a child be able to produce a coherent narrative, but infants and young children (and even older children at times) cannot provide a "narrative" in verbal form. Along similar lines, providers of EBT may not be educated regarding the stress arousal continuum and the need to observe during each session for changes in function due to arousal. Clinicians following a protocol may inadvertently exacerbate the child's dysregulation, leading to disruption or early termination of treatment.

Fidelity to a particular EBT protocol may overlook the needs of families. Parents may be placed in a 10-week class yet may require 15 sessions to understand the material. Similarly, a protocol for children that culminates in writing a trauma narrative may be just the beginning of the trauma work that needs to be done, and symptoms may quickly return. Thus, the content, duration, intensity, and frequency of the treatment or program may not be sufficient to be effective with a particular family.

Limitations of Randomized Controlled Trials

Often, diagnoses and other measures do not adequately describe clinical situations. RCTs may show positive outcomes for specific diagnoses yet not necessarily in functional domains, making the relevance of the intervention less certain. For example, research with an autistic spectrum intervention (Dawson et al. 2010) showed improvement in IQ but not in other functional domains. "These shifts [in IQ] were not matched with clinically significant improvements in terms of…severity scores or measurements of repetitive behaviors" (Warren et al. 2011, p. e1308).

Thus, using RCTs alone may narrow clinical vision, restrict the use and development of varied and more appropriate treatment, and drive professionals to attend to suboptimal, if not irrelevant, outcomes. Published research rarely addresses the relevance of an EBT across complex amalgams of service delivery setting, child chronological and developmental age, parent and parent-child attachment status, child and parent history, neurorelational functioning, cultural variation, parental capacities, and levels of case complexity (Mullen and Streiner 2004). Clinical decision making requires choices based on limited knowledge, whereas EBTs often give the impression of completeness and mastery of a problem.

Evidence-Based Practice

EBP is an integrative decision-making process intended to provide better, more efficient clinical treatment. It takes research into account while emphasizing the importance of clinical judgment to match the intervention to the specific situation at hand. Clinicians consider the range of relevant research about a condition and its treatment and, based on clinical judgment and experience, offer families a range of options and provide guidance about what options make sense; families then make decisions about how to proceed based on their own family values and culture. EBP offers families the opportunity for more fully informed consent. Treatment recommendations are not based solely on specific studies, because these might not make sense in the clinical situation and specific family, and no treatments are recommended that have no real basis in science. The three parts of the EBP process combine to support informed consent: 1) relevant research, 2) clinical judgment, and 3) family culture and values (Figure 18–1).

The concept of EBP, which emerged in the late 1980s (Bennett et al. 1987), was conceptually advanced by Sackett et al. (1996), who described EBP as "the conscientious, explicit, and judicious use of current best evidence in making decisions about the care of individual patients. The practice of evidence-based medicine means *integrating* individual clinical expertise with the best available external evidence from systematic research" (pp. 71–72, emphasis added). EBP was adopted by the American Academy of Sciences' Institute of Medicine in 2001 as a central approach to health care and a prerequisite to true informed consent.

Buysse and Wesley (2006) apply EBP in the early childhood field and the context of working with infant caregivers. These authors underscore the dilemma that clinicians face: "The word 'integration' suggested, for the first time, that clinical decisions would be based on more than a single source of knowledge. Moreover, these sources of knowledge would have to be integrated when making a decision about a particular course of treatment" (Buysse et al. 2012, p. 26).

Addressing the Limitations of Evidence-Based Treatment Through the Use of Evidence-Based Practice

The three parts of EBP (see Figure 18–1) provide solutions to the concerns surrounding EBTs. In the following subsections, we discuss each aspect of EBP and its relatedness to clinical care, policy, and cost-effectiveness.

Relevant Research

One approach to the limitations of EBTs is to broaden the type of research that is considered an evidence-based methodology. Publications by the Institute of Medicine discuss the importance of using a variety of research modalities and approaches beyond the RCT as appropriate and relevant research to consider in EBP (Olsen et al. 2010). Additional research methodologies include comparative effectiveness research, acceptability studies, survival studies, and others.

As an example, *comparative effectiveness research* measures the benefits produced by interventions in routine clinical practice, with the aim of determining what works best for which clients. Comparison studies also highlight common predictors of outcome in multisite approved intervention programs. For example, in research comparing multiple early intervention programs using different approaches for children who have or are at risk for

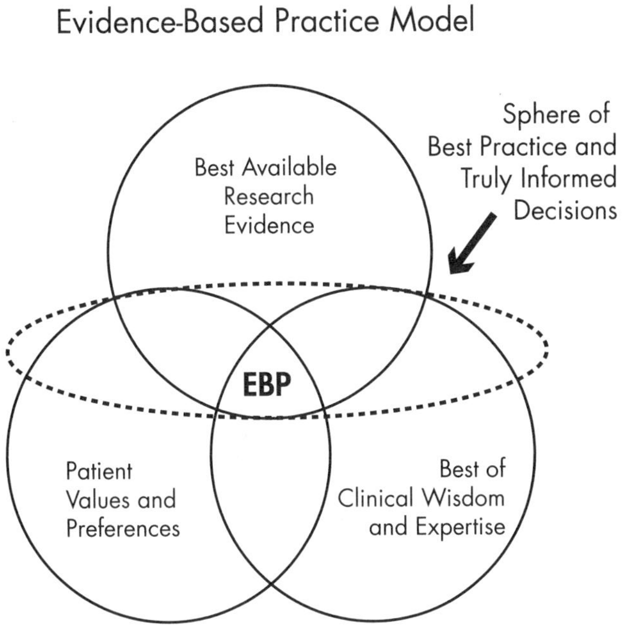

Evidence-Based Practice Model

FIGURE 18–1. Evidence-based practice and sphere of best practice.

Source.   K.Brandt. Adapted from Haynes et al. 2002; Sackett et al. 2000.

developmental disabilities, the mother's level of responsiveness toward her child was the only variable associated with positive developmental outcomes in the children (Mahoney et al. 1998).

Clinical Expertise and Reflective Practice

Clinical expertise includes the development of "clinical wisdom" and the clinician's ability to track his or her own reactions to patients and their needs. After long experience in practice, clinicians develop a capacity for implicit pattern recognition that allows for quick decisions in complex situations related to their work. This ability is developed and refined through extensive experience and practice, in the health professions as in other work. The speed and utility of rapid pattern recognition are evident in a range of fields, from professional sports and military work to trauma surgery and crisis counseling, although the value of implicit wisdom has often been downplayed in the face of more explicit empirical reasoning. In situations where there is less press for immediate action, such processes can be examined and even taught.

Despite its utility, clinical intuition may be biased, however, as demonstrated, for example, by risk avoidance in specialties with substantial litigation risk. Reflective practice is therefore essential to providing good care. In addition, specific biases, fears, and visceral reactions often mirror the family's process. For example, a clinician's feeling of fear or danger may indicate that there is something to be anxious about and to be explored with the family. Alternatively, anxiety may lead clinicians to overaccommodate, leading to resentment toward the family. Other stress responses include agitation and anger at clients, or numbing experiences where one feels detached from a client or family. Containing these visceral reactions and utilizing them for the benefit of the family often require the help of another professional. Attention to these implicit and reflective processes gives EBP an ability beyond EBT to respond to complex human situations (Lillas and Turnbull 2009).

Family Culture and Values

Providers face additional challenges in balancing cultural issues with EBT approaches. Consider a family in which the 8-year-old child presents with extreme suicidal behavior. Although immediate psychiatric intervention may well be indicated, the family may reject psychiatric help. No EBT can be effective if it is not implemented, and conflicts between family culture or values and the fidelity guidelines for EBT approaches can pose ethical dilemmas for the provider. Additionally, certain cultural practices may be unappreciated or poorly understood, and overfidelity to the EBT can challenge the therapeutic alliance. For example, the clinical practice of playing with the child or role-playing may be unfamiliar and put off some families.

Advantages of Evidence-Based Practice in Policy and Practice

Like EBT, EBP is part of the movement toward the use of science to drive better outcomes and control costs in government policy and health insurance regulations. EBP, however, is intended to moderate the rigid adherence to specific studies or treatment methods, respecting scientific values while promoting more flexible and efficient treatment, and ensuring better informed consent. EBP language can be incorporated into laws and used by governmental agencies to guide policy, so that instead of limiting intervention to a list of approved treatments, there are guidelines for using treatments in an EBP process. California Assembly Bill 9 of 2009, for example, wrote EBP into legislation revising the state's approach to developmental disorders.

Currently, lists of specific EBTs are often used by funding or oversight bodies to establish a set of exclusionary criteria. This can be confusing: A treatment appearing on one list is often not on others, and standards for inclusion may be narrow and restrict access to a practice that has demonstrated effectiveness. Lists may also exclude certain patients (e.g., by allowing treatment for autism but not for those showing risk for autism). Some lists reflect conflicts of interest as their advisory groups seek funding for research, conduct training, or practice specific approaches. Some entities that forward lists of EBTs fail to fully disclose criteria for inclusion, expertise and conflicts of reviewers, and funding sources. They may fail to disseminate information on applying for or submitting a treatment for consideration, may not provide a clear description of why treatments are not deemed eligible, and may not offer a fair appeals process.

As the clinical knowledge base grows rapidly, laws and policies may be written more flexibly so that they do not need to be amended as new treatments are studied or the limitations of existing ones are better understood. When EBP is embedded in decision-making processes, it offers a built-in dynamic process that demands the consideration of current relevant research, affords autonomy to the clinician to make decisions about what might make sense within his or her scope of practice and in relation to families' cultural values, and, most important, honors the rights of families to make fully informed decisions.

Applying the Broad Evidence-Based Practice Framework to Evidence-Based Treatments

The framework of EBP suggests a series of reflective questions to help assess a treatment or program that has evidence-based research supporting it. Clinicians can ask about the range of relevant research, consider their own experience with similar situations and their reactions to this situation, and look at how the treatment or intervention fits the specific family. Factors that clinicians might look at in deciding whether a treatment is appropriate include the duration, intensity, and frequency of treatment; cultural appropriateness; flexibility and adaptability of the treatment modality to diagnostic complexity, race, culture, and socioeconomic status; and the match between the EBT's assessment schemes and the target population (Mattox and Kilburn 2012; Seibel et al. 2012). For example, a colleague who visited a rural community in sub-Saharan Africa had planned to do developmental testing with toddlers, only to find that in this community toddlers were never separated from the community and thus could not be assessed in the usual Western manner.

Clinical work in mental health care is often guided by frameworks that support critical thinking to sort through and organize the material and that lead to rational intervention. We describe three frameworks in early childhood mental health.

- *The Touchpoints Model of Development* (Brazelton 1992; Brazelton et al. 1997) lays out an understanding of typical developmental processes in service to building therapeutic alliances. Touchpoints describes patterns of disorganization and functional regression before each step in a child's development, helps providers discern typical developmental events from worrisome deviations, and addresses the meaning of these to the parent. Using the model's relational components, parent and provider coconstruct a therapeutic direction (see Chapter 4, "Brazelton's Neurodevelopmental and Relational Touchpoints and Infant Mental Health").
- *The Neurorelational Framework* (Lillas and Turnbull 2009) provides a comprehensive and efficient map of biopsychosocial complexities. This framework is used to assess variances between adaptive and toxic stress and stress recovery patterns; the quality of parent-child engagement; and individual differences in vulnerabilities and resilience resources across

multiple dimensions and four brain systems (regulation, sensory, relevance, and executive). From a "micro" point of view, distinctions between "bottom-up" developmental processes (e.g., nonverbal processes, implicit memories, automatic reactions to stress and relationships) and "top-down" developmental processes (e.g., verbal processes, explicit memories, abilities to inhibit behavior) provide guidance and assistance in matching clinical modalities to the client's particular developmental functioning. These distinctions allow clinicians to functionally describe individuals, thereby matching EBTs and relevant clinical practices to the neurodevelopment of each child and family (see Chapter 5, "The Neurorelational Framework in Infant and Early Childhood Mental Health").

- *The Neurosequential Model of Therapeutics* (Perry 2006; Perry and Hambrick 2008) is grounded in an understanding of the sequencing of neurodevelopment that is dependently embedded in the experiences of the child. This approach uses biologically and relationally informed assessment, therapeutic approaches, and practices, programs, and policies. This global model uses a brain-mapping matrix to guide providers to identify specific areas for therapeutic work, including EBTs, within its comprehensive therapeutic plan (see Chapter 2, "The Neurosequential Model of Therapeutics").

Conclusion

EBP suggests that clinicians use clinical judgment to weigh all relevant research and provide families with the information they need to make their own fully informed decisions. In doing so, EBP may lead to more efficient care and better outcomes (Yong et al. 2010) by including the rigor of the EBTs but allowing for innovation and humane care while more fully including family culture and values, all of which can reduce the time and resources spent on approaches that have a poor fit and thus less likely efficacy. Reflective practice supports this process in an ongoing and iterative fashion. By equally engaging all three parts of EBP (Figure 18–1), a practitioner can provide an individualized, effective process for each family, such that "evidence does not make decisions, people do" (Haynes et al. 2002, p. 1350). As we have noted elsewhere, "the commitment of the provider to think globally and developmentally about each child, [to] work thoughtfully and respectfully with caregivers, to share professional wisdom, and [to] jointly create a developmentally grounded therapeutic plan is at the heart of EBP" (Brandt et al. 2012, p. 44).

KEY POINTS

- Evidence-based treatments (EBTs) are discrete therapeutic approaches that have met unstandardized scientific criteria established by the entity creating and publishing such criteria.
- Evidence-based practice (EBP) is a process internal both to the clinician and to the relationship between the clinician and the client, and may include thoughtful and collaborative use of one or more EBTs.

- Strict adherence to an EBT does not allow the individualized treatment diversification typically needed to address multiple issues in one treatment plan.
- Despite its utility, clinical intuition may be biased by such things as risk avoidance in specialties with substantial litigation risk. Reflective practice is therefore essential to providing quality care.
- EBP requires clinicians to use clinical judgment to weigh all relevant research and provide families with the information they need to make fully informed decisions.

References

Addis ME, Krasnow AD: A national survey of practicing psychologists' attitudes toward psychotherapy treatment manuals. J Consult Clin Psychol 68:331–339, 2000

American Psychiatric Association: Diagnostic and Statistical Manual of Mental Disorders, 5th Edition. Washington DC, American Psychiatric Association, 2013

Bennett KJ, Sackett DL, Haynes RB, et al: A controlled trial of teaching critical appraisal of the clinical literature to medical students. JAMA 257:2451–2454, 1987

Bonisteel P: The tyranny of evidence-based medicine. Can Fam Physician 55:979, 2009

Brandt K, Diel J, Feder J, et al: A problem in our field: making distinctions between evidence-based treatment and evidence-based practice as a decision-making process. Zero Three 32:42–45, 2012

Brazelton TB: Touchpoints: The Essential Reference—Your Child's Emotional and Behavioral Development. Boston, MA, Addison-Wesley, 1992

Brazelton TB, O'Brien M, Brandt KA: Combining relationships and development: applying Touchpoints to individual and community practices. Infants Young Child 10:74–84, 1997

Buysse V, Wesley PW: Evidence-Based Practice in the Early Childhood Field. Washington, DC, Zero to Three, 2006

Buysse V, Winton PJ, Rous B, et al: Evidence-based practice: foundations for the CONNECT 5-step learning cycle in professional development. Zero Three 32:25–29, 2012

California Assembly Bill 9 of 2009. Available at: http://www.leginfo.ca.gov/pub/09-10/bill/asm/ab_0001-0050/abx4_9_bill_20090728_chaptered.pdf. Accessed July 16, 2013.

Cohen JA, Mannarino AP: A treatment outcome study for sexually abused preschool children: initial findings. J Am Acad Child Adolesc Psychiatry 35:42–50, 1996

Dawson G, Rogers S, Munson J, et al: Randomized, controlled trial of an intervention for toddlers with autism: the Early Start Denver Model. Pediatrics 125:e17–e23, 2010

Gray-Little B, Kaplan D: Race and ethnicity in psychotherapy research, in Handbook of Psychological Change: Psychotherapy Processes and Practices for the 21st Century. Edited by Snyder CR, Ingram RE. New York, Wiley, 2000, pp 591–613

Haynes RB, Devereaux PJ, Guyatt GH: Physicians' and patients' choices in evidence based practice: evidence does not make decisions, people do (editorial). BMJ 324:1350, 2002

Institute of Medicine: Crossing the quality chasm: a new health system for the 21st century. March 2001. Available at: http://www.nap.edu/html/quality_chasm/reportbrief.pdf. Accessed April 1, 2013.

Lieberman AF, Ghosh Ippen C, Van Horn P: Child-parent psychotherapy: 6-month follow-up of a randomized controlled trial. J Am Acad Child Adolesc Psychiatry 45:913–918, 2006

Lillas C, Turnbull J: Infant/Child Mental Health, Early Intervention, and Relationship-Based Therapies: A Neurorelational Framework for Interdisciplinary Practice. New York, WW Norton, 2009

Mahoney G, Boyce G, Fewell RR, et al: The relationship of parent-child interaction to the effectiveness of early intervention services for at-risk children and children with disabilities. Topics Early Child Spec Educ 18:5–17, 1998

Mattox T, Kilburn MR: Understanding evidence-based information for the early childhood field. Zero Three 32:4–10, 2012

Miller WR, Zweben J, Johnson WR: Evidence-based treatment: why, what, where, when, and how? 29:267–276, 2005

Mullen EJ, Streiner DL: The evidence for and against evidence based practice. Brief Treatment and Crisis Intervention 4:113–121, 2004

Nixon RD, Sweeney L, Erickson DB, et al: Parent-child interaction therapy: a comparison of standard and abbreviated treatments for oppositional defiant preschoolers. J Consult Clin Psychol 71:251–260, 2003

Olsen LA, McGinnis JM, Roundtable on Value and Science-Driven Health Care, et al: Redesigning the Clinical Effectiveness Research Paradigm: Innovation and Practice-Based Approaches: Workshop Summary. 2010. Available at: http://www.nap.edu/catalog.php?record_id=12197. Accessed April 1, 2013.

Perry BD: The Neurosequential Model of Therapeutics: applying principles of neuroscience to clinical work with traumatized and maltreated children, in Working With Traumatized Youth in Child Welfare. Edited by Webb NB. New York, Guilford, 2006, pp 27–52

Perry BD, Hambrick EP: The Neurosequential Model of Therapeutics. Reclaiming Children and Youth 17:38–43, 2008

Sackett DL, Rosenberg WM, Gray JA, et al: Evidence-based medicine: what it is and what it isn't. BMJ 312:71–72, 1996

Sackett DL, Straus SE, Richardson WS, et al: Evidence-Based Medicine: How to Practice and Teach EBM, 2nd Edition. London, Churchill Livingstone, 2000

Sanders MR, Markie-Dadds C, Tully LA, et al: The Triple P-positive parenting program: a comparison of enhanced, standard, and self-directed behavioral family intervention for parents of children with early onset conduct problems. J Consult Clin Psychol 68:624–640, 2000

Seibel NL, Bassuk E, Medeiros D: Using evidence-based programs to support children and families experiencing homelessness. Zero Three 32:30–35, 2012

Strain PS, Dunlop G: Recommended practices: being an evidence-based practitioner. Center for Evidence Based Practice: Young Children With Challenging Behavior. 2013. Available at: http://www.challengingbehavior.org/do/resources/documents/rph_practitioner.pdf. Accessed April 1, 2013.

Upshur RE, Tracy S: Chronicity and complexity: is what's good for the diseases always good for the patients? Can Fam Physician 54:1655–1658, 2008

Warren Z, McPheeters ML, Sathe N, et al: A systematic review of early intensive intervention for autism spectrum disorders. Pediatrics 127:e1303–e1311, 2011

Weisz JR, Gray JS: Evidence-based psychotherapy for children and adolescents: data from the present and a model for the future. Child Adolesc Ment Health 13:54–65, 2008

Yong PL, Olsen LA, Roundtable on Evidence-Based Medicine, Institute of Medicine: The Healthcare Imperative: Lowering Costs and Improving Outcomes: Workshop Series Summary. 2010. Available at: http://www.nap.edu/catalog.php?record_id=12750. Accessed April 1, 2013.

Zero to Three: Diagnostic Classification of Mental Health and Developmental Disorders of Infancy and Early Childhood, Revised (DC:0-3R). Washington, DC, Zero to Three, 2005

CHAPTER 19

Transforming Clinical Practice Through Reflection Work

Kristie Brandt, C.N.M., M.S.N., D.N.P.

Reflection, Reflective Process, and Reflective Practice

One of the primary concerns in the infant-family and early childhood mental health field is to know more about how clinicians gain expertise, enhance skills, and continually transform their clinical practice—and then how to foster methods that sustain these processes. For beginning clinicians, the entry to independent practice is typically marked by a passage (e.g., graduation, passing board exams) indicating the acquisition of a body of knowledge sufficient to place them at the threshold of safe and competent practice in their profession. However, in this learning, have the newly minted professionals learned to learn? Have they learned skills for acquiring and incorporating new knowledge throughout their career and for staying on the leading edge of their field as the field advances and as experience fuses with new knowledge, which in turn creates more advanced knowledge for practice? How is it that these new clinicians trained in one area of expertise will be able to expand their knowledge and work into other related specialty areas over time? Also, among their many skills, have these new clinicians cultivated their ability to consciously recognize how past experiences impact current work, and to examine what is touched emotionally in them and how such affective activation impacts their work? Are these new clinicians—indeed, are all clinicians—able to construct knowledge through contextualized meaning while continually ordering, reordering, and examining information and experiences?

The process of ongoing professional development lies at the heart of high-quality clinical practice and improved outcomes for those served. Essential in all fields, this continuing development is particularly crucial for clinicians in infant and early childhood mental health, where a sense of urgency suffuses the work, fueled by continuous advancements in neu-

293

roscience related to pregnancy, infancy, and early childhood; a keen awareness of the rapidity of child development that is shaping key relationships from the moment of birth, with a layering of experience and meaning as development progresses; and recognition of the significance of the child's early environment (including caregiving) to his or her lifelong health and well-being. This urgency looms large as clinicians try to explore the nature and efficacy of therapeutic work, operationalize new knowledge in the field, process what is thought and felt about the work, and attempt to determine what to do to make things better for a given dyad.

For the purposes of this chapter, *reflective process* is defined as a means of professional development wherein the practitioner continually uses internal knowledge and external knowledge to examine and advance practice. *Reflective practice* involves not only use of this synthesized knowledge in practice but also active engagement in the synthetic process while in clinical encounters (Schön 1983). The *internal* element of this process depends on the inner processes of ideas, thoughts, awareness, experience, insight, intuition, empathy, points of activation or triggers, projection, transference, recognition of patterns and themes, and so on, whereas the *external* is reliant on such things as research, publications, best practice standards, observations, analysis, and feedback from others. When both are actuated in a reflective process, the ability to imagine, think, and plan generates new awareness and construction of new understandings, and the potential to transform practice.

Reflective work is multidirectional (resembling an electrodynamic field that is simultaneously linear, circular, elliptical, and diffuse), offering only a context for examining, testing, and probing the work, not a direct path to discovery or change. This constructive examination and discovery enables active transformation of clinical practice, and is a messy, complex, nonlinear task (Van de Ven et al. 1999), eclipsed only, perhaps, by the arduousness of the change process itself. Inevitably, too, moral dilemmas will be unearthed that cannot be solved, but must be tolerated or lived with in order for the clinical work to move on (Bishop and Scudder 1990; White 1995).

Ideally, reflective *activities* lead to reflective *practice,* resulting in improved clinical work and better outcomes for those served. The compelling basis for reflective work in the infant mental health field is the desire for professional excellence and/or the hope of making things better for children and families. If the usual set of clinical methods and approaches were sufficient for all situations, consistent improvement and positive outcomes for clients, as well as professional satisfaction, would be universal. However, the uniqueness of each child and family, acquired self-awareness on the part of the clinician, and the onward progression of new findings and discoveries in the field more than suggest that what a clinician does today is not sufficient for the rest of his or her career, or even for the next child or family to be seen.

Reflective thinking is "an active, persistent, and careful consideration of any belief or supposed form of knowledge in the light of the grounds that support it and the further conclusions to which it tends" (Dewey 1933, p. 9). This introspection depends on pragmatic consideration and activation of what the clinician believes, or more specifically what the clinician *knows,* and obliges exploration of the support for any contention, conviction, assumption, or knowledge—exploring particularly what is practiced or done without examination and for which there is relative certitude. In reflective work, "there is recognition that one's expertise is a way of looking at something which was once constructed and may be reconstructed" (Schön 1984, p. 296). In a simplistic illustration for students, Dewey (1933) had them ponder the sociopolitical-religious context of Europe in the 1400s and the prevailing pressure not only to believe but also not to question the certitude that the world was flat. Through deliberation and pursuit of evidence, the certitude was dispelled and the individual came to "know" something through active construction and reconstruction of knowledge that was absent for those individuals who acquired this knowledge as unquestioned fact.

The Influence of Certitude on Clinical Work

Certitude abounds within the interdisciplinary field of infant mental health, and within the related disciplines. For example, a common certitude in the field is that the 50- to 60-minute therapeutic encounter once a week is the way in which most therapeutic work (e.g., home visits, psychotherapy, occupational therapy, speech-language therapy) should be—or is most effectively—carried out. The 50-minute "hour" is typically how contacts are scheduled, billed, and reimbursed. Many industries, including scheduling and billing systems, and reimbursement schematas are built around this custom. How is it *known* that this schedule is the most "therapeutic"? In therapeutic work, this variable is rarely questioned and is assumed to be a given. In the 1950s, Jacques Lacan was soundly criticized for questioning such certitude in the psychoanalytic field, and the resulting upheaval led to a major split in the French Psychoanalytic Society (Clement 1983). Such is the strength of unquestioned and unexamined practices within professional cultures and the socialized intolerance for reflecting on the original or current relevance. The order and timing of psychoanalytic sessions were a certitude constructed on an unexamined historical base, absent both a curiosity about this custom and data to support the precedent as being superior to other session scheduling. When anchored to such convictions, these become intrinsic, irrefutable, and defensible. Such certitude imperceptibly shapes clinical practice as beliefs or assumptions go unquestioned or unchallenged over time and then creep into personal practice, disciplinary culture, policies, education of professionals in the field, and mentorship of new clinicians. Other examples of common "certitudes" include the following: substance-using mothers do not love their babies; it is best not to have young children get too attached to foster parents; families are better off in the long run if they see their stillborn infant, even if they do not want to; a father cannot be a primary caregiver; sexualized behavior in a 4-year-old is evidence of sexual molestation; every woman must breast-feed her baby; childhood obesity is caused by poor parenting; psychotherapy is the only way to achieve long-term change; substance exposure in utero results in very specific patterns of behavior in the young child; cosleeping can cause sudden infant death syndrome; and some clients cannot be helped. Disturbingly, such certitudes reside in professional cultures and work settings, as well as within individual practitioners, as so basic a known or so imperceptible a conviction that they are unquestioned even as they profoundly influence clinicians' work. Schön proposed that an ongoing process of questioning beliefs and previous understanding and of examining both thinking and practice is a source of professional vigor and renewal, as the clinician becomes a researcher-in-action and constructs new understandings and knowledge (Schön 1984).

Role of a Facilitator

Not all reflective work is facilitated, and ultimately all reflective work (even when facilitated) depends on the individual's ability to reflect. The art of facilitation is discussed below in the section "Reflective Facilitation," but a brief description of the facilitator's role is provided here. In some settings a facilitator is either provided for the clinician by the organization or sought by the individual to support professional advancement. Facilitation is a process in which a facilitator uses a variety of interpersonal and other relevant skills to support individuals or groups to enhance their practice (Kitson et al. 1998). This role includes supporting practitioners in moving evidence into practice and advancing their work through other means. The facilitator role is about helping and supporting rather than telling or persuading (Harvey et al. 2002, p. 585). Expert facilitators are proficient in assisting others in the reflective process; they are both skilled and comfortable in working with what emerges in a session, across the range of intellectual to affective aspects of the work. Facilitators are not providing psychotherapy but rather focus directly on the exploration and advancement of clinical practice and on scaffolding clinicians in answering their own questions about their work. To achieve these objectives, facilitators possess an expert understanding of the activation and regulation of the stress arousal continuum, skills for reflecting-in-action and mindful self-regulation, and the ability to use environmental and other strategies for coregulating facilitatees.

Neurobiology and Reflection

The neurobiological implications for reflective work are often overlooked by those engaging in solo, group, or one-to-one reflective activities, and even by reflective facilitators and supervisors. To reflect at the level being considered here, one must have access to the neocortex (the thinking brain), specifically the prefrontal cortex, while also having access to emotional and affective content through the limbic system, with the ability to recognize, even recall, body sensations.

Perry's (1998) conceptualization of the functional brain (Figure 19–1) demonstrates the clustering of the brain's major structures and functions into four primary hierarchical categories, from the brain stem at the bottom to the neocortex at the top. Although an oversimplified model, it can help in understanding two key concepts: 1) the brain has greater plasticity in the neocortex and limbic systems, whereas the brain stem is less malleable, and 2) stress arousal influences one's functional developmental age, and the functional or operant availability of systems in the brain. Typically, the higher the stress arousal, the less available the higher centers become as the functional-operational base descends into the lower centers in the brain. This concept may be better visualized in Table 19–1.

To imagine, plan, think, dream, and wonder, one needs access to neocortical functioning. To recall in-context emotional content, activation, triggers, and body sensations, one must have access to limbic structures. Others might describe this from a right and left brain perspective, but the content and processing availability remain the same. To reflect as a means of transforming practice requires bringing both thoughts and feelings (thinking and feeling) into awareness. Quieting the stress arousal system through whatever manner is satisfactory to the practitioner thus becomes a key component of solo, group, or individual reflective work. There is no place in this process for strategies on the part of facilitators to provoke or intentionally activate the stress arousal system, as might be used in some forms of therapeutic work. Instead, skilled facilitators employ environmental and co-regulatory strategies that support clinicians in managing their arousal level between rest and vigilance, thus gaining access to limbic, neocortical, and body information to facilitate and inform reflective activities. It is in this neurobiological space where the conditions exist for insight, exploring reactions and responses, examining thoughts and feelings, imagining, planning, and integrating knowledge and theories (Brandt 2009). This is also very much a parallel process as practitioners enhance their self-regulatory skills and in turn enhance their ability to provide co-regulatory supports for clients during clinical encounters.

Engaging in Reflection

Dewey (1933) contended that people do not learn from experience but rather from reflecting on their experiences, and he believed that past experience heavily influenced current ways of being. Throughout his career, Schön (1984), who wrote his dissertation on Dewey's work, probed the essence of professional excellence and viewed technical knowledge and artistry as the catalysts for professional excellence. He also espoused two critical steps in reflective practice: 1) "reflection *on* action," during which practitioners allow themselves to find places of puzzlement, surprise, confusion, and so forth in their work and to examine this directly with an eye to transforming practice, and 2) "reflection *in* action," during which reflection actively transpires in the course of a direct client contact (Schön 1984). Later, Greenwood (1998) introduced the practice of "reflection *before* action," wherein the practitioner engages in active reflection prior to the client encounter to more efficiently facilitate the movement of knowledge into clinical practice. Amulya (2011) offers three key questions on which to reflect: 1) What do you do? 2) What does it touch in you? and 3) What does this mean for those being served? A more succinct reason for reflection is simply to follow Brazelton's counsel to practitioners: "Recognize what you bring to the interaction" (Brazelton et al. 1997, p. 79). Schön expanded the focus in asking practitioners to reflect on these two questions: "What, in my work, really gives me satisfaction?" and "How can I produce more experiences of that kind?" (Schön 1984, p. 87).

There are many ways to engage in the reflective process, and essentially no comparative evidence is available to suggest that solo work (nonfacilitated), individual (one-to-one)

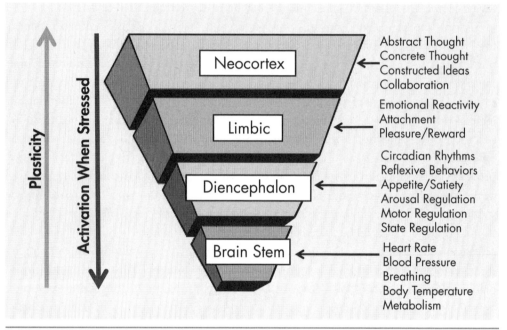

FIGURE 19–1. Perry's conceptualization of the functional brain.

Source. Bruce D. Perry, M.D., Ph.D. All rights reserved. Used with permission.

facilitation (whether with a facilitator or peer), or group work (whether with peers or facilitator) is any more or less beneficial than any other form; nor is there compelling evidence to suggest that a group of one facilitator with 8 facilitatees, for instance, is any more or less effective than a group with 3 or 20 facilitatees. However, various state and professional organizations around the United States have firmly established ratios of facilitators to facilitatees (supervisors to supervisees) as well as the number of hours of reflective work or prelicensure supervised clinical hours (regardless of whether reflective in nature or not) necessary to achieve licensure, endorsement, renewal, grant requirements, and so on. Dewey himself would likely suggest that these unexamined ratios and standards deserve to be reflected upon as a way of understanding whether or not such standards are effective, whether other formulas are equally or more effective, from where such standards were derived, and what were the promulgating entities' attachment to and motives for establishing and enforcing such unexamined standards. Regardless of such ratios or hours, however, a primary intent of *any* facilitated reflection should be to cultivate in the facilitatee a rich "culture of reflection" such that when the facilitated relationship ends, the facilitatee has "learned to learn" and can carry on a process of productive solo or peer-with-peer reflective work throughout his or her career.

There are many goals or objectives for the reflective process (Brandt 2009; California Infant-Family and Early Childhood Mental Health Training Guidelines Workgroup 2011; The Reflective Practitioner 2013b), but regardless of the reflective setting (solo, one-to-

TABLE 19–1. Perry's progression of stress arousal

Adaptive response	Rest	Vigilance	Freeze	Flight	Fight	Terminal dissociation
Sense of time	Extended future	Days Hours	Hours Minutes	Minutes Seconds	Loss of sense of time	Blocked
Dissociative continuum	Rest	Avoidance	Compliance	Dissociation	Loss of consciousness	Complete
Mental state	Calm	Alert	Alarm	Fear	Terror	Surrender
Brain areas	Neocortex Subcortex	Subcortex Limbic	Limbic Diencephalon	Diencephalon Brain stem	Brain stem ANS	ANS Shock
Cognition	Abstract	Concrete	Emotional	Reactive	Reflexive	Halted
Functional age (months)	>15	8–15	3–8	1–3	0–1	0

Note. ANS = autonomic nervous system.

Source. Bruce D. Perry, M.D., Ph.D. 1998. All rights reserved. Used with permission. Revised by Perry and Brandt, 2013.

one, or group), reflective work should share a common purpose of supporting the clinician to 1) explore his or her experience more deeply in order to recall and examine intentions, motivations, meanings made, judgments, assumptions, reveries, resistance, neurobiological states, moments of activation, and so on; 2) genuinely contemplate the experience of others/clients, including their perspectives, experience and expression of culture, wishes, hopes, goals, intentions, and so on; 3) examine harmonious and disharmonious states and how both were negotiated; 4) attend to successes, professional satisfaction, challenges, clinical errors, and moments of insight in the work, and consider the antecedents of each with the aim of using this knowledge to enrich practice; 5) search and contemplate current knowledge bases in the field, including research, publications, practices, and standards of care that were used in this encounter, could have been used in this encounter, or should be used in future similar encounters (Johns 1994); and 6) synthesize and actuate the knowledge of self, other, clinical practice, and relevant knowledge bases to reshape practice.

Opportunities for Reflection

The reflective activities below can contribute to reflective practice when engaged in "for the purpose of examining the work, achieving greater levels of understanding and competence, and transforming practice" (Brandt 2009, p. 35). Some methods may require substantial time to fully realize the benefits to practice.

- *Reflective consideration:* Independently thinking about, meditating on, or contemplating the work and engaging in a mindful process of examination of either content that emerges in the process or content that was specifically chosen for reflective consideration.
- *Reflective expression:* The use of poetry, painting, drawing, dance, music, collage, montage, clay work, or other forms of creative expression to explore thoughts, feelings, experiences, beliefs, motivations, and so forth that influence the clinician's work.
- *Reflective analysis:* Listening to or watching audio or video recordings of clinical encounters and reflectively analyzing the content as a means of exploring the work. The intent is to more deeply understand the interactional process, the *actions* of the clinician and client; the *interactions* between the clinician and client; and opportunities presented, missed, noted, acted on, and so forth. Such analysis may also be a part of a reflective discussion, facilitation, or supervision process.
- *Reflective journaling:* An exploration of challenges, emotional content, insights, successes, confusing elements, and other content related to the work, and not simply a chronological narrative of events (Stickel and Waltman 1994).
- *Reflective discussion:* Informally or formally discussing professional encounters with one's peers or other colleagues, without a designated facilitator for the discussion. This may occur face-to-face or by phone, e-mail exchanges, electronic video conferencing, or other electronic means.
- *Reflective facilitation (mentorship, guidance, or coaching):* A formal relationship between an individual or group and a facilitator skilled in supporting others in the reflective process

who meet regularly for the purpose of professional development by reflectively examining and exploring the work.

- *Reflective supervision:* Although often used casually, the term *supervision* in psychotherapy work is a legally defined term in many jurisdictions and is used here to refer to a formal pre- or postlicensure relationship of a psychotherapist and a clinical supervisor who is approved by a licensing board and who, in prelicensure contexts, is legally responsible for protecting the welfare of the client (third-party protection); overseeing and mentoring supervisees in their professional development, including determining fitness for licensing and/or licensing examination; and protecting both the public at large and the interests of the profession (DeTrude 2001; Todd and Storm 1997). For those not in the psychotherapy disciplines, the word "supervision" may refer to one's superior in an organizational structure or system (literally, who signs your time card) or to someone who provides clinical support, consultation, or direction. It is worth noting here that not all "supervision" (of either type) is reflective in nature. For the balance of this chapter, the term *facilitation* is used to infer both facilitation and supervision.

There are many ways to reflect, and it is unfortunate that some entities and projects assume that reflective facilitation either is the only way to achieve high-quality reflection or is superior to other methods. Essentially no comparative evidence is available to support the notion that reflective work with a facilitator is consistently more effective or of a higher quality than that achieved by the practitioner alone (e.g., reflective analysis, reflective journaling) or in less formal relationships (e.g., reflective discussion). The multidisciplinary influences on current concepts of reflective practice in the United States have likely contributed to certitudes about related ratios, frequency of encounters with facilitators, value or disregard for solo reflective work, and so on. For readers so inclined, it would be worthwhile to examine the influences on current reflective practice concepts and approaches using the figure presented here (Figure 19–2): 1) psychodynamic and psychoanalytic theories and practices have contributed substantially to the intent, goals, approaches, and philosophical underpinnings; 2) psychotherapy (particularly psychology) prelicensure supervision has influenced concepts related to ratios (supervisor to supervisees), requirements regarding hours of supervision for achievement of a status such as licensing or endorsement (Association of State and Provincial Psychology Boards 2012); 3) education, particularly through the foundational work of Schön, has contributed a modernist perspective, theoretical base, research, and operational testing of applications; and 4) nursing has contributed numerous models for reflection, supported robust dialogue on the topic, and has a substantial literature. The model presented offers additional influencing concepts and theories.

Models for Reflection

A wise cautionary statement is that "if you're going nowhere, you are sure to get there." Such is the case in reflective work. Although valuable, reflecting on practice, without having any structure, is at risk of being random and episodic (The Reflective Practitioner 2013a). The style of reflection being discussed here, whether facilitated or not, is directed at transforming practice and improving outcomes for those served, through a deliberate process of examining the work; considering what the clinician brings to the work (including thoughts and emotions); understanding how this impacts the work; and adding both this knowledge (internal knowledge) and external knowledge, such as new research findings or models of care, to one's practice model or conceptual framework.

Facilitated reflection is frequently assumed to be a process limited to appreciative inquiry (Kinni 2003), unconditional positive regard (Rogers 1961), motivational interviewing (Miller and Rollick 1991), or similar valuable approaches, but these lack the express aim of transforming practice through a process of knowledge development. Various models for facilitation and solo work have been developed for moving the process toward these intended goals, including 1) Boud et al.'s (1985) three steps for reflection, 2) Atkins and Murphy's (1994) six-step Cycle of Reflection, 3) Johns' (1994) model of structured reflection, and 4) Kolb's (1984) reflective model for transformation of information into knowledge. For the most part, these can all be used in solo, individual, or group reflective work.

Reflective Facilitation

Skilled facilitators guide and support reflection through their presence, thoughtful listening, comments and questions, summarizing and wondering, awareness of behavioral cues, monitoring and helping to manage stress arousal, noticing and commenting on points of activation or triggers in the facilitatee that are worthy of consideration, and maintaining directional intent with reasonable flexibility. Effective facilitators also possess a diverse range of other skills and personal attributes (Royal College of Nursing 1990), but there is little agreement in the literature related to the mix or importance of specific skills necessary to be successful (Harvey et al. 2002). A facilitator acts to co-regulate a facilitatee or group after first reflecting in action to mindfully self-regulate and appreciate the process occurring between and within the facilitator and the facilitatee or group, and can use body gestures, posture, carefully chosen questions or comments, prosody of speech, silence, and so on to support the process.

Consider this facilitatee's statement: "I mean, I was just undone by this, it was so overwhelming …just too much to think about and do. I wanted to just throw in the towel and walk away. I want to scream…to just quit. I can't stand it anymore." While bearing in mind that this process is not psychotherapy, the facilitator is focused on scaffolding the practitioner in the process of transforming practice by incorporating new knowledge of self and/or new knowledge for the field into one's practice model. The facilitator has many choices for a direction at this point, such as these: 1) say nothing and wait to let the facilitatee take the next step in choosing a direction; 2) choose a comment or question to linger more with the emotional content and inner experience of the clinician, such as "This case has really touched something very powerful in you"; 3) use Brazelton's concept

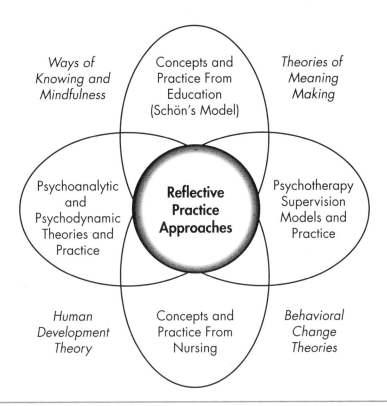

FIGURE 19–2. Current influences on reflective practice approaches in the United States.

Source. Kristie Brandt, C.N.M., M.S.N., D.N.P., 2009. All rights reserved. Used with permission.

of explicitly acknowledging and valuing the passion expressed (Brazelton et al. 1997) by saying, for example, "It's obvious how much you care about this case"; or 4) choose a comment or question to gently bring the facilitatee in a neocortical direction, such as "As you talk about this case, what do you think has been the most challenging part?" When too limbically laden, the content is emotionally driven, and when too neocortically laden, the content is overintellectualized, yet feelings and cognition are both necessary for such learning (Davies 1995). Striking a balance supports the reflective process, as well as the quality and usefulness of the outcomes derived. Facilitated reflection may be perceived here to have a slight advantage over solo reflection due to the co-regulatory potential and directional questions or comments, although these are at the facilitator's discretion and may not always take the facilitatee to where he or she wants or needs to go.

The following is an example of reflective facilitation.

A facilitatee was discussing a case in which she described the mother and father in the family as being in a "role reversal." When asked about the meaning of this description, the facilitatee said the mother was the disciplinarian and the father was "like a kid himself." When asked more about how she came to think of this as a role reversal, she said, "Well, you know, in most families the father lays down the law, he sets the limits, but in this family the mother is setting all the limits on the children on the dad." This opened a space for wondering to-gether about her beliefs regarding family structure and roles, how this belief about what is typical or normal influences her work with families, what implications her beliefs have for her work with single parents or same-gender parents, and what experiences she believes shaped and solidified this belief. [*Author's note:* This is directly related to the work of Dewey (1933) in examining a belief or supposed form of knowledge, the grounds that support it, and the further conclusions to which this belief tends.] The session ended with a plan for her to journal about this, including the influence of strongly held ideas about family roles on her work. In a later session, she said she was able to realize that she was resenting the father in this family for not "stepping up to the plate" and doing his fair share of the hard work of parenting. She said she also had found herself blaming the mother for not being firmer with the father in making him take on more of the "parenting work." As a result, much of her work with the family had stalled as she felt and acted clinically on her increasing exasperation with the mother and her previously unrecognized desire for the mother to be more assertive with the father. This led to many rich discussions on what she felt was "parenting work," the "hard work of parenting," her beliefs on gender roles, and advancing her skills for un-derstanding parents' perspectives and values.

In this example, the facilitator followed Johns's (1994) model of guided reflection and used a sophisticated set of skills and knowledge for scaffolding discussion, supporting crit-ical thinking, and enabling the learning process. By offering a thoughtfully co-regulated environment and an open, nonjudgmental stance, the facilitator crafted the space for hon-est wondering and potential advancement of clinical efficacy. Such a presence of mind and body, as well as willingness to deal with what emerges, is the hallmark of good facilitation. In summary, "quality reflective practice facilitation is not a random, casual or accidental process. It is a deliberate, conscious blend of artistry and skill, nested in a conceptual frame-work, within an actively managed environment wherein this relational, empathic, impro-visational work unfolds" (Brandt 2009, p. 85).

Conclusion

Schön (1984) argued that the reflective process starts with practitioners allowing them-selves to experience surprise, confusion, puzzlement, uncertainty, unfamiliarity, and so on in their work and then reflecting on this experience, including how similar situations were understood in the past and what implicitly influenced how the practitioner responded. With this new awareness, the practitioner can reflect on other possible approaches and plan for their implementation. Professionals may find it unfamiliar or uncomfortable to acknowledge moments of confusion or puzzlement, and to identify deeply held feelings and beliefs associated with the work. Yet, according to Schön, such experiences offer the promise of transforming practice.

In the dynamic infant mental health field, providers are increasingly encountering new neuroscientific information, changing family and social structures, fluctuating funding and political influences, challenging and sometimes seemingly hopeless cases, and so forth, while simultaneously having strong beliefs of their own and experiencing powerful emotions related to the work. Certainly, "reflective practices offer us a way of trying to make sense of the uncertainty in our workplaces and the courage to work competently and ethically at the edge of order and chaos" (Ghaye 2000, p. 7). Developing reflective practice skills supports clinicians in continually renewing their professional satisfaction and incorporating new findings into their work with integrity and fidelity, while thoughtfully processing the emotions and other experiences related to the work—a progression that can transform practice and improve outcomes for those served.

KEY POINTS

- Reflective process is defined as a means of professional development wherein the practitioner continually uses internal knowledge and external knowledge to examine and advance practice. Reflective practice involves not only the use of this synthesized knowledge in practice, but also active engagement in the synthetic process while in clinical encounters.

- Reflective work is multidirectional, offering only a context for examining the work, not a direct course. This constructive examination and discovery enables imagining and planning for active transformation of clinical practice, and is a messy, complex, nonlinear task, eclipsed only, perhaps, by the arduousness of the change process itself.

- Disturbingly, certitudes reside in professional cultures and work settings, as well as within individual practitioners, as so basic a known or so imperceptible a conviction that they are unquestioned even as they profoundly influence work.

- There are many ways to engage in reflection. To imagine, plan, think, dream, and wonder, one needs access to neocortical functioning. To recall in-context emotional content, activation, triggers, feelings, intuition, and body sensations, one must have access to limbic structures. Professional learning is both affective and cognitive.

- Reflective facilitation is a form of reflective work in which a professional is supported by a facilitator whose role is to scaffold, guide, and advance the reflective process. Good reflective facilitation is a highly complex, nonprescriptive, improvisational endeavor in which the facilitator scaffolds the facilitatee to find what she or he is seeking.

References

Amulya J: What is reflective practice? May 2011. Available at: http://www.community-science.com/images/file/What%20is%20Reflective%20Practice.pdf. Accessed April 1, 2013.

Association of State and Provincial Psychology Boards (ASPPB) Handbook of Licensing and Certification Requirements: Supervised Experience Requirements by Jurisdiction. 2012. Available at: http://www.asppb.org/HandbookPublic/Reports/default.aspx?ReportType=SupervisedExperience. Accessed April 1, 2013.

Atkins S, Murphy K: Reflective practice. Nurs Stand 8:49–56, 1994

Bishop A, Scudder J: The Practical, Moral, and Personal Sense of Nursing. Albany, State University of New York Press, 1990

Boud D, Keogh R, Walker D: Reflection: Turning Experience Into Learning. London, Kogan, 1985

Brandt KA: Facilitating the Reflective Process: An Introductory Workbook for the Infant-Parent and Early Childhood Field. Napa, CA, PICI Press, 2009

Brazelton TB, O'Brien M, Brandt K: Combining relationships and development: applying Touch-points to individual and community practices. Infants Young Child 10:74–84, 1997

California Infant-Family and Early Childhood Mental Health Training Guidelines Workgroup: California Training Guidelines and Personnel Competencies for Infant-Family and Early Childhood Mental Health, Revised. Sacramento, California Center for Infant-Family and Early Childhood Mental Health, 2011

Clement C: The Lives and Legends of Jacques Lacan. New York, Columbia University Press, 1983

Davies E: Reflective practice: a focus for caring. J Nurs Educ 34:167–174, 1995

DeTrude J: The supervision process: complications and concerns. Professional Issues in Counseling On-Line Journal, Summer 2001. Available at: http://www.shsu.edu/~piic/summer2001/detrude.html. Accessed April 1, 2013.

Dewey J: How We Think: A Restatement of the Relation of Reflective Thinking to the Educative Process. Boston, MA, DC Heath, 1933

Ghaye T: Into the reflective mode: bridging the stagnant moat. Reflective Practice 1:5–9, 2000

Greenwood J: The role of reflection in single and double loop learning. J Adv Nurs 27:1048–1053, 1998

Harvey G, Loftus-Hills A, Rycroft-Malone J, et al: Getting evidence into practice: the role and function of facilitation. J Adv Nurs 37:557–558, 2002

Johns C: Nuances of reflection. J Clin Nurs 3:71–75, 1994

Kinni T: The art of appreciative inquiry. Harvard Business School Working Knowledge for Business Leaders, September 22, 2003. Available at: http://hbswk.hbs.edu/archive/3684.html. Accessed April 1, 2013.

Kitson A, Harvey G, McCormack B: Enabling the implementation of evidence-based practice: a conceptual framework. Qual Health Care 7:149–158, 1998

Kolb DA: Experiential Learning: Experience as the Source of Learning and Development. Englewood Cliffs, NJ, Prentice Hall, 1984

Miller WR, Rollnick S: Motivational Interviewing: Preparing People for Change. New York, Guilford, 1991

The Reflective Practitioner: professional mastery through model building: path to mastery. 2013a. Available at: http://www.reflectivepractitioner.com/path_to_mastery.htm. Accessed April 1, 2013.

The Reflective Practitioner: professional mastery through model building: seminars. 2013b. Available at: http://www.reflectivepractitioner.com/seminars.htm. Accessed April 1, 2013.

Rogers C: On Becoming a Person. Boston, MA, Houghton Mifflin, 1961, pp 283–284

Royal College of Nursing: Quality Patient Care: The Dynamic Standard Setting System. London, Scutari, 1990

Schön D: The Reflective Practitioner: How Professionals Think in Action. London, Temple Smith, 1983

Stickel SA, Waltman J: A practicum in school counseling: using reflective journals as an integral component. Paper presented at the annual meeting of the Eastern Educational Research Association, Sarasota, FL, 1994

Todd T, Storm C: The Complete Systemic Supervisor: Context, Philosophy, and Pragmatics. Needham Heights, MA, Allyn & Bacon, 1997

Van de Ven AH, Polley DE, Garud R, et al: The Innovation Journey. New York, Oxford University Press, 1999

White J: Patterns of knowing: review, critique, and update. ANS Adv Nurs Sci 17:73–86, 1995

CHAPTER 20

Attachment, Intersubjectivity, and Mentalization Within the Experience of the Child, the Parent, and the Provider

Stephen Seligman, D.M.H.

In this chapter, I present a "relational-representational-transactional" approach to infant-parent psychotherapy and infant intervention. This perspective is rooted in the notion that all interventions depend on the relationship systems within which they occur, including complex interactions between different elements within those systems. In addition, several specific dimensions of infant-parent interventions will be surveyed, including nonverbal and emotional aspects, intersubjectivity, attachment, mentalization, and the intergenerational transmission of trauma. In general, a psychodynamic perspective is emphasized, including the importance of the therapist's attention to her own reactions and personal and professional background.

Relationships as Fundamental Motivators and Organizers: Mutual Regulation and Mutual Influence in the Dyadic Field

The relationship between infant and parent is the fundamental unit for development, and the creation and maintenance of ties to other people are central motivations. Over time, through evolving sequences of signals and responses, infants and caregivers continually influence and regulate one another's internal states and behaviors. These early interaction patterns have been shown to exert an influence into adulthood (Beebe et al. 2010; Main 2000; Seligman 2012).

A 7-month-old and her father play face-to-face. The father smiles. An instant later, the baby lifts her head, coos, smiles, and fixes her eyes on his face. His brows lift and his eyes brighten as he says, "Hiiii, Luuucie!" Cooing even more brightly and loudly, she lifts her arms enthusiastically. Dad lifts her into the air, and she laughs and waves her arms in rhythm with the pace at which her father carries her upward and forward. Their vocalizing follows a similar rhythm.

Here, Lucie and her father are *cocreating* a relationship in which each of them becomes more himself or herself. They are involved in mutual regulation of their intertwined senses of their dyad and of each of their individual bodily mental states, "negotiating" what they mean to each other and within each of their "selves." Kristie Brandt (personal communication, November 2012) has characterized such everyday interactions as "concurrent, overlapping, and intersecting processes wherein the inner life of human beings both influence and are influenced by the inner life of other human beings, in an organic, dynamic, and improvisational confluence."

Brandt also notes that such interchanges are "unique within each moment, yet supported by fixed templates and representations." Indeed, even as a "good-enough" mother is responding sympathetically to her baby, she is reacting in such a way as to reflect her own character, constitution, and personal history. It is the intricate working out of these different dimensions—ranging from details of infant endowment, through individual parental psychology, family dynamics, socioeconomic circumstances, cultural influences, and so on—that determines the course of each person's emergence.

Nonverbal and Affective Dimensions of Early Experience

Infant-parent interactions such as that of Lucie and her father highlight the centrality of nonverbal communication (Trevarthen 2009). The infant relies on motor activity, affect, sensation, and autonomic experience to communicate with and make sense of her relationship with her caregiver: Researchers and therapists have often underestimated or oversimplified these basic dimensions of experience. In fact, nonverbal systems can be complex and highly organized, and are integrated into an early sense of self in infancy and throughout the life cycle. The infant communicates by movements of arms, legs, head, and neck; by facial expression; and by vocalizing—crying, cooing, and babbling. The caregiver responds in corresponding modalities, through body temperature, skin tension, heart and respiratory rate, and so on. Even when the caregiver speaks, it is the nonverbal, aural components of speech—tone, volume, pace, and rhythm—that register.

Nonverbal interactions organize into different patterns between infant and caregiver (many of which can also be observed in adult relationships). These include moments of mutual regulation, coordination and discoordination, sequences of call and response, disruption and repair, and many others (Beebe et al. 1993; Stern 1977; Tronick 2007). Terms such as *procedural knowledge* and *implicit relational knowing* have been used to capture how nondeclarative interpersonal patterns shape everyday behavior (Grigsby and Schneiders 1991; Lyons-Ruth 1998). These patterns involve interpersonal, action or affect schematas ranging from riding a bicycle or stopping at a red light to patterns for seeking interpersonal equilibrium in a marriage, a business partnership, or psychotherapy.

The Transactional Perspective: Nonlinear Dynamic Systems at the Core of Development

The *transactional perspective* places complex relationships at the center of both developmental and clinical theory, proposing that living systems, especially humans, organize themselves in complex, shifting, *dynamic and nonlinear patterns,* synthesizing an array of different factors. For infant-parent systems, such factors include genetics, epigenetics, intrauterine effects, affect, sensorimotor growth and development, temperament, the social surround, parental sensitivity or psychopathology, caregiving, and countless others (Sameroff and Emde 1989; Seligman 2005). The effect of any single factor cannot be understood or predicted without reference to the others with which it is "transacting."

Here is a hypothetical and oversimplified (but realistic) illustration: Consider a mildly depressed single mother with two babies, one of whom is constitutionally persistent. Her depression would likely have a less damaging effect on the persistent infant because the baby who gives up quickly may never evoke the engagement she needs from her mother, whereas the persistent one might eventually succeed. Over a series of interactions, the less persistent infant might withdraw, amplifying the depressed mother's sense of rejection, leading to further withdrawal on both sides. In contrast, the persistent infant might disconfirm the mother's expectations, encouraging her to respond in the future so as to reinforce the baby's ongoing efforts.

Intersubjectivity as Core Motivator and Organizer

Infant researchers have shown how individual identity and the sense of connection with others are related; apparently paradoxically, individuality depends on being understood by attentive others. *Ideally, even as it is rooted in individual history and personality, personal experience becomes what it is by being shared with someone different.* The infant researchers have shown that the infant's sense of self occurs much earlier in development than has been imagined and is social at its core (Stern 1985).

Another infant-parent interaction shows how partners in relationship *cocreate* meanings and experiences of self-with-other. An 8-month-old begins biting his mother's nose, harder each time. She shrieks in delight, and eventually pain, as the baby squeals responsively. Sometimes they break into peals of laughter, which the baby interrupts by biting again. After a number of increasingly fierce bites, Mom playfully exclaims, "Stop!" while finally re-straining him more definitively and trying to distract him. The baby laughs, and Mom fol-lows. This duo is constructing something that has never existed before that also reflects each person's individuality (Winnicott 1971).

An intersubjective perspective focuses on how infant and parent "negotiate" specific behaviors as well as how they regard one another. If the mother had taken the baby's biting as hostile aggression, for example, she would have responded differently, with more re-straint, anxiety, or even fear. If the mother had lost track of his age-related limitations and stimulated him even more, the baby might have felt overwhelmed rather than enjoying the play. Overall, this episode shows the central role of the *recognition process* (Sander 2008): Both baby and mother are becoming themselves as they become more than themselves, inter-acting with one another. Elaborating Sander's thinking, Tronick (2007) has described "the dyadic expansion of consciousness."

Attachment Theory and Research

As infant-parent relationships develop consistent patterns of mutual and self-regulation of action, emotion, and bodily state, infants usually develop a relatively stable set of expec-tations about the extent to which the interpersonal world is a protective place that offers the physiological and emotional support necessary to promote adequate and secure devel-opment. Through the correlation of external and internal processes, core patterns of achiev-ing emotional security and proximity/distance with caregivers develop, in a range of more or less threatening circumstances.

The terms *attachment* and *attachment theory* refer to a specific body of theory and research concerned with such processes. Drawing on primate research and direct observation of young children, Bowlby (1969/1982) asserted that a child's tie to caregivers is a primary, autonomous system essential for species survival. He went on to reformulate the psycho-analytic theories of motivation, separation and loss, and defense in accord with emerging regulatory systems models, stressing the importance of affects, especially fear. Subsequently, Mary Ainsworth (Ainsworth et al. 1978) developed the Strange Situation, an assessment in which infants are briefly separated from their mothers and then reunited so as to determine their attachment behaviors. Ainsworth validated three attachment classifications—*secure, insecure/avoidant,* and *insecure/resistant-ambivalent*—and demonstrated that attachment is a cross-cultural phenomenon. Her work launched a worldwide network of academic re-searchers, constituting a formidable subfield of developmental psychology. Their retrospec-tive and prospective studies correlating infant and adult attachment classifications have provided substantial support for the proposition that early interpersonal experience has en-during effects. Attachment researchers have reliably predicted the sense of security in adult-hood as well as attachment classification across generations (Main 2000).

In addition, more recent attachment researchers have validated a fourth classification, *disorganized/disoriented,* which is applied to infants, children, and adults with attachment organizations primarily characterized by mixtures of incoherence, fear, controlling behaviors, and the like (see, e.g., Hesse and Main 2000). Disorganized attachment is associated with both early relationship trauma and adult borderline psychopathology (Fonagy and Bateman 2008; Gabbard et al. 2008; Main and Solomon 1990). Overall, findings from research in other areas—the study of long-term effects of early neglect, trauma, and maltreatment on the brain and functional magnetic resonance imaging demonstrating patterns of brain dysfunction in adult disorders (Hollander and Berlin 2008)—suggest a convergence of attachment and neuroscience research (Schore 2003).

Mentalization and Development

Bowlby's (1969/1982) initial proposal and Ainsworth's (Ainsworth et al. 1978) elaborations are regarded as the first two stages of attachment theory. The third phase, "the move to the level of representation," follows Bowlby's (1988) interest in internal working models of attachment. Following Bowlby's proposal, these theorists describe the "internal working models" of each attachment classification as stable representational structures that regulate the sense of personal security. In a major breakthrough, Main et al. (2005) developed the Adult Attachment Interview, a semistructured interview that classifies adults into groups correlated with the infant categories. In a crucial addition, they correlate the sense of personal security with *coherent reflection* on one's own memories and experience, rather than the actual historical events. As interest in the internal world has been further developed and discussed, using terms such as *mentalization* and *reflective functioning,* it is particularly encouraging for psychodynamic therapists. The experience of being understood appears to be basic to feeling secure (Fonagy et al. 2002; Main 2000).

Mentalization refers to an emerging mental capacity, achieved in a crucial process in development during which the child comes to understand that her immediate experience, compelling as it may seem, is a *personal* experience different from other people's. This capacity thus implies a number of distinctions: the distinction between one's own mind and the minds of others; the distinction between intentions and effects; and the ability to imagine that one's own experience of "reality" may be one among many. The child is coming to know that she has a mind of her own, in a world of her own that includes other people, who see the "same world" from a different perspective. A key feature here is that these all-important senses of there being an "objective reality," and other minds coexisting in that reality, are constituted in relationships, rather than being discovered. *In adequate development, then, the mentalization process involves the child seeing herself seen in the eyes (and mind) of someone who cares for her, at the same time that she sees that that person has a view of her that is not the same as her own sense of herself from the inside.* In tandem with this, she can share attention to other objects with such caregivers, coming to the complex experience that the same object is seen from different vantage points (Fonagy et al. 2002; Stern 1985). The child who can take on multiple perspectives can grasp how her own internal experience could be different from what someone else understands about her.

Early Developmental Failures, Projection, and Subsequent Psychopathology

Thinking reflectively and making meanings that make sense are thus a crucial aspect of feeling secure in the world and experiencing a sense of personal coherence. When such developments are impaired, basic psychopathology, especially character disorders, will likely ensue; such outcomes are commonly associated with early relationship trauma, especially abuse and neglect in infancy (Gabbard et al. 2008, among others). Other people cannot be relied on to provide the basic senses of personal security, organization, vitality, effectiveness, and self-worth, and the developing child is stranded in unmanageable mental and emotional states, such as fear, despair, detachment, listlessness, and impaired attention, and possibly impaired bodily coordination, especially because physiological, affective, and interpersonal regulation are so intertwined in infancy and early childhood. The unprotected, overwhelmed child must rely on adaptive strategies that are psychosocially and physiologically costly, at best; these include emotional and even physical numbness and other forms of disconnection and dissociation, hyperactivity and/or inhibition of activity, hypervigilance, withdrawal, indiscriminate affection for strangers and others, and dysregulated aggression, all amidst overall feelings of uncertainty and anxiety.

Under such stressful circumstances, projections often come to play a special role for children. Some stability is gained by imagining emotional threats as external, supporting the belief that they can be managed by flight, inattention, or altering external factors. Such relief, however, is often vulnerable and transient, as the distress recurs (albeit in an altered or even distorted form). At times, projections and other defenses break down, with the recurrence of overwhelming emotionally encoded memories and other related mental states that are prone to hyperarousal. Mentalization deficits are often linked to personal isolation and fear, labile self-organization and self-esteem, and a sense of emotional emptiness, along with pathological idealizations, contempt, and oscillations between these. In addition, an array of compensatory reactions may be observed, including acute and resentful disappointment, frenetic action, resentment, irritability, and even rage, and in problematic cases, other forms of coping such as substance abuse, patterns of unreliable relationships with frequent abandonment, and violence. (Socioeconomic and cultural stressors often exacerbate these tendencies, and should be taken into account in case formulation and intervention.)

Intergenerational Transmission of Trauma and Neglect: Parental Projections and Deficits

The parents of a child in an infant mental health case carry the influence of their own childhood with them into the current generation, in their roles as parents (Figure 20–1).

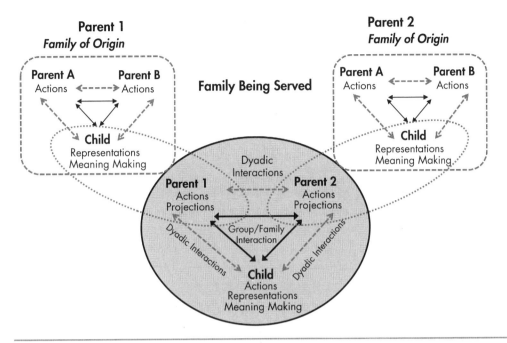

FIGURE 20–1. Influences on parenting through parental childhood representations from family of origin.

This figure shows how the parents of a child in an infant mental health case carry the influence of their own childhood with them into the current generation, in their roles as parents. Very schematically, the rectangular boxes ("Parent 1" and "Parent 2") show the history of the current parents' relationships with their parents ("Parent A" and "Parent B") as they are carried forward in their internal representations of their pasts. These then affect the current generation (*in the large ovals*) and are expressed with their own children through their own actions and ways of making meaning with their children, in both dyadic interactions and in the overall family interactions. *Source.* Adapted in part from Stern 1995.

Many infant mental health cases involve intergenerational transmission of trauma and neglect. The parents have themselves been cared for inadequately, were traumatized as children, or both, such that difficulties managing their own inner worlds impair their ability to care for their babies. Sometimes these problems are subtle, but often the presentation includes a more or less explicit projective repetition of early abuse. Other situations include patterns of chronic neglect, insufficient responsiveness, chaotic family life, and other manifestations of personal and family difficulty and psychosocial distress.

The first of two case vignettes illustrates a rather direct repetition in the moment-to-moment interaction of parent and infant.

> During the first meeting with an infant-parent therapist, Robert, an inner-city gang member who had been beaten as a young child, held his 3-day-old daughter, Hannah, just below her neck, forcefully bringing her face within an inch of his own with a frightened look that seemed to convey some tenderness along with fear. Next, he tried to force her to drink

from a bottle, while she desperately signaled that she was satiated by tensing up and keeping her mouth closed, and then going limp. Robert rebuffed both his wife's and the therapist's inquiries. As the baby seemed to collapse into a droopy, withdrawn state, he lifted her high in the air, saying, "That's enough of your garbage!" (See Seligman 1999 for an extensive discussion of projective identification and the intergenerational transmission of trauma.)

Selma Fraiberg et al. (1980) reported the following vignette, in which "the ghosts in the nursery" were projected onto the therapist.

Annie, the young mother of a 5-month-old boy, was beginning to open up to her psychotherapist in an infant-parent psychotherapy that had initially focused on her difficulty touching and holding her baby. In the sixth session, Annie began to describe her experiences of physical abuse at the hands of her father, and in the seventh, an even more painful meeting, she began to talk about her mother's abandoning her at age 5. After this, however, Annie was unavailable for 2 months of home-based sessions. Sometimes she was not there and sometimes she would not answer the door. The therapist believed that she herself had become a figure in Annie's transference such that, in Annie's mind, she was a potential abandoner. Annie was thus avoiding experiencing her more excruciating, emotionally overwhelming memories of the abuse and abandonment.

The Therapist's Experience

Even the most ordinary encounters with babies can produce especially strong reactions—both positive and negative—in therapists. These reactions are amplified when the infants are in distress, as in most treatment situations. Therapists are exposed to the same influence processes that are so essential to infant-parent communication—faces, body positions, gestures, rhythms, and other patterns of nonverbal interaction that are often awkward, jagged, and even tormenting—along with extended moments when the infant's cries for help and protection go unheard or are treated as an occasion for punishment and even revenge. Complex feelings about the parents themselves are common for therapists, especially when parents appear to be the source of their babies' agonies. The range of therapist reactions is very broad, including extremes of sympathy, frustration, blaming, and even hatred, with self-criticism, guilt, and other forms of self-doubt even more acute when interventions are not effective. Other professionals may evoke strong reactions, especially in the face of bureaucratic tangles, puzzling situations, or cultural, disciplinary, or other differences. Infant-parent work can be exhausting and provocative, and leave providers bewildered and depleted.

Sometimes, therapists have to choose between an array of apparently unsatisfactory and even torturous responses. Empathizing with the inner worlds of the parents (which may be similar to those of the babies), the therapist may be narrowly constrained in a confining matrix of intrapersonal experiences and interpersonal choices, such as coercion and abandonment, torture and neglect, abuser and abused, and the like. In the case of Annie, described in the previous section, the therapist realized that she could not avoid falling into one or another of the painful roles presented by Annie's enacted representations of her past—that is, abandoner or abusive intruder. Still, the therapist wrote Annie that she would feel compelled to report her to the child protective services agency if she would not meet with her. She was concerned that the transferences would engulf the infant-parent relationship, leaving the baby at profound risk. Although deeply upset by this "threat," Annie agreed to meet. The therapy then proceeded for 2½ years. Annie eventually recovered painful memories and became an adequate and even affectionate mother (Fraiberg et al. 1980).

Impact of the Professional's Own Personality and Professional Situation

Professionals of all disciplines bring their own backgrounds and personalities to their work. Although most professional training emphasizes technical and goal-directed dimensions, every intervention relies on the collaborative relationship between the family members, the individual providers, and the various organizations involved (Seligman 1994; Seligman and Pawl 1984). A great deal goes on beyond each discipline's specific focus, whether it is psychopharmacology, developmental pediatrics, or parenting education, among others. These crucial dynamics are largely unconscious and prereflective. All of this is further complicated by therapists' own personalities, personal histories, sociocultural stances, attitudes about professional roles, and the like. For example, one psychotherapist may feel put off or disorganized by an angry client, whereas another might welcome this anger as a sign of renewed emotional contact. Such differences might be influenced by the therapist's own personal experiences of aggression and interpersonal protest as a child, in current intimate relationships, or in the work milieu (say, if aggression was typically coupled with warmth and support in the second therapist's family of origin). Specific circumstances may evoke parallel reactions in professionals; in one case of sexual abuse, a therapist recalled her own uncle's inappropriate erotic attention. Cultural and disciplinary factors are similarly evocative.

Tolerating and Using Emotional Reactions in Service of Therapeutic Goals

Emotional reactions are inevitable in therapy and should not be viewed as undesirable. Instead, they should prompt some important questions: How are these reactions helping or hindering the therapeutic task at hand? What can be learned from them? When care providers and their organizations sustain an atmosphere of open discussion and acceptant attention to these reactions, both clients and providers will benefit. Increasingly, best practice standards in the infant intervention field include "reflective practice," so as to provide nonjudgmental, mutual support and introspection at every level of a service organization. Mental health workers often have special expertise in this area, which can be offered reflectively and tactfully to other professionals, when appropriate.

For example, when a resilient and resourceful social worker knocked on the door of a client's apartment for an initial appointment in a tough housing project, she was met with a long silence. When a gruff female voice finally said, "Who the hell are you?" the social worker felt angry, self-doubting, and even inferior. But the therapist realized that the mother's insult showed how bruised the mother felt by all that was happening to her now and in the past, an instance of "identification with the aggressor" (Freud 1936/1966), where inner emotional distress is inflicted on others. With this in mind, the therapist said, through the door, "You seem ready to fight. You must feel pushed around." Using a combination of explicit thinking, intuition, and self-observation, she crafted an empathic intervention that started things off on the right foot.

Therapists' self-reflective efforts can thus transform negative reactions into explicit formulations and more effective and empathic responses. For example, a therapist who finds herself feeling irritated with a mother's rough handling of her baby might say, "Maybe you feel that it's just too hard to get your baby to understand what will make her feel better." Reorienting one's own reactions into emotionally evocative information can often have especially positive effects.

Contemporary Psychodynamic Models and Infant Mental Health Work

Contemporary psychoanalytic clinical theory emphasizes such transference-countertransference dynamics. From the contemporary Bionian-Kleinian perspective, for example, the analyst's first task is to "contain" what the patient cannot bear, leading over time to the prospect of greater understanding and personal growth. Relational and interpersonal analysts see the transference-countertransference field as a "playground" for reworking the wounds of the past. Developmentally oriented therapists draw even closer analogies to the infant-parent relationship, seeing the therapeutic relationship as potentiating new experiences that can enhance affect regulation, reflective functioning, and other adaptations.

These formulations also add new dimensions to the classical approach, in which the analyst interprets the repetition of the past in the problematic maneuvers of the present. The original models of infant-parent psychotherapy featured this, although Fraiberg's (1980) interest in direct support and "nondidactic developmental guidance" also highlighted the direct effects of the new intervention relationships. In "updating" the Fraiberg model in light of work with unconventional populations and the new emphasis on relationship dynamics and transactional processes, I wrote,

> The...supportive therapeutic relationship...can...disrupt the influence of prior relationships ...by providing a contrast to the parent's more problematic expectations.... The therapeutic relationship...is in continuous and simultaneous interaction with the actual current relationships...as well as with the parents' internal representations of prior relationships. It may be useful to conceptualize all interventions in the context of a triad of relationships—those between the therapist and the parent, the intervenors and the infant, and the infant and the parent, all...substantially determined by the parents' conscious and unconscious defenses, wishes, and internal representations of earlier relationships. (Seligman 1994, pp. 485–486)

Recognition Process and the Emergence of Developmental Potentials

Louis Sander (2008), in his seminal perspective, describes the central role of the "recognition process" in the development of effective, flexible, and inclusive adaptive life patterns. Following biological systems theory, Sander sees recognition as a basic element of life processes at many levels of how organisms function, from such small-scale processes as cells "recognizing" one another to form tissues, to such large-scale forms as international commerce. Infant-parent interactions and therapist-caregiver interactions might be thought of as somewhere in the middle of this scale. Elaborating this, Sander (2008) wrote,

> The idea of recognition as a process provides a bridge over which the increasing complexity and diversity in the development of different systems can be integrated with biologic processes, and both with the developing organization of infant consciousness, to provide continuity in the necessary specificity of connection that is essential for the construction of coherence in systems as they gain increasing inclusiveness.... I was beginning an interview with one of our new mothers some weeks after the delivery of her first baby. Things seemed not to be going too well. The mother, unsure of herself with the baby, felt that she was not doing the right thing, that the baby was not eating as well as it should, that it seemed fussy and was difficult to quiet, and that she just didn't know how to manage it.
>
> As we sat down in the interviewing room, I had taken the baby from her to hold, and, as we were talking, I had placed him supine on my lap where I could make visual contact with him as the interview proceeded. After a few minutes of my glancing at the baby's eyes, the baby's eyes suddenly met mine. At this instant the baby kicked out with his legs, threw out his arms, and broke into a wide and engaging smile. The mother gasped in astonishment: "He can see!" she exclaimed. "Oh, yes," I said, "indeed he can see." "Oh," she replied with an excited tone. "Now I know he will know who is being good to him!"
>
> The mother now realized that she was known by her infant, and, sure enough, at the next visit she and the infant had their act together. The difficulties had vanished, and things were going well. Here was specificity at two levels: a level of simplicity—the meeting of my eyes, the eyes of a perfect stranger, with the eyes of the infant; and a level of complexity—the specific meaning to the mother of being seen by her infant as being "known" by him. The experience of knowing herself as mother could come together with the specificity of her infant's behavior in a new coherence of relationship. I am suggesting how the subtleties of the experience of being "known" by a significant "other" describe a moment of recognition and how the experiencing of such moments provides an organizing principle in the developmental process. (pp. 33–34)

Sander's (2008) fundamental formulations integrate basic biology, neuroscience, psychoanalysis, and infant development research. The overall theme here (and, indeed, throughout this chapter) is that reciprocal contact between people can lead to new syntheses of previously unavailable and unexperienced potentials. Overall, therapists' flexible, attentive responsiveness is essential to all interventions, the "platform" from which specific techniques can be effective. There are basic parallels between the conditions that facilitate child development and therapeutic progress.

Thinking Transactionally in Infant Mental Health Work

Therapeutic efforts, from whatever discipline, must be understood as interventions into complex relationship systems within which the infant's care is being provided, the course of which is affected by multiple factors in dynamic flux, whose patterns and outcomes fluctuate as social, economic, and physical conditions change over time, especially when the infant is growing so rapidly. The birth of a child is a world-changing event and shifts relationships with nuclear and extended family members, jobs, friends, the physical living space, neighborhoods, the family's economic situation, and so on. Simultaneously, the new baby evokes powerful internal representations, fantasies, and longings to an extent almost unparalleled in the life cycle. Parents often find themselves with special potentials to grow psychologically but also face substantial pitfalls of repeating old, counterproductive, and even traumatic patterns of behavior and feeling. Early childhood is thus a time of both great opportunities and risks. Sometimes small interventions will be amplified by the evolving developmental systems so as to have great effects, whereas at other times the destructive momenta overwhelm whatever skills and good intentions are brought to bear. In general, the effects of specific interventions are hard to predict, especially because the various factors and forces can amplify and/or dampen their effects.

Infant intervention theory proposes that there are multiple "ports of entry" in most cases: the internal world of the parents, the details of the infant-parent interactions, family dynamics, the broader social surround, non–mental health services supporting the family, and so on. In the complex, nonlinear dynamics of infant development, these apparently distinct strands are intertwined; interventions into one are likely to have effects throughout the others. Each can shift the emerging developmental system, and potentiate changes in other dimensions and overall. Multiple interventions and therapeutic actions may often be synergistic, with the aggregate effects greater than the effects of each. In any case, a working alliance with the family will be essential to any effort to enhance the child's development (Seligman and Pawl 1984).

KEY POINTS

- The relationship between infant and parents is the fundamental unit for early development, and the creation and maintenance of ties to other people are central motivations. Through evolving sequences of signals and responses, infants and caregivers continually influence and regulate one another's internal states and behaviors. These early interaction patterns exert an influence into adulthood.

- Early neglect, trauma, and maltreatment have long-term pathogenic effects, including effects on brain dysfunction and related psychosocial difficulties.

- Problems in infant emotional development often involve parents' difficulties managing their own inner worlds, difficulties that impair their ability to care for

their babies. Parental psychopathology and psychosocial strains are often implicated. Many parents have suffered from a range of inadequate emotional care,
chaotic family life, maltreatment, and childhood trauma of varying severity. These
individuals' parenting difficulties can range from explicit repetition of early abuse
to quite subtle distortions and deficits in parenting.

- Professionals of all disciplines bring their own backgrounds and personalities to
their work. Although most professional training emphasizes technical and goal-
directed dimensions, every intervention also relies on the collaborative relationship between the family members, the individual providers, and the various organizations involved.

- Early childhood is a time of both great opportunities and risks. Sometimes, small
interventions will be amplified by the evolving developmental systems so as to
have great effects. At other times, the destructive momenta overwhelm whatever skills and good intentions are brought to bear. In general, the effects of specific interventions are hard to predict, especially as the various factors and forces
can amplify and/or dampen their effects.

References

Ainsworth M, Blehar M, Waters E, et al: Patterns of Attachment: A Psychological Study of the Strange Situation. Hillsdale, NJ, Erlbaum, 1978

Beebe B, Jaffe J, Lachmann F: A dyadic systems view of communication, in Relational Perspectives in Psychoanalysis. Edited by Skolnick N, Warshaw S. Hillsdale, NJ, Analytic Press, 1993, pp 61–81

Beebe B, Jaffe J, Markese S, et al: The origins of 12-month attachment: a microanalysis of 4-month mother-infant interaction. Attach Hum Dev 12:3–141, 2010

Bowlby J: Attachment and Loss, Vol 1: Attachment. (1969). New York, Basic Books, 1982

Bowlby J: A Secure Base: Parent-Child Attachment and Healthy Human Development. New York, Basic Books, 1988

Fonagy P, Bateman A: Mentalization-based treatment of borderline personality disorder, in Mind to Mind: Infant Research, Neuroscience, and Psychoanalysis. Edited by Jurist EL, Slade A, Bergner S. New York, Other Press, 2008, pp 139–166

Fonagy P, Gergely G, Jurist E, et al: Affect Regulation, Mentalization, and the Development of the Self. New York, Other Press, 2002

Fraiberg S (ed): Clinical Studies in Infant Mental Health: The First Year of Life. New York, Basic Books, 1980

Freud A: The Ego and the Mechanisms of Defense (1936). New York, International Universities Press, 1946

Gabbard G, Miller L, Martinez M: A neurobiological perspective on mentalizing and internal object relations in traumatized borderline patients, in Mind to Mind: Infant Research, Neuroscience, and Psychoanalysis. Edited by Jurist EL, Slade A, Bergner S. New York, Other Press, 2008, pp 204–224

Grigsby J, Schneiders JL: Neuroscience, modularity and personality theory: conceptual foundations of a model of complex human functioning. Psychiatry 54:21–38, 1991

Hesse E, Main M: Disorganized infant, child & adult attachment. J Am Psychoanal Assoc 48(4):1097–1127, 2000

Hollander E, Berlin HA: Neuropsychiatric aspects of aggression and impulse-control disorders, in The American Psychiatric Publishing Textbook of Neuropsychiatry and Behavioral Neurosciences, 5th Edition. Edited by Yudofsky SC, Hales RE. Washington, DC, American Psychiatric Publishing, 2008, pp 535–565

Lyons-Ruth K: Implicit relational knowing: its role in development and psychoanalytic treatment. Infant Ment Health J 19:282–289, 1998

Main M: The organized categories of infant, child, and adult attachment: flexible vs. inflexible attention under attachment-related stress. J Am Psychoanal Assoc 48:1055–1099, 2000

Main M, Solomon J: Procedures for identifying infants as disorganized/disoriented during the Ainsworth Strange Situation, in Attachment in the Preschool Years: Theory, Research, and Intervention. Edited by Greenberg MT, Cicchetti D, Cummings EM. Chicago, IL, University of Chicago Press, 1990, pp 121–160

Main M, Hesse E, Kaplan N: Predictability of attachment behavior and representational processes at 1, 6, and 19 years of age: the Berkeley Longitudinal Study, in Attachment From Infancy to Adulthood: The Major Longitudinal Studies. Edited by Grossmann KE, Grossmann K, Waters E. New York, Guilford, 2005, pp 121–160

Sameroff AJ, Emde RN: Relationship Disturbances in Early Childhood: A Developmental Approach. New York, Basic Books, 1989

Sander L: Living Systems, Evolving Consciousness, and the Emerging Person: A Selection of Papers From the Life Work of Louis Sander. Edited by Amadei G, Bianchi I. New York, Analytic Press, 2008

Schore AN: Affect Dysregulation and Disorders of the Self. New York, WW Norton, 2003

Seligman S: Applying psychoanalysis in an unconventional context: adapting infant-parent psychotherapy to a changing population. Psychoanal Study Child 49:481–500, 1994

Seligman S: Integrating Kleinian theory and intersubjective infant research: observing projective identification. Psychoanal Dialogues 9:129–159, 1999

Seligman S: Dynamic systems theories as a metaframework for psychoanalysis. Psychoanal Dialogues 15:285–319, 2005

Seligman S: The baby out of the bathwater: microseconds, psychic structure, and psychotherapy. Psychoanal Dialogues 22:499–509, 2012

Seligman S, Pawl J: Impediments to the formation of the working alliance in infant-parent psychotherapy, in Frontiers of Infant Psychiatry, Vol 2. Edited by Call JD, Galenson E, Tyson R. New York, Basic Books, 1984, pp 232–237

Stern DN: The First Relationship: Infant and Mother. Cambridge, MA, Harvard University Press, 1977

Stern DN: The Interpersonal World of the Human Infant. New York, Basic Books, 1985

Stern DN: The Motherhood Constellation: A Unified View of Parent-Infant Psychotherapy. New York, Basic Books, 1995, p 31

Trevarthen C: The intersubjective psychobiology of human meaning: learning of culture depends on interest for co-operative practical work—and affection for the joyful art of good company. Psychoanal Dialogues 19:507–518, 2009

Tronick E: The Neurobehavioral and Social-Emotional Development of Infants and Children. New York, WW Norton, 2007

Winnicott DW: Playing and Reality. London, Tavistock, 1971

Index

Page numbers printed **in boldface** type refer to tables or figures.

Appendix 2-1

Excerpts of Initial Report for Suzy[1]

---

[1] For full report, see http://test.childtrauma.org/Appendix_BDP_2012_redact.pdf.

Neurosequential Model of Therapeutics : Clinical Practice Tools

A Brief Introduction:

The Neurosequential Model of Therapeutics (NMT) is an approach to clinical work that incorporates key principles of neurodevelopment into the clinical problem-solving process. The NMT Metrics are tools which provide a semi-structured assessment of important developmental experiences, good and bad, and a current "picture" of brain organization and functioning. From these tools estimates of relative brain-mediated strengths and weaknesses can be derived. This information can aid the clinician in the ongoing therapeutic process.

The results from the NMT Metrics should not be viewed as a stand-alone psychological, neuropsychological, psychiatric or psychoeducational evaluation. These reports are intended to supplement the clinical problem solving process and provide broad direction for the selection and sequencing of developmentally appropriate enrichment, therapeutic and educational activities.

Client Data

Client: SuzySample
Age: 4 years, 1 month
Gender: Female
Case ID: CTA_Teach

Report Data

Clinician: Bruce Perry
Report Date: 8/28/2012
Time: 1
Site: CTA_Teach

Developmental History

A brief introduction

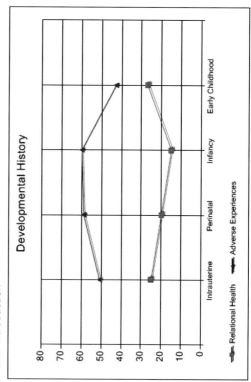

Developmental History

Developmental History Values

	Adverse Events	Relational Health	Developmental Risk
Intrauterine	51	25	26
Perinatal	59	20	39
Infancy	60	15	45
Early Childhood	43	27	16

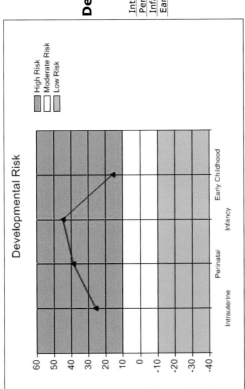

Developmental Risk

High Risk
Moderate Risk
Low Risk

Intrauterine   Perinatal   Infancy   Early Childhood

Adverse Experience Confidence: Moderate
Relational Health Confidence: Moderate

Plate 2   *Appendix 2–1: Excerpts of Initial Report for Suzy*

Current CNS Functionality

	Brainstem	Client	Typical
1	Cardiovascular/ANS	4	11
2	Autonomic Regulation	6	12
3	Temperature regulation/Metabolism	6	12
4	Extraocular Eye Movements	8	12
5	Suck/Swallow/Gag	6	11
6	Attention/Tracking	3	10

	DE/Cerebellum		
7	Feeding/Appetite	4	10
8	Sleep	3	10
9	Fine Motor Skills	5	8
10	Coordination/Large Motor Functioning	4	7
11	Dissociative Continuum	2	9
12	Arousal Continuum	3	9
13	Neuroendocrine/Hypothalamic	6	10
14	Primary Sensory Integration	4	9

	Limbic		
15	Reward	4	10
16	Affect Regulation/Mood	3	9
17	Attunement/Empathy	2	9
18	Psychosexual	5	7
19	Relational/Attachment	3	7
20	Short-term memory/Learning	6	9

	Cortex		
21	Somato/Motorsensory Integration	5	8
22	Sense Time/Delay Gratification	2	6
23	Communication Expressive/Receptive	5	9
24	Self Awareness/Self Image	4	6
25	Speech/Articulation	4	8
26	Concrete Cognition	4	7

	Frontal Cortex		
27	Non-verbal Cognition	5	6
28	Modulate Reactivity/Impulsivity	2	6
29	Math/Symbolic Cognition	1	6
30	Reading/Verbal	1	6
31	Abstract/Reflective Cognition	2	6
32	Values/Beliefs/Morality	2	6
	Total	**124**	**271**

Current CNS Confidence Level: Moderate

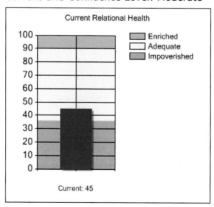

Current Relational Health Confidence Level: Moderate

Functional Brain Map(s) and Key

Client (4 years, 1 month)   Report Date: 8/28/2012

2	1	5	2	1	2
4	5	5	2	4	4
3	2	4	3	5	6
	6	2	3	4	
	5	4	3	4	
		6	3		
		6	8		
		4	6		

Age Typical - 4 to 5

6	6	6	6	6	6
8	9	8	6	6	7
7	9	10	9	7	9
	10	9	9	9	
	8	10	10	7	
		11	10		
		12	12		
		11	12		

Functional Item Key

ABST (31)	MATH (29)	PERF (27)	MOD (28)	VERB (30)	VAL (32)
SPEECH (25)	COMM (23)	SSI (21)	TIME (22)	SELF (24)	CCOG (26)
REL (19)	ATTU (17)	REW (15)	AFF (16)	SEX (18)	MEM (20)
	NE (13)	DISS (11)	ARS (12)	PSI (14)	
	FMS (9)	FEED (7)	SLP (8)	LMF (10)	
		SSG (5)	ATTN (6)		
		MET (3)	EEOM (4)		
		CV (1)	ANS (2)		

Functional Brain Map Value Key

DEVELOPMENTAL
Functional

12	DEVELOPED
11	TYPICAL RANGE
10	
9	EPISODIC/EMERGING
8	MILD Compromise
7	
6	PRECURSOR CAPACITY
5	MODERATE Dysfunction
4	
3	UNDEVELOPED
2	SEVERE Dysfunction
1	

Functional Domains Values

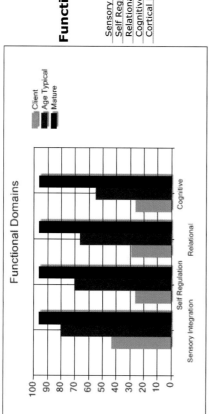

Functional Domains

	Client Age	Age Typical	Mature	% Age Typical
Sensory Integration	43	80	96	53.75
Self Regulation	26	70	96	37.14
Relational	29	66	96	43.94
Cognitive	26	55	96	47.27
Cortical Modulation Ratio	0.42	2.42	49	17.35

General Summary

Recommendations are based upon data provided by the clinician when completing the NMT online metrics. Based upon the data provided, cut off scores are used to indicate whether activities in each of the 4 areas are considered essential, therapeutic or enrichment. Activities selected for each category should be age appropriate, positive and provided in the context of nurturing, safe relationships.

Essential refers to those activities that are crucial to the child's future growth in this particular area. In order to fall into the essential category the child's score must be below 65% of the age typical score. It is our belief that unless functioning in the essential area is increased the child will lack the foundation for future growth and development in this and other areas.

Therapeutic refers to those activities aimed at building in strength and growth in the particular area. Scores that fall within 65 to 85 percent of those typical for the child's age are considered appropriate for more focused treatment. Therapeutic activities are viewed as important for the child's continued growth and improvement in the area.

Enrichment refers to activities that provide positive, valuable experiences that continue to build capacity in the given area. Children who fall into the enrichment category are at or above 85 percent of age typical functioning. Activities recommended in this category are designed to enhance and reinforce strengths previously built into the particular area of focus.

The information below is designed to provide the clinician with broad recommendations based upon the NMT approach. These recommendations should be used as guidelines for the treating clinician when considering particular therapeutic activities. Final treatment decisions must be based upon the clinical judgement of the treatment provider. The CTA cannot be held responsible for any of the treatment decisions made by the clinician based upon their own interpretation of NMT principles or recommendations.

Sensory Integration

Client Score: 43   Age Typical: 80   Percentage: 53.75

Essential: (below 65%) – Scores below 65% of age typical functioning indicate poorly organized somatosensory systems in the brain. The introduction of patterned, repetitive somatosensory activities weaved throughout the day have been shown to lead to positive improvements. These activities should be provided multiple times each day for approximately 7-8 minutes at a time for essential reorganization to occur. Examples of somatosensory activities include massage (pressure point, Reiki touch), music, movement (swimming, walking/running, jumping, swinging, rocking), yoga/breathing and animal assisted therapy that includes patterned, repetitive activities such as grooming.

Self Regulation

Client Score: 26   Age Typical: 70   Percentage: 37.14

Essential: (below 65%) – Scores below 65% of age typical functioning suggest the child has poor self-regulatory capabilities. These children may have stress response systems that are poorly organized and hyper-reactive. They are likely impulsive, have difficulties transitioning from one activity to another, and may overreact to even minor stressors or challenges. Children in this category require structure and predictability provided consistently by safe, nurturing adults across settings. Examples of essential activities in this category include: developing transitioning activity (using a song, words or other cues to help prepare the child for the change in activity), patterned, repetitive proprioceptive OT activities such as isometric exercises (chair push-ups, bear hugs while child tries to pull the adult's arms away, applying deep pressure), using weighted vests, blankets, ankle weights, various deep breathing techniques, building structure into bedtime rituals, music and movement activities, animal assisted therapy and EMDR.

Relational

Client Score: 29   Age Typical: 66   Percentage: 43.94

Essential: (below 65%) - Scores below 65% of age typical functioning suggest the child has poor relational functioning. Children who have a history of disrupted early caregiving, whose earliest experiences were characterized as chaotic, neglectful, and/or unpredictable, often have difficulties forming and maintaining relationships. In order to make sufficient gains in relational functioning, essential activities must include interactions with multiple positive healthy adults who are invested in the child's life and in their treatment. Examples of essential relational activities include: art therapy, individual play therapy, Parent Child Interaction Therapy (PCIT), dyadic parallel play with an adult, and when mastered, dyadic parallel play with a peer. Once dyadic relationships have been mastered supervised small group activities may be added. Other examples of essential activities include animal assisted therapy and targeted psychotherapy.

Cognitive

Client Score: 26   Age Typical: 55   Percentage: 47.27

Essential: (below 65%) - Scores below 65% of age typical functioning suggest the child has poor cognitive functioning. As in other areas of focus, essential cognitive activities must take place in the context of safe, nurturing relationships with invested adults. It is in the context of safe, relationally enriched environments that essential healing and growth can occur. Examples of essential cognitive activities include: speech and language therapy, insight oriented psychodynamic treatment, cognitive behavioral therapy, and family therapy.

Cortical Modulation refers to the capacity of important cortical networks to regulate and modulate the activity and reactivity of some of the lower neural systems. As the brain organizes and matures, this capacity increases and the Cortical Modulation Ratio (CMR) increases. The CMR reflects both cortical "strength" and over-reactivity in lower neural systems involved in the stress response. Any Cortical Modulation Ratio below 1.0 suggests that the individual has minimal capacity to self-regulate. Ratios between 1.0 and 2.0 indicate emerging but episodic self-regulation capacity. This item can prove useful when determining whether a client is "ready" to benefit from traditional cognitive interventions.

Appendix 2–2

Initial Recommendations for Suzy

Plate 5 *Appendix 2–2: Initial Recommendations for Suzy*

Initial Recommendations: Therapeutic Web

A central element of NMT recommendations includes recognition of the importance of the therapeutic, educational and enrichment opportunities provided in the broader community, especially school. In this section, samples of the sites, activities and relational opportunities that may be important in helping a child heal are listed. These sample listings may be helpful as the clinical team creates its reports and recommendations.

School/Childcare	Rating	Action	Notes
Psychoeducation	Essential	Discuss S. with school staff and provide ongoing consultation	key areas to cover: 1. State dependent functioning, 2. Relational sensitivity and the intimacy barrier, 3. reassurance re: pros/cons psychopharmacology
Special modifications	Essential	ignore traditional structure to day and minimize transitions	use in room aide as primary relational anchor
In-room aide	Therapeutic	select one primary aide	remember present, parallel, patient and positive
Create somatosensory nest and opportunities	Therapeutic	depending upon OT eval, enrich OT/SS activities	pending report, however provide opportunities for motor vestibular and somatosensory exploration and regulation times
Extracurricular	Rating	Action	Notes
DEFER extracurricular at this time	Enriching	At present defer any extra transitions or out of home or school activities	S. is not yet able to manage this level of transition and novelty
Culture/Community of Faith	Rating	Action	Notes
Psychoeducation	Essential	provide psychoeducation to anticipate future engagement	At some point, Family will include S. in church and church-related activities; essential to prepare them to create gradual and positive transitions
Other	Rating	Action	Notes
DEFER additional relational complexity at this time	Essential	do not yet add complexity to S. life	help family understand the need for "simple" relational environment for S. right now. Ultimately all of these enriching activities can be added

Initial Recommendations: Family

The family is often the key to the therapeutic approach. In many cases, the parent's history will mirror the child's developmental history if chaos, threat, trauma or neglect is involved. Transgenerational aspects of vulnerability and strength in a family play important roles in the child's educational, enrichment and therapeutic experiences. When the caregivers and parents are healthy and strong, their capacity to be present, patient, positive and nurturing is enhanced and maintained. When the parent's needs are unmet it is unrealistic to ask them to play a central role in the child's healing process.

Mother/Female	Rating	Action	Notes
Psychoeducation	Essential	Go over NMT metrics and recommendations	focus on the "Rs" - developmentally relevant, rewarding, repetitive, rhythmic, relational, respectful
Respite	Essential	FM needs to create a regulatory map for herself	self care plan with opportunity to work and 'play' is essential - as is finding time for FM and FF to be alone
Physical hygiene	Therapeutic	FM needs to develop self-care plan	exercise, sleep, nutrition all essential to keep FM 'in the game'
Social Supports	Therapeutic	FM needs to resume her social activities	FM quit many of her activities when S. came and was so demanding. She needs to understand the importance of relational supports for herself
Father/Male	**Rating**	**Action**	**Notes**
Psychoeducation	Essential	As with FM, meet and go over recommendations	FF is likely harder sell but suspect he will be helped by NMT Map
Physical hygiene	Therapeutic	As with FM, same core recommendations	As FM above, Respite, self-care plan, focus on need for sleep, exercise and relational supports
Siblings	**Rating**	**Action**	**Notes**
Psychoeducation	Therapeutic	have family meeting to review impressions	Sibs can be great source of positive interactions for S. If they understand her, they will be more empathic, patient and positive.
Extended Family	**Rating**	**Action**	**Notes**
Engage and recruit	Therapeutic	try to get FF and FM extended family to help with respite and social support	there are multiple older cousins, aunties and uncles in the community who can be a positive presence for S.
Psychoeducation	Enriching	Hold large family meeting to share impressions and answer questions	find dates to hold meeting from FM

Initial Recommendations: Individual

The selection and timing of various enrichment, educational and therapeutic experiences should be guided by the developmental capabilities and vulnerabilities of the child. This listing suggests some, but not all, activities that can help the clinician select various activities and experiences that can provide patterned, repetitive and rewarding experiences as recommended by the NMT Metric. As the clinical team prepares final recommendations, use this listing (and related activities) to help create therapeutic experiences that are sensitive to developmental status in various domains, and to state regulation capacity.

Sensory Integration	Rating	Action	Notes
Healing touch/massage	Essential	refer to KB for therapeutic massage	KB to teach FM several simple techniques to be used during transition; focus on pattern - 4 to 5 minutes, multiple times/day
Primary somatosensory	Therapeutic	create SS schedule - and try to find S.'s preferences	use NMT Somatosensory mapping tool to figure out the timing
Rocking/Swing	Therapeutic	continue with rocking - but build in schedule	do not let S use rocking to "stay" in comfort zone. Slowly transition to scheduled and predictable rocking patterns during the day
Transitional plan to return to pre-school	Essential	pre-school is too overwhelming at this point	keep at home; and work with us to create a gradual transition plan with somatosensory regulatory "bridges" to help with transitions; after one or two months begin slow transitions to expose to PK - then add 15 min at PK etc.
Modify medications	Therapeutic	taper Risperdal and Ritalin off	no evidence that these are effective in this age-range with this set of problems. Slowly taper these off and closely observe for any behavioral effects.
Self Regulation	Rating	Action	Notes
OT directed activities	Essential	need sensory profile from OT assessment	schedule OT eval
Sleep hygiene	Therapeutic	build in sleep rituals	again - focus on slow and gradual transitions away from FM bed (X work on plan with FM)
Walk, run, exercise	Therapeutic	begin scheduled walks around the yard	as tolerated start to venture out of yard; parallel with FM, hand in hand; as tolerated, let her explore (do this at least 15 min 3x/day)
Music-◻ movement	Therapeutic	let her use the headphones to listen to music	rather than trying to leverage this as reward or punishment view this as an important regulatory tool
Relational regulatory time	Therapeutic	continue to allow FM to be the relational anchor for her	over time sibs and FF wil be able to do this as well - but for now let FM be the primary relational regulator

Relational	Rating	Action	Notes
Parallel play - dyadic adult	Therapeutic	use FM as above and as tolerated, introduce others	S is very relationally 'sensitive' - for her, intimacy is an evocative cue - as is "abandonment" - so she is sensitized to both relational interactions that are intimate and perceived rejection - remember - present, attentive, attuned and responsive - and stay parallel - don't expect words to do too much
Psychotherapy (specify)	Enriching	not sure individual Tx is yet likely to be helpful	use therapeutic time to support and guide FM and school - at a later point, S will be ready for a therapeutic relationship - too dysregulated now to do much effective work
DO NOT push peer interactions	Essential	DO NOT overload S with peer relationships yet	S is not ready for dyadic relationships yet. This will come - remember she is more like an infant in this regard.
Cognitive	Rating	Action	Notes
Speech and Language Tx	Enriching	Needs S/L eval (but not yet)	S is too dysregulated to tolerate either an S/L evaluation or Tx
BE PATIENT about cognitive development	Essential	Do not expect too much from traditional cognitive interactions yet	S. is so dysregulated that she will not be able to either express her current cognitive capabilities nor easily internalize new cognitive experiences. Work on SS/SR domains - and the cognitive needs and strengths can be identified and addressed at a later point in the treatment process.

Appendix 2-3

Reevaluation Report for Suzy

Neurosequential Model of Therapeutics : Clinical Practice Tools

A Brief Introduction:

The Neurosequential Model of Therapeutics (NMT) is an approach to clinical work that incorporates key principles of neurodevelopment into the clinical problem-solving process. The NMT Metrics are tools which provide a semi-structured assessment of important developmental experiences, good and bad, and a current "picture" of brain organization and functioning. From these tools estimates of relative brain-mediated strengths and weaknesses can be derived. This information can aid the clinician in the ongoing therapeutic process.

The results from the NMT Metrics should not be viewed as a stand-alone psychological, neuropsychological, psychiatric or psychoeducational evaluation. These reports are intended to supplement the clinical problem solving process and provide broad direction for the selection and sequencing of developmentally appropriate enrichment, therapeutic and educational activities.

Client Data

Client: SuzySample
Age: 5 years, 5 months
Gender: Female

Report Data

Current Clinician: Bruce Perry
Report Date: Redacted

Developmental History

A brief introduction

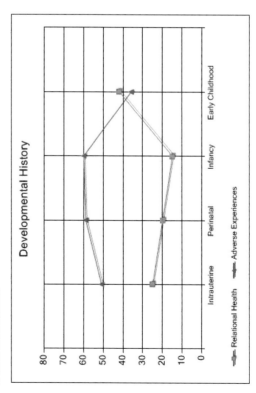

Developmental History Values

	Adverse Events	Relational Health	Developmental Risk
Intrauterine	51	25	26
Perinatal	59	20	39
Infancy	60	15	45
Early Childhood	36	42	–6

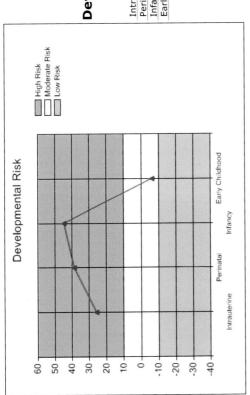

Developmental Risk

High Risk
Moderate Risk
Low Risk

Intrauterine Perinatal Infancy Early Childhood

Adverse Experience Confidence: Moderate
Relational Health Confidence: Moderate

Plate 9 *Appendix 2–3: Reevaluation Report for Suzy*

Current CNS Functionality

	Brainstem	Time 1	Current	Typical
1	Cardiovascular/ANS	4	7	11
2	Autonomic Regulation	6	7	12
3	Temperature regulation/Metabolism	6	7	12
4	Extraocular Eye Movements	8	8	12
5	Suck/Swallow/Gag	6	6	11
6	Attention/Tracking	3	6	10

	DE/Cerebellum			
7	Feeding/Appetite	4	6	10
8	Sleep	3	6	10
9	Fine Motor Skills	5	6	8
10	Coordination/Large Motor Functioning	4	5	7
11	Dissociative Continuum	2	6	9
12	Arousal Continuum	3	5	9
13	Neuroendocrine/Hypothalamic	6	6	10
14	Primary Sensory Integration	4	6	9

	Limbic			
15	Reward	4	6	10
16	Affect Regulation/Mood	3	6	9
17	Attunement/Empathy	2	6	9
18	Psychosexual	5	6	7
19	Relational/Attachment	3	5	7
20	Short-term memory/Learning	6	7	9

	Cortex			
21	Somato/Motorsensory Integration	5	6	8
22	Sense Time/Delay Gratification	2	4	6
23	Communication Expressive/Receptive	5	6	9
24	Self Awareness/Self Image	4	5	6
25	Speech/Articulation	4	4	8
26	Concrete Cognition	4	5	7

	Frontal Cortex			
27	Non-verbal Cognition	5	5	6
28	Modulate Reactivity/Impulsivity	2	4	6
29	Math/Symbolic Cognition	1	3	6
30	Reading/Verbal	1	4	6
31	Abstract/Reflective Cognition	2	4	6
32	Values/Beliefs/Morality	2	4	6
	Total	**124**	**177**	**271**

Client (5 years, 5 months) Report Date: 8/31/2012

4	3	5	4	4	4
4	6	6	4	5	5
5	6	6	6	6	7
	6	6	5	6	
	6	6	6	5	
		6	6		
		7	8		
		7	7		

Age Typical - 4 to 5

6	6	6	6	6	6
8	9	8	6	6	7
7	9	10	9	7	9
	10	9	9	9	
	8	10	10	7	
		11	10		
		12	12		
		11	12		

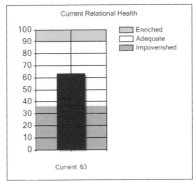

Current Relational Health

- Enriched
- Adequate
- Impoverished

Current: 63

Functional Item Key

ABST (31)	MATH (29)	PERF (27)	MOD (28)	VERB (30)	VAL (32)
SPEECH (25)	COMM (23)	SSI (21)	TIME (22)	SELF (24)	CCOG (26)
REL (19)	ATTU (17)	REW (15)	AFF (16)	SEX (18)	MEM (20)
	NE (13)	DISS (11)	ARS (12)	PSI (14)	
	FMS (9)	FEED (7)	SLP (8)	LMF (10)	
		SSG (5)	ATTN (6)		
		MET (3)	EEOM (4)		
		CV (1)	ANS (2)		

Functional Brain Map Value Key

DEVELOPMENTAL

Functional

12	DEVELOPED
11	TYPICAL RANGE
10	
9	EPISODIC/EMERGING
8	MILD Compromise
7	
6	PRECURSOR CAPACITY
5	MODERATE Dysfunction
4	
3	UNDEVELOPED
2	SEVERE Dysfunction
1	

Client (4 years, 1 month)   **Report Date: 8/28/2012**

2	1	5	2	1	2
4	5	5	2	4	4
3	2	4	3	5	6
	6	2	3	4	
	5	4	3	4	
		6	3		
		6	8		
		4	6		

Age Typical - 4 to 5

6	6	6	6	6	6
8	9	8	6	6	7
7	9	10	9	7	9
	10	9	9	9	
	8	10	10	7	
		11	10		
		12	12		
		11	12		

Current Functional Domains Values

	Client Age	Age Typical	Mature	% Age Typical
Sensory Integration	51	80	96	63.75
Self Regulation	44	70	96	62.86
Relational	44	66	96	66.67
Cognitive	38	55	96	69.09
Cortical Modulation Ratio	0.78	2.42	49	32.27

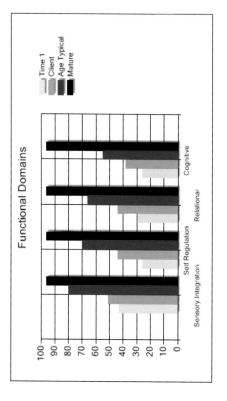

Functional Domains

Legend: Time 1, Client, Age Typical, Mature

Categories: Sensory Integration, Self Regulation, Relational, Cognitive

General Summary

Recommendations are based upon data provided by the clinician when completing the NMT online metrics. Based upon the data provided, cut off scores are used to indicate whether activities in each of the 4 areas are considered essential, therapeutic or enrichment. Activities selected for each category should be age appropriate, positive and provided in the context of nurturing, safe relationships.

Essential refers to those activities that are crucial to the child's future growth in this particular area. In order to fall into the essential category the child's score must be below 65% of the age typical score. It is our belief that unless functioning in the essential area is increased the child will lack the foundation for future growth and development in this and other areas.

Therapeutic refers to those activities aimed at building in strength and growth in the particular area. Scores that fall within 65 to 85 percent of those typical for the child's age are considered appropriate for more focused treatment. Therapeutic activities are viewed as important for the child's continued growth and improvement in the area.

Enrichment refers to activities that provide positive, valuable experiences that continue to build capacity in the given area. Children who fall into the enrichment category are at or above 85 percent of age typical functioning. Activities recommended in this category are designed to enhance and reinforce strengths previously built into the particular area of focus.

The information below is designed to provide the clinician with broad recommendations based upon the NMT approach. These recommendations should be used as guidelines for the treating clinician when considering particular therapeutic activities. Final treatment decisions must be based upon the clinical judgement of the treatment provider. The CTA cannot be held responsible for any of the treatment decisions made by the clinician based upon their own interpretation of NMT principles or recommendations.

Sensory Integration

Client Score: 51　　Age Typical: 80　　Percentage: 63.75

Essential: (below 65%) – Scores below 65% of age typical functioning indicate poorly organized somatosensory systems in the brain. The introduction of patterned, repetitive somatosensory activities weaved throughout the day have been shown to lead to positive improvements. These activities should be provided multiple times each day for approximately 7-8 minutes at a time for essential reorganization to occur. Examples of somatosensory activities include massage (pressure point, Reiki touch), music, movement (swimming, walking/running, jumping, swinging, rocking), yoga/breathing and animal assisted therapy that includes patterned, repetitive activities such as grooming.

Self Regulation

Client Score: 44　　Age Typical: 70　　Percentage: 62.86

Essential: (below 65%) – Scores below 65% of age typical functioning suggest the child has poor self-regulatory capabilities. These children may have stress response systems that are poorly organized and hyper-reactive. They are likely impulsive, have difficulties transitioning from one activity to another, and may overreact to even minor stressors or challenges. Children in this category require structure and predictability provided consistently by safe, nurturing adults - across settings. Examples of essential activities in this category include:: developing transitioning activity (using a song, words or other cues to help prepare the child for the change in activity), patterned, repetitive proprioceptive OT activities such as isometric exercises (chair push-ups, bear hugs while child tries to pull the adult's arms away, applying deep pressure), using weighted vests, blankets, ankle weights, various deep breathing techniques, building structure into bedtime rituals, music and movement activities, animal assisted therapy and EMDR.

Relational

Client Score: 44　　Age Typical: 66　　Percentage: 66.67

Therapeutic: (65% - 85%) - Scores between 65 and 85 percent suggest that the child has some difficulty with relational functioning. It is important to remember that unless and until re-organization takes place in the lower parts of the brain, specifically self-regulation, therapeutic efforts on more relationally related problems in the limbic system will likely be unsuccessful. In order to make sufficient gains in relational functioning, relational stability with multiple positive healthy adults who are invested in the child's life and in their treatment is required. Examples of relational therapeutic activities include: parallel play, first with an invested adult and/or therapist and when mastered, parallel play with a peer. Once dyadic relationships have been mastered, small group activities may be added. Other examples include animal assisted therapy.

Cognitive

Client Score: 38　　Age Typical: 55　　Percentage: 69.09

Therapeutic: (65% - 85%) – Scores between 65 and 85 percent suggest that the child has some difficulty with cognitive functioning. Once fundamental dyadic relational skills have improved, therapeutic techniques can focus on more verbal and insight oriented or cortical activities. Examples of therapeutic activities include: insight oriented treatment, cognitive behavioral therapy, reading enhancements, and structured storytelling.

Cortical Modulation refers to the capacity of important cortical networks to regulate and modulate the activity and reactivity of some of the lower neural systems. As the brain organizes and matures, this capacity increases and the Cortical Modulation Ratio (CMR) increases. The CMR reflects both cortical "strength" and over-reactivity in lower neural systems involved in the stress response. Any Cortical Modulation Ratio below 1.0 suggests that the individual has minimal capacity to self-regulate. Ratios between 1.0 and 2.0 indicate emerging but episodic self-regulation capacity. This item can prove useful when determining whether a client is "ready" to benefit from traditional cognitive interventions.